The Guide to Living with HIV Infection

The Guide to Living with HIV Infection

Developed at the
Johns Hopkins AIDS Clinic

REVISED EDITION

John G. Bartlett, M.D.
Ann K. Finkbeiner

The Johns Hopkins University Press
Baltimore and London

Note to the Reader

This book is not meant to substitute for medical care of people with HIV infection, and treatment should not be based solely on its contents. Instead, treatment must be developed in a dialogue between the individual and his or her physician. Our book has been written to help with that dialogue.

Copyright © 1991, 1993 The Johns Hopkins University Press
All rights reserved
Printed in the United States of America on acid-free paper

First edition, 1991

The Johns Hopkins University Press
2715 North Charles Street
Baltimore, Maryland 21218-4319
The Johns Hopkins Press Ltd., London

Library of Congress Cataloging-in-Publication Data

Bartlett, John G.
    The guide to living with HIV infection : developed at the Johns
Hopkins AIDS Clinic / John G. Bartlett, Ann K. Finkbeiner.—Rev.
ed.
        p. cm.
    Previously published: 1991.
    Includes index.
    ISBN 0-8018-4663-3 (acid-free paper).—ISBN 0-8018-4664-1 (acid-
free paper : pbk.)
    1. HIV infections—Handbooks, manuals, etc. 2. HIV infections—
Psychological aspects—Handbooks, manuals, etc. 3. HIV infections—
Patients—Rehabilitation—Handbooks, manuals, etc. I. Finkbeiner,
Ann K., 1943–   . II. Johns Hopkins AIDS Clinic. III. Title.
RC607.A26B376   1993
362.1'969792—dc20   93-18324

A catalog record for this book is available from the British Library.

Contents

Prologue

To People with HIV Infection and to Their Caregivers

Joseph "Jody" Maier

I'd like to begin by offering some "Directions for Use" for what I'm about to say. First, I speak from my experience alone. Other persons with AIDS may have different experiences. I respect that diversity of experience. While my personal perspective may be quite instructive, it is not offered here as the Truth—capital T—about AIDS. I'm a white, gay male. This is only one of the many profiles that make up [people] with AIDS. So keep in mind that what you are about to hear is only one of the tales that could be told.

Second, I am only one of a handful of persons with AIDS in Maryland who has "gone public." Some time ago, I decided that the best way not to be a pariah with AIDS was not to act like one. An extraordinary combination of love from friends and family, enlightened support from my employer, and cooperation among my care providers has made this possible. These are not typical circumstances, and this is not the usual response. Third, it has been nearly a year since I was diagnosed with AIDS. Today, you catch me at a time of stability, energy, and mental clarity. I'm acutely aware of being a survivor. Half of the people diagnosed with AIDS in Maryland in 1986 are already dead. Indeed, two of my four roommates in the hospital have died. AIDS is nothing if not constant flux. Things change.

Jody Maier, foreign editor of the Population Information Program, School of Hygiene and Public Health, Johns Hopkins University, delivered this speech on April 28, 1987, before the participants in the Institute on the Ministry to the Sick, Johns Hopkins Hospital, Baltimore, Maryland.

Perspectives change. So let's call these remarks "Work in Progress."

That said, I want to share with you a few lines by a contemporary American poet whom I have long admired, A. R. Ammons. Rediscovering these lines last fall and reflecting on my situation, I felt in them a new and powerful resonance.

> Outside the window the leaf in a hedge breeze
>
> spins at the end of an invisible web, a lure
>
> to the present from the nothingness it came from
>
> and goes to . . . in the knowledge of our death already
>
> in some way dead, we know, as leaves do not . . .
>
> the contemplation of our spinning keeps us, though
>
> separated, here, shocked awake, sharp with ruin.
>
> (from "For Andrew Wyeth")

"Here, shocked awake, sharp with ruin." That's what it's like to learn you have AIDS and to live with that knowledge. I was as well prepared for the news as anyone can be, I suppose. I worked in a public health-related field . . . and I had read most of the scientific literature on AIDS since the first case reports in 1981. I was working as a volunteer for [an] AIDS information, education, and support organization . . . ; I answered AIDS Hotline calls, I edited the first issues of their newsletter, I used my lunch hour to visit fellows with AIDS in [the hospital]. I became a buddy for two people with AIDS and watched both of them wither away. I went to the support group meetings and for eighteen months watched people with AIDS, their lovers, friends, and families come and go. I was—and still am—a participant in a major study . . . that follows the natural history of infection with the virus that causes AIDS. So, I knew I was infected.

A year and a half ago, when the blood reports were no longer reassuring and showed the virus's silent work of ruin, I asked myself, "What's it going to be: the glass half-empty or the glass half-full?" Since I felt healthy, I chose to come down on the side of living rather than focus on disease and decline. In fact, apart from some fatigue, my body gave no hint of what was to come. The onset of life-threatening pneumonia in May of last year was unexpected and sudden. Within a matter of days, I went from enduring what I thought was a bad cold to monstrous fevers and sweats, gasping for breath and coughing the dry wracking cough that every article and pamphlet I'd ever read told me was the sign of AIDS-related pneumonia. I had a pretty good idea what was going on. As a result, the diagnosis of pneumocystis pneumonia was more of a relief than a shock. I knew that, barring treatment failure, it would be possible to survive that initial infection. Shocked awake, sharp with ruin: here I am in my late thirties reaching the end of my life and knowing, as I say it now, I'm still very much alive.

I *live* with AIDS. I'm a person *living* with AIDS, not an AIDS *victim* or an AIDS *sufferer* and mercifully only from time to time an AIDS *patient*. Why is this the case? Why do some people with AIDS do better than others? What attitudes help determine the quality of life after diagnosis? If I may steal a bit of Dr. di Giovanni's professional thunder, I'd like to share with you the results of an interesting study, carried out at UCLA, that involved fifty gay men with AIDS. The men who fared the worst were those who avoided thinking about AIDS altogether. They had the highest levels of concern about their health and about dying. They had the highest levels of depression and the lowest self-esteem.

Avoiding the issue, the researchers point out, does not protect people with AIDS from feeling distressed or concerned about their condition. Ignorance is not bliss, and denial is far from constructive—though there were certainly enough people who tried to convince me otherwise. The first was my mother, who blithely related the story of a woman who was living in her retirement community and was suffering from a horribly disabling illness. It wasn't until the woman died that Mother and the other residents found out that she had also been suffering from lung cancer. Said my mom, "She was so wonderful about it. Nobody knew." And there was a friend who really didn't want to hear a thing about AIDS and thought I should just blank out my five years' worth of reading about the subject. She kept citing the case of a friend of hers who had been diagnosed three years ago, didn't know a thing about AIDS or his treatments, ignored it completely, kept working, and was doing just fine. I was obsessing about AIDS, she said. Why couldn't I do something else with my life? She wanted the "old Jody" back.

It was hard not to succumb to the wishes of the ones I

loved most. I could hardly bear to be the cause of so much pain and distress in so many people. Being deathly ill doesn't bolster one's self-confidence. I was ready to give in. "What if they're right?" I kept asking myself. AIDS troubles clear waters; it encourages self-doubt; it takes away firm footing; in relationships, the balance tips quickly to dependency. In the barrage of unexplained symptoms, the unexplained fevers, the unexplained headaches, the unexplained skin eruptions, the constant and fearful change, I needed to find the right path with the people I loved, and I wanted to be loved with AIDS as much as I'd been loved without it.

A month and a half after the bout with pneumonia, I was hospitalized again, this time with central nervous system toxoplasmosis, which is a serious brain infection. I lost all fine motor control of the right side of my body. I couldn't write. I had trouble putting sentences together. I suffered short-term memory lapses. I started having seizures in my right arm. This hospital stay was short, but during the long recovery that followed, there occurred a change in my attitude about having AIDS. I'm not certain how this change occurred, but I can describe it. I began by shedding some of my self-doubt and started trusting the firmness of my convictions. This meant that I trusted my assessment of what was happening in my body, that I was right on the money about symptoms, and that I wanted to be less a passive patient and more an active participant in treating and gathering knowledge about my illness. It meant helping family and friends deal with their denial, for which I now have infinite patience.

I had to examine myself and ask if I really had an emotional investment in being sick, that is, if I was making a vocation out of symptoms and decline—professional tears, sadness, and illness, I call it. I remember the advice of the fellow with AIDS whom I'd "buddied" a year before I got sick. "Get over your sorrow," he said, "it serves no useful purpose." By which he meant: don't deny your sadness, just don't wallow in it. He was right. In the hospital, when I explained to a friend how sorry I was that what we had shared in a decade of very close friendship would be coming to a halt, he would have none of it. "Nonsense," he said, "your life was rich and filled with music before you got AIDS and you'll find the way for it to be rich and full of music regardless of the nasty cards and handicaps you'll be dealt." *That* was a jolt. I decided to come down firmly on the side of life and of affirmation. I said "yes" to life. The possibility of death didn't have to terrorize my every waking moment. . . .

There is a useful and life-affirming kind of denial as well as the more usual self-destructive kind. In fact, I don't even call it denial. Rather, I call it bracketing: death is plainly marked and present, but suspended from consideration, so I can get on with living. The UCLA researchers, by the way, found this to be the most helpful strategy in coping with AIDS. They called it "the fighting spirit."

These same researchers found that the most common reaction among the gay men studied involved an attempt to find some meaning in their dismal situation. People who used this technique in dealing with AIDS prayed for a good ending to the situation, thought about positive changes in themselves since they developed the disease, and trusted in their belief in God. The researchers found this often resulted in obsessive thoughts and feelings, which in turn did not help the men cope with AIDS. . . . We are, ourselves, I believe, the primary agents of our own health. Passively putting trust in something or someone out there that is not connected to us yields little. Waiting for pills or drugs to work a magic cure all by themselves is not optimum treatment. In large measure, we allow health to happen. Better to work at health than pray that things will work out all by themselves. Better to acknowledge the Divine within each of us than to wait for an estranged and separated God to intercede.

[And what can the caregiver do?] Help those of us who are troubled with AIDS to love ourselves, lesions and all. Helping us find that love within is the first step in empowering us to be as healthy as we can be.

Last Friday, a friend of mine went to [a hospital] to take an older black man with AIDS to his foster home. It was early afternoon. No nurse or aide had yet done morning care on the gentleman. He was disheveled. There was dried vomit on his face. The man was despondent. He kept saying that God no longer loved him, and certainly [the hospital] was supplying ample evidence in support.

What steps would you take to minister to this man? Here are my suggestions. There is no particular technique that gets applied to persons with AIDS. We are helping people to find that spark, that love within. I'd say listen to him. Take your cues from what he has to say. Touch him. Hug him. Hold on to him for dear life, as it were. You aren't going to get AIDS from holding hands or a hug. Be forgiving and be merciful, that is, be loving. Compassion is not enough—you have to demonstrate that you care. Better always to be loving than just compassionate. Better to show that you love than just mouth the words. Be respectful of difference. We are trying to help people with AIDS themselves, not make them over. . . .

What else can you do? . . . Take action. If I've learned anything in the last twelve months, it's "words are one thing, action is another." Take this loving response to the people with AIDS in your communities. Take community action. Don't limit your activities to institutions such as the church or the hospital. There is usually plenty of support in the hospital, and very little outside of it, where it matters most, where it makes a difference who does well and who does not. The fellow with AIDS with whom I was a buddy used to complain bitterly that everyone from his church would flock to him whenever he was hospitalized, but no one came to visit him at home where he needed it most. No one persisted in support, either. During his fourth and fifth hospitalizations, the visitors dwindled to a handful. No one understood that AIDS is a long haul and that the loving response has to be vigilantly maintained. . . .

Lend support to these people. It doesn't have to be complicated and sophisticated to be effective. If the person with AIDS is living alone, check in daily by telephone to see how he or she is doing. Are they eating regular meals? Are they bathing? Do they have adequate supplies of medications? Are they taking them regularly? This kind of loving action is probably more important for the health of someone with AIDS than, say a short visit now and then . . . or a monthly trip to the movies.

Remember that the loving response to AIDS is not about helping people with the disease to die poetically or enabling them to become martyrs or making them over into saints. The loving response is a way of empowering persons with AIDS so that they can do the best they possibly can, maximize their health, and cope with their problems at any time during their illness. . . .

I am fortunate in that I have the love of my family and an army of friends. Their loving response sustains me, and that sharing of love is the stuff of a life.

separated into the knowledge of our death . . .

giving way neither to easy dream nor helpless ruin . . .

we make a life that keeps, a time that going holds . . .

a motion that moving stays.

(from "For Andrew Wyeth")

Celebrate the love that we share, I tell my friends when they're sad. Rejoice: I'm still alive.

The Guide to
Living with
HIV Infection

Introduction:
About This Book

- Medical issues you need to understand first
- Psychological and social issues
- Questions and answers about HIV infection
- About this book

HIV infection puts extraordinary stresses on people's lives. Most of these stresses are unusual, and people are unsure how to handle them. This book guides people through HIV infection, lets them know what they're up against, and helps them deal thoroughly and positively with the medical and emotional problems the infection presents. The book is about how to live with HIV infection, that is, how to live as long and full and satisfying a life as possible.

This book will cover the parts of people's lives that HIV infection affects: their physical health, their emotional health and social difficulties, and their financial and legal problems. Sometimes these issues will be kept separate—one chapter is only about medical care, one only about financial and legal problems. Sometimes the issues will be merged—the chapter on what to do when first diagnosed covers both medical and emotional issues.

Medical Issues You Need to Understand First

A few things you need to know right away. Some of these things may not be uppermost in your mind, but you need to know them to protect yourself and others. All these things are discussed in more detail in Chapter 1; we include them in this introduction to alert you to their necessity.

1. What HIV infection and AIDS are: AIDS stands for acquired immune deficiency syndrome. *Acquired* means that AIDS is not inherited (many diseases of immune deficiency *are* inherited), but

1

acquired from some substance or microbe outside the body. *Immune deficiency* means that the immune system has been weakened. A *syndrome* is not so much a disease as it is a collection of symptoms. In the case of AIDS, the syndrome is a collection of conditions or complications that result from immune deficiency.

AIDS is often used incorrectly as a catch-all term for infection with the AIDS virus. The name of the AIDS virus is HIV, the human immunodeficiency virus, so called because HIV infects the immune system and weakens it. People with HIV infection do not necessarily have AIDS. AIDS is only one stage of a whole series of stages in HIV infection. When people are first infected with HIV, they show no obvious symptoms for a long period called the *asymptomatic period*. When they begin to show symptoms of a weakened immune system, they are said to be in the *early symptomatic period*. (This period has also been called *ARC*, or *AIDS-related complex*.) When the immune system is weakened severely, people begin having certain specific infections and tumors called *opportunists* or *AIDS-defining diagnoses* (see Chapter 3). It is only at this stage that people have AIDS. The AIDS stage is also called the *late symptomatic period*.

2. What the prognosis is: The studies done so far have shown that half of those with HIV infection will develop AIDS within eight to ten years after becoming infected, and most of the rest will have laboratory evidence of weakened immune systems. The same studies showed that people lived a year or more after they were diagnosed with AIDS. These studies were done before any treatment was available. We now know that with early treatment, the whole course of the disease can be slowed down, and that the statistics from these early studies now do not mean much. We also know that new drugs and new treatments are being developed so fast that it is not possible to predict the average time between infection with HIV and AIDS; we know only that the time is longer. Most people with HIV infection, if untreated, will eventually develop AIDS, but we do not know if all people will. We only know that the time before development of AIDS should continue to lengthen. Nor is it possible to predict how much longer the new drugs and treatments will allow people to live after a diagnosis of AIDS. As above, we only know that the time is now longer and will get even longer yet. One day, treatments may conceivably prolong good health for people with HIV infection indefinitely. HIV infection should eventually become a chronic and manageable disease, managed the way diabetes and hypertension are.

3. When you can transmit the virus to others: You must consider yourself infectious from the time you are infected. Once HIV is in a person's body, it is virtually impossible to become "uninfected." Once infected, you can transmit the virus for the entire course of the disease.

4. How to avoid transmitting the virus (see Chapter 2):
• Use safe sex or safer sex. Safe sex means sex with no exchange of semen, vaginal fluids, blood or menstrual blood; safer sex means intercourse (oral, vaginal, or anal) with a condom and spermicide.
• If you use drugs intravenously, try to stop. If you cannot, stop sharing needles and works. Rinse the needles and works with chlorine bleach after every use.
• Do not donate blood, body organs, semen, or other body tissue or fluids.
• To be extra cautious about transmitting HIV through blood, avoid sharing toothbrushes and razors.
• Casual contact—shaking hands, sharing a toilet, sharing eating utensils, sneezing on others—does not transmit the virus.

5. Whom you must notify: You must notify anyone you may have exposed to the virus. That includes anyone with whom you have had unprotected sex (without condoms and spermicide), or with whom you have shared needles or works. If you know when you were infected, tell anyone you may have exposed since then. If you do not know (though no one knows absolutely how far back in time you should go), the common recommendation is to notify anyone you may have exposed in the last one or two years. You should also tell your physician and dentist of the diagnosis.

Important: Other than sex or needle-sharing partners, and your physician and dentist, you need not tell anyone else. An exception: health care workers should notify their supervisors or employers according to local policy.

6. Whether to get medical help: Everyone with HIV infection requires regular medical evaluation. And medical treatment will make your life more comfortable and longer.

Psychological and Social Issues

Parts of this book are about dealing with the extraordinary stresses that HIV infection puts on people's minds. The stresses are not limited to people with HIV infection; their caretakers often feel the same stresses.

In general, people with HIV infection and their caretakers do not easily divide themselves into sick people and people who have escaped sickness: they are all affected by the disease. They say, over and over, that they are in this together. For that reason, this book is addressed both to people with HIV infection and to their caregivers—that is, this book is addressed to all the people affected by HIV infection.

People affected by HIV infection face greater emotional strain than most people ever do. Furthermore, many face it at an unconscionably young age. Those affected by the disease are shocked or angry or depressed or afraid or guilty or confused or have any number of these emotions at once. They worry about revealing the diagnosis, about being dependent, about expressing sexuality, about relations with the people they love. They worry about dying. The rest of society not directly affected by the disease reacts with fear and prejudice, making those affected by the disease also feel like outcasts, isolated and lonely.

In general, people affected by HIV infection tend to run into three periods of particular emotional difficulty. One is at the initial diagnosis of infection with HIV: people feel uncertain about what the diagnosis means, about whether they will infect other people, how long they will live, what their lives will be like. The next difficult period comes with the first illness that defines a diagnosis of AIDS: people begin to face the reality of a disease that includes an array of illnesses, hospitalizations, medications, and medical procedures. The third period comes with the second AIDS-defining illness: people are troubled by feelings of hopelessness, dependency, and awareness of death.

With time, people come to deal with each period, using the same strategies that have worked for them in all their previous periods of difficulty. Their strategies for dealing with their problems are usually effective and usually different. Many of their strategies contradict those used by others. Some people talk out their problems, others work them out alone. Some people immerse themselves in work, others quit and go to Tahiti. Some people refuse to think of themselves as sick, others make out their wills. Some contemplate, some act. Some go to mental health professionals, others rely on their friends and themselves. Strategies can be opposite and still be equally effective. People tend to use whatever strategies have worked best in handling past problems. In fact, they use whatever strategies work at all.

Mental health professionals who deal with people affected by HIV infection agree that the best strategies are whatever works. Nevertheless, mental health professionals recommend a few general guidelines. The first is to protect your physical health. That includes eating healthful foods, cutting alcohol and smoking down or out, and exercising. Take good care of your body, give it a chance to fight the infection. In addition, protect the health of others: practice safer sex; don't share needles; avoid passing blood, semen, or vaginal fluids to another person.

The second guideline is to cultivate emotional health. Value yourself and be around others who value you. Try to see accurately who you are and what you feel. Enlist your sources of support and try to communicate with them truthfully and thoughtfully. If a problem seems too severe or does not go away, or if you are seriously considering suicide, or if you simply want someone to whom you can talk freely, see a mental health professional. Therapy may concentrate on the overwhelming problems people must face and feel they cannot solve: How can I face rejection? How can I deal with my anger? Can I come to feel less guilt? Are there ways to have sex without hurting myself or anyone else? Why me? Why now? What will I do with the rest of my life? What will happen to my kids? My parents? The people I love? Will I die? How will I die? Am I a good person?

The third guideline is to take control of your life. In spite of much that is unavoidable or unchangeable, the decisions about your life are yours to make. Consider and accept the consequences of your actions. Once that's done, you know what's best for you. You are in charge.

Satisfy these and any other principles you hold yourself to. Then trust yourself and live the way you feel you must. People affected by HIV infection say the same thing this way: be kind to yourself and others, come to terms with yourself, love yourself, trust yourself.

Questions and Answers about HIV Infection

People whose lives are so drastically affected by HIV infection naturally have questions about the disease. But because it is a new disease, medical scientists still have much to learn about its effects on the body and how to treat those effects. What medical scientists know depends on what kinds of studies they have done.

One kind of study examines *virology*, or the virus itself: what genes make it up, how it reproduces, how it attaches to cells, what effect it has on the cell. These studies will ultimately suggest new drugs for controlling or destroying the virus. Another kind of study, called a *clinical trial*, tests drugs to see if they are effective both against HIV and against the infections that accompany a weakened immune system.

The third kind of study is *epidemiological;* that is, it charts the course of HIV infection through whole populations. In the early 1980s, epidemiological studies were responsible for identifying and defining the disease and for finding out how the disease was transmitted, even before the virus was discovered. Currently, a federal agency, the Centers for

Disease Control, or CDC, does epidemiological studies that keep track of the spread of the infection. From those studies, we now know the number of cases of AIDS, the populations that are affected, the way the virus is transmitted, the average course of the disease, and the average life expectancy.

To further help epidemiologists keep track of it, AIDS was made a "reportable disease," meaning that health care providers are required to report, by name, all people with AIDS to their state's department of health. Ultimately, the states report these cases to the CDC, but not by name. (HIV infection is reportable by name in some states but not in others.) As a consequence, the CDC has excellent information on AIDS. Information on other stages of HIV infection, however, is much more fragmented and incomplete.

In short, the answers to questions about HIV infection are limited by how far medical science has progressed in its studies. Knowledge of how the virus operates in the body depends on the progress made in the virological studies. Knowledge of what drugs are most effective depends on the progress made in the clinical trials. Knowledge of the natural course of the disease in the body depends on the progress made in epidemiological studies. Information coming out of these studies is discussed throughout this book.

As a result, some questions people have about HIV infection can be answered completely and substantially. Other questions will have answers that are, for the present anyway, closer to educated guesses.

About This Book

This book is meant as a reference and a companion. It is unfortunately not a complete guide to living with HIV infection. One subject left out is home nursing care—you can get specific details about this subject from nurses or home health care workers. Another subject omitted is the care of children with AIDS. Both of these topics warrant books of their own. Any other information omitted or dealt with only sketchily is accompanied by a referral to a reliable source for the information.

This book was not written to be read from start to finish. Read the book in whatever order you please: read one chapter at a time, one section at a time; read about whatever problems you face now, or about whatever questions you currently want answered; skip chapters or sections and go back to them when you're ready, or don't go back to them at all. Each chapter is intended more or less to be read as though it stands alone. As a result, some information gets repeated in several chapters. If the repetition is irksome, please ignore it.

The book discusses emotional and social issues in human voices, that is, in the words of the people affected by the infection. The reason is that many of the ways of dealing with those issues come not only from mental health professionals but from the people affected by HIV. In some of the following chapters are the voices of six people: their names are Dean Lombard, June Monroe, Steven Charles, Helen Parks, Alan Madison, and Lisa Pratt. Together, these people are meant to represent the population of people affected by HIV. They are men and women, have different financial resources, are different ages, have different jobs, are caretakers and people who need care. Those with HIV have become infected a number of different ways and are in all stages of infection. Though their names and certain characteristics are fictional, what they say is not. In every case, the words are quotes of real people affected by HIV; the quotes are nearly verbatim.

This book is full of medical terms, some of them familiar, some complicated and unfamiliar. We explain these terms as they appear. But we also know the reader will not remember every new word or every aspect of its meaning. So the last chapter in the book is a glossary of all these words, and the reader can refer to it as needed. The glossary includes, among other words, the names of the conditions associated with HIV infection, the tests to diagnose them, and the drugs used to treat them.

And finally, we avoid, where possible, addressing separate groups of readers in separate sections. For the same reason that we avoid separate sections for people with HIV infection and their caregivers, we also avoid having separate sections for women, gay men, or IV drug users. The reason is that most of the issues and problems faced by all these people are the same. Women, gay men, hemophiliacs, transfusion recipients, and IV drug users are surely all concerned about their children. Everyone worries about the legal rights of an unmarried partner. Everyone is made unhappy by social isolation. Condoms and spermicide should be used during sex regardless of who the partners are.

Some issues, however, are truly unique to one group. Women have medical problems men do not; and they can transmit the virus, through pregnancy and breast-feeding, in ways men cannot. Gay men can face problems because revealing their HIV status can mean also revealing homosexuality; transfusion recipients do not necessarily face a similar problem. Our policy is to discuss issues unique to one group in the section devoted to those issues. So gynecological problems are in the chapter on medical problems; pregnancy and breast-feeding are in the chapter on transmitting HIV; problems talking about homosexuality are in the section on problems with talking about HIV status. Again, like the people with HIV infection and their caregivers, we're all in this together.

Chapter 1

When First Diagnosed: Understanding and Communicating about HIV

- **What you need to know**
- **Reacting to the diagnosis**
- **Telling people about the diagnosis**

The first thing on a person's mind after a positive HIV (human immuno-deficiency virus, sometimes called the AIDS virus) test is probably not a list of practical things to know and do. Nevertheless, a person with HIV infection should begin doing some things immediately, and this chapter will talk about these things first. After these practicalities are covered, the discussion will turn to the emotional and social concerns people have when first diagnosed.

What You Need to Know

The Accuracy of the Test

The HIV blood test, like all tests in medicine, is subject to human and laboratory error. Nevertheless, this test is one of the most accurate in medicine. A positive test almost always means you are infected; a negative test almost always means you are not infected. Further information about the test and its results is provided in "Understanding Tests for HIV," which begins on page 299.

The Prognosis

A blood test that shows the presence of antibodies to HIV means that HIV itself is also in the blood. Unlike antibodies for other infections, the antibodies for HIV cannot kill the virus. This means that once HIV is in the blood, it will always be in the blood.

There have been occasional reports of individuals with positive tests that subsequently became negative—in other words, reports indicate that the virus was once present and then was somehow eliminated. So far, these reports have nearly always turned out to be the result of errors in the test. We are aware of possibly three cases of a person who was once infected becoming uninfected. This is disappointing, but it should be faced. People with positive tests should consider themselves infectious to others for the indefinite future.

HIV infection causes the gradual weakening of the body's immune system. This process takes years or even decades. The person with HIV infection usually feels entirely well and has no symptoms of infection for years. When symptoms of a weakened immune system begin to occur, the person is said to be in the early symptomatic stage, sometimes called AIDS-related complex, or ARC. When the immune system becomes even weaker, certain opportunistic infections—common infections usually fought off by the immune system—appear, and the person is said to be in the late symptomatic stage, or to have AIDS. All stages of HIV infection are discussed in more detail in Chapter 3.

Current studies indicate that about half the people with positive blood tests for HIV will develop AIDS within eight to ten years after infection takes place, and that people diagnosed with AIDS live a year or longer. This is an estimate based on studies of people who became infected with HIV in San Francisco as early as 1978. Some of these people who were studied have weakened immune systems but remain well ten or twelve years later. So no one knows how long any individual person with HIV will take to develop AIDS; the upper limit is clearly well over ten years.

The most important thing to understand is this: what we know about the progression of the whole course of HIV infection comes from those studies, and those studies were done when no one knew much about the benefits of therapy.

We do not understand all the factors that govern how fast HIV infection progresses or how fast the immune system weakens or how fast AIDS itself progresses. But paying attention to wellness—good nutrition, exercise, regular medical check-ups—apparently helps to slow down the progression of the course of HIV infection through the body (see Chapter 12).

We do know that people with AIDS live substantially longer than they once did, and that current treatments delay the average time between initial infection with HIV and the development of AIDS. We think medical treatment will eventually prevent HIV infection from leading almost inevitably to AIDS. We think HIV infection will become a chronic and manageable disease. Like diabetes, HIV infection will be a persistent medical problem that will always need attention, but it will not drastically interfere with quality or length of life. With early detection and new treatments, we believe, many people will be able to count on an indefinite period of good health.

How to Avoid Transmitting the Virus

A positive HIV blood test means that the virus is present and may be transmitted to others. Once infected, people remain infectious to others for the rest of their lives.

In most cases, HIV is transmitted to others by sexual contact or by intravenous drug use. The blood supply has been screened ever since 1985. Extensive studies since then of people who knew how they became infected show that sex, IV drug use, or transmission from mother to fetus have accounted for 99.9 percent of all cases. Most of the remaining 0.1 percent of cases (1 in every 1,000 infected people) are health care workers who had needlestick injuries, people who received organ transplants, and people who received blood transfusions. It is important for you to know that this virus is not transmitted to others by casual contact—by shaking hands, sharing a toilet, sharing eating utensils, sneezing on others, and the like.

The best way to avoid sexual transmission is to abstain from sex. The next best way is to use "safer sex," that is, use condoms and spermicides for all genital contact, or have the kind of sexual contact that does not involve transferring semen, vaginal fluids, menstrual blood, or blood from one person's body into another's. Women with HIV should avoid getting pregnant because of the risk of transmitting the virus to the fetus. Women with HIV who have a baby should not breast-feed. The best way for intravenous drug users to avoid transmission is to stop using drugs. If this is impossible, intravenous drug users must absolutely stop sharing needles and works. The next best way is to use chlorine bleach to clean the needles and works after every use.

To be extra cautious, avoid sharing toothbrushes and razors. It is also necessary to avoid donating blood, body organs, semen, or other body tissue or fluids. Anyone with HIV infection who has a universal donor card for organ transplantation should destroy this card.

Preventing transmission of HIV is discussed more thoroughly in Chapter 2.

Whom to Notify

People with HIV infection have an ethical and, in many places, a legal requirement to notify people they may have exposed to HIV. Those with HIV infection must also tell people with whom they are having the kind of contact that might transmit HIV. These are two of the hardest things someone with HIV infection has to do (see the following sections on who to tell).

People with HIV infection are obliged to notify anyone they have exposed to the virus. This means anyone with whom they have had nonsafe sex (that is, sex without a condom, or sex that involved exchange of body fluids) and with whom they have shared needles or works. This applies to past as well as present and future relationships.

For past relationships, the major problem is knowing how far back in time to go. Most people with HIV do not know when they acquired the infection. Since the infection may be silent for a long time, they may conceivably have been placing others at risk for several years. For practical purposes, most authorities recommend notifying all contacts for the past one or two years. This is the absolute minimum.

People who have been exposed should be notified and advised to take the test to find out if they are infected. They might also want to ask a physician about the probability of infection, the necessity for medical evaluation beyond simple testing for HIV, and the desirability of subsequent testing (see "Understanding Tests for HIV," which begins on page 299). It may be at least somewhat reassuring to know that the virus is not easily transmitted. Studies of heterosexual couples show that the risk of infection is estimated to be less than 1 in 100 for a single sexual contact. The same studies show that, even for those who have had regular sexual contact over extended periods, the risk of infection is less than 50 percent. This includes hemophiliac men's wives, who have infection rates of 10 to 30 percent, despite having had unprotected sex for years. Similar studies have not yet been done for gay men; the risks are probably higher.

There are two reasons for notifying people you may have exposed to HIV. One is so they can obtain health care and counseling themselves; they will also need to take precautions not to spread the infection further. This is the only way, right now, that the epidemic can be controlled. The other reason for notification is that doing so is probably a legal requirement; depending on where you live, notification may be the law. Though legal requirements vary from state to state, most states now have laws that mandate notification.

Moreover, physicians may be obliged to notify anyone you do not notify. There is debate about this. On the one hand, the patient-physician relationship is privileged, or private. On the other, the physician has an obligation to society. A legal precedent was established with the case of *Tarasoff v. Regents of the University of California*, in which a psychologist who learned of a patient's intent to murder a young woman was held liable for not taking appropriate steps to protect her. This decision established that the physician has what is called a "duty to warn" unsuspecting people who are engaged in behavior that puts them at risk. As a result, the physician will usually advise a patient to notify people who have been and continue to be placed at risk of infection. If the patient is unwilling to do this, the physician appears to have the authority and even the responsibility to do it, either directly or through public health authorities.

Notifying others of the possibility of HIV infection is extremely difficult. People who simply cannot do it are advised to discuss their concerns with their physicians. They might also benefit from consulting a psychiatrist or a psychologist, or by participating in support groups, or by talking to friends and relatives.

Those who remain unable to tell others directly might do it indirectly, through another individual such as a physician. An alternative is for the person or the physician to notify public health authorities, who will then make the necessary notification. Neither physicians nor public health authorities have to identify the source of their information. The person who may be exposed is simply told of the possibility of exposure without ever being told the specific source. Any of these alternatives is acceptable. The important thing is for the person exposed to be notified, tested, and counseled—and as soon as possible.

Deciding Who Else to Tell

Beyond those you must inform, deciding who and who not to tell is difficult. For someone who is newly diagnosed, the first advice is to limit the number of people. Tell those you must: physicians, dentists, and anyone who has been or will be exposed by sexual contact or shared needle use. If you are a health care worker, you should notify a superior or a medical adviser where you work, following local guidelines.

No one else need know. Almost all the people who had AIDS in the early 1980s could recount a seemingly endless array of war stories about how their medical care, employment, and relationships with friends and relatives changed when their diagnoses became known. Until you have sorted out your own reactions to the diagnosis, and have thought through which people you want to tell and what you want to tell them, you are probably better off not saying anything. Put it off for a while. Limit those you tell.

Finding a Stable and Congenial Source of Medical Care

Everyone with HIV infection requires regular medical care. Medicine cannot yet cure HIV infection, but it can treat it. Early treatments slow the infection down, and people do not get sick as fast. Later treatments ease troublesome symptoms and stop each opportunistic infection. (Chapter 6 discusses each opportunistic infection by symptom; Chapter 8 advises how to choose physicians.) Find a physician or a group of physicians or a clinic which you find congenial, in which you have trust, and which you will continue to visit.

What's at Stake in Becoming Pregnant

Women who have HIV and then become pregnant can transmit this virus to their babies. Women who become infected with HIV while they are pregnant can also transmit the virus to their babies. The risk of transmission is around 30 percent to 35 percent, meaning that about one-third of the babies born to mothers with HIV will also have the virus.

A woman who becomes infected with HIV after she has had a baby has less to worry about. Any woman with HIV infection, regardless of when she became infected, must not breast-feed her baby.

HIV infection is different in children than in adults. In children, the disease progresses more rapidly. Most children with HIV infection will have medical problems by age four or five years, although some children with HIV remain well until they reach eight, nine, or ten years of age.

Because the chances of transmitting HIV to a fetus are high, and because children with HIV have little hope of cure, women with HIV are usually advised to avoid pregnancy. They are counseled to use effective methods of birth control: not only condoms, but also additional kinds of contraception, like the pill. The same applies to women who are having sex with infected men. Nonsafe sex with an infected man can make you pregnant and can expose you to the virus at the same time. The pill will help prevent pregnancy, but will not prevent the transmission of HIV. Condoms are not as fail-safe as the pill for preventing pregnancy, but are a pretty good barrier to the transmission of HIV.

For women who are already pregnant, the consequences of delivering the baby and the option of abortion should be thought out carefully. Women with HIV infection often say that since the chances that the baby will not be infected with HIV are 65 percent or better, they should not consider abortion. But even a healthy baby can be devastated by HIV infection if the mother or father or brother or sister is infected. You must think carefully about who will care for your baby if your own health should worsen. These things are best considered during the first three months of pregnancy; if you want an abortion, this is the time when abortion is safest.

If a woman has already given birth without prior testing and subsequently learns she has HIV, she should have all her children of preschool age tested. Older children who have remained healthy and developed normally are unlikely to have HIV infection, but some mothers will still want the reassurance of a negative blood test.

Reacting to the Diagnosis

Most people react to learning of their diagnosis of HIV infection with acute confusion, shock, and disbelief. Steven Charles is twenty-five years old, and infected by HIV but asymptomatic. He is a gay man who lives alone in an apartment. Steven talks openly about his first reaction: "I got the diagnosis the day after my birthday. I went for the test, hoping to confirm I was negative. When the doctor told me, I ran out of the office and stood in the hall. I didn't know whether to cry or not. I couldn't believe it. I didn't know what my priorities should be. Do you start gearing yourself up to leave the world, or to live?

Lisa Pratt's husband, Glen, a sixty-year-old man who had received an infected blood transfusion, would not believe the test results. Like Steven Charles, Lisa's husband reacted to the diagnosis of HIV infection with shock and disbelief: "He kept saying, 'Those idiots don't know what they're doing.' He made them test him again and again," Lisa said later. Some people, because they are gay or use drugs intravenously, have anticipated the diagnosis. In either case, the diagnosis confronts people, usually for the first time, with the possibility of getting sick and dying.

This possibility has no normal place in our lives. No one is ready to hear this news, or to assimilate it all at once: "What do you *do* with that kind of information," said Steven Charles, "that you have this kind of disease?" It assaults our plans for the future, the principles by which we make decisions, who we think we are. As a result, people go into shock. Some people continue their lives almost unthinkingly: "For a few days after my diagnosis," Steven said, "if it wasn't automatic, it wasn't getting done." Others say they "freeze up" or "go on hold": Lisa said that for a while, "Glen simply quit getting out of bed, quit eating."

Shock and disbelief are the normal reactions to this diagnosis. So are problems with eating and sleeping. Alan Madison is thirty-five years old, also infected with HIV, is gay, and lives in a condominium with a long-time partner. "I didn't sleep at first," said Alan. "It was a lot of emotions for one thirty-six-hour period."

With shock and trouble eating and sleeping comes an assortment of related reactions. People blame themselves and lose their good opinion of themselves. They are agitated and anxious and entirely preoccupied with the diagnosis. They are depressed, sad, unable to enjoy or take pleasure in things. They isolate themselves: "At first," said Alan, "I unplugged the phone and said no visitors. I put up roadblocks on purpose." When people first hear the diagnosis, they lose hope for the future and think about suicide. They are also furious: "My husband stood in our living room, swearing," said Lisa Pratt. "He yelled, 'Damn it, damn it, how did I hit odds that small?' "

When they first hear of their diagnosis, people with HIV are frightened by the prospect of sickness and death. Most are confused and don't know what to expect or how to make plans: Will I be alive in ten years? Will I be alive for my next birthday? Can I eat in a restaurant? Will my partner leave me? Should I stay in my job? Will I live to see a cure? Will I run out of money? How should I behave? What should I feel? How am I different? People close to the person who is newly diagnosed may also be confused: "I didn't understand what it meant," said Lisa. "I thought he'd die in six months."

Though these feelings are terrible, and though they will recur, their acuteness is shortlived. They last from a few weeks to a few months— typically around six weeks. People deal with these feelings the way they have dealt with all other crises in their lives. They use the same skills, the same strategies they always have. "My husband cried when he told me about it," said Lisa. "I told my husband, 'Don't be sorry. I love you. We'll handle this the way we handle everything else.' "

Strategies for Handling the Feelings

Different strategies for handling the feelings work for different people. In general, people try to fit the infection into their lives, to see what the infection does mean and what it does not mean.

Because people are so different, their strategies for coping are different—in fact, sometimes completely opposite. Any strategy that allows you to accept the diagnosis and stay emotionally intact is a good one.

Use whatever strategies have worked on other problems. Use whatever strategies your needs and personality seem to dictate.

Some people talk about it: "When I got the diagnosis of AIDS," said Steven, "I called my cousin and she flew in. Then I talked to my parents. My father was hysterical, my mother was in shock. For a while, we were all moderately hysterical together." By sharing news of the diagnosis, people surround themselves with the warmth and comfort of those who care about them. In these surroundings, they find it easier to let the fact of the diagnosis sink in, and easier also then to put that fact into perspective. Other people want to handle it alone. Lisa used to sit for hours with her head between her knees, giving herself time, she said, to "just feel what I felt" before she had to put a public face on her feelings. The "roadblocks" Alan said he put up between himself and other people gave him time to deal with his own reactions to the diagnosis before taking on anyone else's. If you want the sense of companionship that talking will bring you, talk. If you want time to sort out your feelings alone, don't talk. If you want both, have both.

Some people read books on HIV infection and talk to doctors, to educate themselves about every aspect of the infection. This gives them a sense of knowing what they are up against, a sense of control over what affects them. Others accept information about the infection bit by bit, as they are ready for it. They want to keep their defenses intact and not feel overwhelmed by the diagnosis.

Some abolish their bad feelings: "For a long while now," said Steven, "I've squelched anxiety. I put it out of my mind. I can't worry about craziness." They find that feeling and acting normally helps them accept the diagnosis gradually and stay in control of their feelings. Others express the bad feelings—to friends, in a private journal, or alone. They have crying spells, like Alan, who says "I cry it out." Expressing these feelings often seems to dilute them, and they hurt less. Many people alternate between expressing and avoiding their feelings.

Some people, like Steven, talk individually to people with HIV infection: "I talked to someone who had AIDS and asked him a lot of questions," Steven said. "It was hard to do, but it seemed necessary." Some look up those affected by HIV infection, not to talk about the infection, but simply to socialize: go to the theatre, to sports events, out to eat. Many join support groups for people with HIV infection (see section on support and therapy groups in Chapter 12). In support groups, they lose their sense of isolation. They see others handling what seems overwhelming. They hear of new strategies for dealing with the diagnosis and decide what would work for them and what wouldn't.

Many talk to mental health professionals—psychiatrists, psychologists, social workers, counselors, and therapists of all kinds—who help people with HIV infection. Mental health professionals help people understand that their reactions are normal. The professionals often offer advice and alternate strategies, and they can be told anything.

Some people turn to their religions: Lisa Pratt said her husband became more spiritual, and that she herself was learning "to trust, not my feelings, but God's promise that I'll find peace in the midst of this." Religion gives people a context in which the diagnosis seems less threatening.

The Turning Point

One way or another, people's strategies usually work, and their acute distress fades. They come to understand they can live with the virus. This understanding often comes as a sudden turning point. Alan Madison, after a few days of isolating himself, talked to his mother, who told him to get over it. "That didn't help," he said. "Then the next day in the shower I said to myself, 'This stinks, but I'm stuck with this virus and would rather have my life happy than sad.' "

Steven Charles had a similar turning point: "After I was diagnosed with the virus, I read up on it, and decided my life expectancy was eight years. So I took my bank account and divided it into eight piles. Then I thought, what if I live nine years? That sort of settled me. I decided to let tomorrow take care of itself."

Lisa Pratt's turning point was more religious: "At first, I let the house go. I let junk pile up. After a while, the facts started sinking in. I said to God, 'You've got your work cut out for you. I'm going to turn a lot of this over to you until I can handle it.' Then I went out and bought one hundred narcissus bulbs because I knew we'd need a reminder of the renewal of life. And it worked. My husband said, 'They make me feel so good.' "

Occasionally, however, nothing works. Even after a few months, people remain extremely depressed: they are still preoccupied, or think seriously about not wanting to live, or persist in having problems eating and sleeping. This more serious type of depression happens to about 5 percent to 15 percent of people with HIV infection (the same percentages of people who become severely depressed after being told that they have cancer or some other serious illness). Some people deny they are infected and persist in behavior that puts the health of both other people and themselves at risk. Some people consider suicide, though less than one percent of those with HIV infection actually commit suicide. People who experience severe depression, denial, or thoughts of suicide need to get help from a psychiatrist, psychologist, or other mental health professional (see Chapter 4). Persistent depression may be best treated with medication, which a psychiatrist can prescribe.

Most people gradually understand and believe that they are not going to die tomorrow. They have time to get used to the infection, to find answers to their questions. They restabilize, and they continue living. "Life changes, then comes back to normal," said Steven. "I'm no longer sitting around waiting to get sick."

People also understand that living with the virus means taking precautions against infecting other people, and guarding their own health. "I had the universal reactions," said Alan Madison, "but I grew out of it. Now I just try to take care of myself and act responsibly."

Some people, at their own pace, begin thinking how they might change their lives. Alan's hobby had always been writing, and now he thought he would like to write a really good book. Steven, who worked as a technician for a scientific laboratory, had always wanted to teach, and volunteered as a teacher in a community adult education course.

Some people begin tidying up relationships: Lisa's husband called his brother more often, and they began going to ball games together. Steven eventually asked his cousin to come stay with him: "We'll spend more time enjoying the things that give us pleasure."

This is not to say that under normal circumstances, fear or depression or isolation go away and stay away. The feelings almost seem to cycle, to come back in waves over and over again. But with each cycle, the feelings become easier to deal with, and the strategies people use to deal with them become almost automatic. "I was fearful and depressed for a whole summer," Alan said. "But now, when it starts washing over me again, I know what to do. I get busy, and then I'm not afraid." Steven said, "At first, my diagnosis was the only thing on my mind. That was a year ago, and I still get pretty depressed, but now it's not the only thing my mind." Chapters 4 and 12 go into more detail about the recurring feelings and about people's strategies for dealing with them.

Telling People about the Diagnosis

One of the first practical, concrete problems most people face after their diagnosis is deciding who to tell. This decision is difficult. Different people decide differently, depending on the situation, their own personalities, and the personalities of those they might tell. "I told my parents," said Steven Charles. "I learned early in life I put nothing over on them. Everybody around me knows, I tell lots of people." Alan Madison, on the other hand, says he is careful whom he tells: "Only my partner. And my mother, my sister, and my young nephew. No one else." Lisa Pratt said, "In the eight months since I've known about my husband, I've told only my daughters, my father, and my stepmother. I have brothers and sisters I have not told."

June Monroe is a fifty-five-year-old mother and housewife who lives in a close-knit neighborhood within a large city. "My son has AIDS," she said. "I told my sister. The neighborhood we live in, the people are nice but I don't think they could be helpful. I don't think we'll tell them." Dean Lombard is a forty-year-old gay man who has AIDS. Dean has a son by an earlier marriage, and now owns a house with a long-term partner. "I told my partner, my parents, brother, sister, my son, and my pastor," Dean said. "I stopped there. It's hard to explain—I'm extremely close to other people and all my relatives. But I don't want to tell them."

In another case, the decision is complicated. With each person, you balance the reasons for telling against the reasons for keeping silent.

Who to Tell and Why

First, decide who you are obliged to tell. That category includes your doctor and dentist, your sexual partners, needle-sharing partners if you use drugs, the health care institution in which you work, and, only if you are filing claims for HIV-related conditions, your insurance company.

Next, decide who you would like to tell. Some people feel that they have a responsibility to tell those they love. They worry that not telling might be seen as lying. Steven Charles and Dean Lombard both feel close to their families and do not want to be seen as secret-keepers. They both think their families would want to know something this important. "I couldn't *not* tell my parents," Dean said, "I owed them at least that."

Many people want to tell those they trust because they need the sympathy and support of these people. "My relatives who knew said, 'Don't tell anyone else,'" said Lisa Pratt, whose husband was then in the final stages of AIDS. "I said, 'I've *got* to. I can't live alone with this.'" People find it hard to be alone with physical illness or emotional distress. They find that talking to someone alleviates that loneliness. Talking also makes problems easier to analyze and to solve. And if the problems have no solutions, talking them over makes them easier to live with.

Some people even want to tell everyone. They find that going public with their problems helps other, more isolated people. These people write articles about AIDS, and have even begun newspapers and newsletters. Lisa eventually talked to a reporter, she said, "because so many people were hurting. And the article did help people who are alone in this." Once the newspaper article on Lisa was published, the rest of her relatives and friends found out about her husband's diagnosis.

To decide who you would like to tell, ask some of the following questions. Who do you feel ought to know? Who do you love? Who will not run away? Who can see past the infection, and love and value you? Who can keep a confidence? Who is practical and sensible and reliable? Who can help you plan your affairs? Who can respond to requests for help? Who can listen to what you have so say? You might also think about which you are more comfortable with: the sense that you have no secrets, or the sense that you take care of your own business.

Lisa initially told her daughters because she babysits regularly for one daughter's children and the other daughter is a practical nurse whose help she might need. Steven told his parents partly so they could prepare themselves in case he got sick, and partly because he couldn't put anything over on them. He told his sister so she could help his parents. Alan told his partner, so his partner could get tested and so they could both take precautions. He also told his counselor and a friend, because "it helps when someone knows you other than as a patient." Later, he told a co-worker, who also happened to be infected with HIV, because "he's a positive, 'up' person to talk to. It does good to hear how someone else handles it, someone who has a good outlook." June told her sister about her son's diagnosis: "She feels as badly as I do. We share the misery." In general, Steven likes sharing his life with everyone he knows. Alan is more comfortable maintaining a sense of his own privacy.

Sometimes people guess the facts and ask. Perhaps they knew of a person's homosexuality or drug use and had been worrying about the possibility of infection. Alan's partner's father asked Alan's partner, "Alan's been sick a lot. Does he have this AIDS?"

In general, like June, most people believe they can trust their own inner senses of who they can tell: "You play it by ear," June says. "You know who's right to discuss it with."

If you would like to talk about your diagnosis and are uncomfortable telling the people you would usually talk to, you might try joining a support group for people with HIV infection.

Deciding who to tell has a complication: telling people about your diagnosis also means telling them how you got the virus. Sometimes that means telling them about a history of blood transfusions or hemophilia, or your spouse's transfusions or hemophilia. Other times, it means telling them things about your sexual habits or drug use they might find difficult to accept.

Homosexuality. Information about sexual habits is hard to say and hard to hear. Along with learning the diagnosis, some people hear for the first time that their son or brother or husband or lover is gay. As a result, relationships often become unhappy or difficult. June had found out by accident that her son was gay: "I felt like someone hit me with a claw hammer. It broke my heart. He said, 'I want to explain.' But I didn't want to know. I was bitter. I cried for a month."

Probably the best way to resolve the estrangement is to talk about it. One Sunday, June began crying in church and had to leave: "My son followed me outside the church and said, 'Don't you still love me? Am I any different?' I told him I wasn't raised to understand gays. I said I didn't understand it, and he said, 'Mom, I didn't choose my sexuality. And I don't understand you and Dad either.' What bothered me was that I'd miss his marriage and children, but that was just selfish. I had to take the parts of me that were my old beliefs and upbringing and set them aside. I had to come to terms with my son's gayness." Like many people, though, June continued to hope her son would change.

Steven's cousin, who is his caregiver, knew Steven was gay: "She said she knew all along," Steven said. "She'd change me if she could. But when I get tired of her arguing about it, I tell her." Steven and his cousin, and June and her son, like many others, discuss their differences, and if they do not understand each other, agree to let it be. No one in these relationships thinks their differences are as important as their bonds. "Loving is loving," June said. "I've always loved my son. I would have a harder time not loving him than loving him."

Discussion does not always lead to resolution, especially for gay or bisexual men and their wives. Sometimes a couple can discuss the husband's sexuality openly. This sometimes results in divorce, sometimes in friendship, sometimes in an agreement that the man and woman will still help each other out. Other times, the couple has an unspoken agreement to ignore the husband's sexuality; it remains his own private business, and no one asks questions. Sometimes, even after a diagnosis of AIDS, the husband denies that he is gay and the wife agrees to believe the denial. All these alternatives work; each couple decides what works best for them. The only resolution that is unhealthy is one in which one person is infected with HIV and the couple does not practice safer sex.

Drug use. Drug users face the same possibility of rejection that gays face. Helen Parks is a divorced, thirty-five-year-old woman with two sons who live with their father. Helen, who is now in the early symptomatic stage of HIV infection, became infected with HIV after using drugs intravenously. She said that once she told her father, from then on, she had to face his suspicions. "My dad means no harm," said Helen, "but he accuses me of being high when I'm not, like when I'm crying or being easy to get along with. He goes through my things. It plays on my nerves, but I don't resent his suspicions. I've put him through a lot this year."

Drug users are also likely to have to face charges, such as, "So that's where you've been," or "So that's where my money went," or "So that's why you got fired." But in fact, drug users do not usually have to tell their parents or their partners about drug use. Unless drug use is recreational, that is, unless it has not changed the person's life and habits, parents and partners always know before they are told.

Reasons for Keeping Silent

Some people who made their diagnoses public have compromised their jobs, their ability to get mortgages, and their ability to keep their insurance. For this reason, many advise people with HIV infection to tell as few others as possible: tell those they are obliged to tell, tell those they love and whose support and help they need, and then tell no others. You are certainly under no obligation to tell your neighbors, your employer, your landlord, or, unless you are filing HIV-related claims, your insurance agent.

The reason most people cite for keeping silent is worry about others' reactions. "I don't make a point of the truth about my son," said June, "but I would answer if asked. So far, no one has. I'm not ashamed of the truth, but it bothers other people."

The particular truth of HIV infection does indeed bother people. When Dean Lombard first told his mother, she stayed out of church for a long time because she was afraid the other members would not talk to her; Dean's sister was afraid of being rejected by her friends. Alan Madison worried that his mother would feel guilty, overreact, and make his life more difficult by "asking me questions and giving me orders." Alan also stopped inviting friends over because he thought that when they found out about his infection, they would worry because they had used his coffee cups. Steven Charles worried that his co-workers would no longer want to work with him. He thought that his sister would no longer invite him to dinner or allow him to play with her children. He was worried about how much he would hurt his relatives and about how much pain he would cause them.

Other people have related reasons for keeping silent. Helen Parks worried that people would find out without her telling them: "Psychologically," she says, "that plays on my nerves." Her sons, she thought, could not keep confidences. She was afraid that those she told would gossip, and she would lose control over who knew and who did not. She even bought the drugs to control her infection in a nearby city rather than risk being seen in her local pharmacy. She worried about having to tell her insurance company. June Monroe did not want to tell her mother-in-law, her son's grandmother; the old woman was in failing health, and June did not want to add to her troubles. Lisa's husband did not want to tell his daughter: "He told me he just couldn't, and started crying," she said. "He said he was so ashamed."

How Others React

Often, these worries are without foundation, and people, when told, react much differently from how we expect them to react. Alan's mother says she feels guilty for not having somehow protected him against the virus, but she is able to talk freely to him and thinks of ways for him to get out of the house. Dean's mother had stopped going to church, but when she noticed that the other members of her church were still talking to her, she began going again. Steven's sister makes a point of leaving her children with him, and his co-workers asked the social worker at the local hospital how to help Steven out if he got sick. Helen's father, who had always been reserved with her, "dropped his mask," she said, "and changed. He became warm and loving." Alan says not to underestimate your family and friends.

Unfortunately, worries about others' reactions are sometimes justified. Just as sympathy and sensitivity are part of human nature, so are fear, discrimination, and avoidance of illness. After the newspaper article on Lisa was published, she talked to her friends about her husband's illness: "I said, 'I want to tell you, I learned my husband has AIDS.' And my friends said, 'Why are you telling us this?' And I said, 'I love my husband, now he's going to die, and I need your help.' But they couldn't help. They couldn't call, not even the priest."

Sometimes, as with Lisa's friends and priest, these unpleasant reactions come from those you most count on. Alan's dentist refused to treat him, and his pastor barred him from church. Dean said, "My dentist told me to go somewhere else. My father went behind me and cleaned the phone with disinfectant. My pastor didn't want me touching anything he had to touch." Helen's stepmother insisted on protective papers over the toilet seat; Helen said, "She acted like my house had a plague in it, like it had devils in it." Lisa went to the hospital for a chest x-ray and found written on the orders for the x-ray, "Husband has AIDS"; the nurses held her hospital gown by their fingertips. When June's son was in the hospital, the staff left meal trays outside the door of his room; the same thing happened to Dean in a different hospital.

In some people, these reactions are only temporary: Lisa's friends finally began visiting and bringing in meals; Dean's father and Helen's stepmother both stopped worrying about the telephone and the toilet seat. For other people, these reactions, in spite of being unpleasant, are probably not going to change. Inevitably, you will tell someone who cannot handle the news.

This starts a series of reactions in you. You may feel rejected, angry, isolated. Sometimes these feelings are reinforced by other worries: that people are right to reject you, that you brought the virus on yourself, that you are to blame for your diagnosis. This series of reactions is understandable; people are especially vulnerable when the diagnosis is still new.

But these reactions confuse issues that are really separate and unrelated. People who cannot handle your diagnosis are probably not rejecting you personally. In any case, their actions toward you have no bearing on your worth or your good opinion of yourself. Instead, people who reject you are rejecting what they fear. HIV infection reminds them of fears they have—about contagion, illness, sexuality, mortality, dependency—which they cannot face. Rejecting you because you remind them of their fears helps them keep at a distance. They are not thinking about you at all; they are concerned only with their own problems, they are only protecting themselves.

Perhaps, while you are still vulnerable to people's reactions, it is best to keep silent. Wait until your feelings stabilize and you feel more sure of yourself. Then decide who to tell. If people disappoint you, the best policy might be to accept them as they are and, if necessary, avoid them.

You Need Not Tell Everyone

Once a nurse said that Helen ought to tell her sons about her diagnosis, and Helen got so angry she asked the nurse to leave. Whether she told her sons, she thought, was her decision alone. Helen was right: you are the best judge of who to tell and who not to tell. Your diagnosis is not everyone's business. In fact, you might find it refreshing to have a group of people—say, co-workers—who treat you as though you were completely healthy. Alan looks healthy and strong, and people tell him he looks good. When his partner asked if this bothered him, Alan replied, "Not at all. I love it."

Alternatives to Outright Telling

People also decide to avoid the problem of who to tell and who not to, and find ways around making the decision. Some people do not tell, but instead let their friends and families ask. These people leave clues, they may talk about friends who have AIDS, leave pamphlets and books on

AIDS where others can find them, buy grave plots and talk about funerals, say someone at work told them a story about a person with AIDS, and talk about TV programs on AIDS and recommend their families watch them. The families and friends sense the truth. Then, if they can handle the information, they will ask; if they can't, they won't.

Some people do trial runs of telling, testing for rejection before telling. One woman was so afraid her children would reject her that she thought she could not tell them without breaking down. So she rehearsed by telling a cousin whose rejection she feared less, and when she finally told her children, she could keep the composure she wanted. Some people, like those who let their friends and families ask, leave clues. Then, they judge by reactions to the clues whether telling will be safe or will result in rejection.

Other people find alternatives to the outright facts. If they become sick, they say they have pneumonia or a lung disease, herpes, leukemia, ulcers, meningitis, or hepatitis, or a cancer, or an infection of the nervous system. They choose whatever disease is most appropriate to their symptoms. Helen said, "I read in a medical book about a blood disease that can be either acute or fatal. As long as I'm alive, I'll say it's acute."

Chapter 2

Preventing Transmission of HIV Infection: Understanding How HIV Is Spread

- **Principles of contagion**
- **Preventing transmission through sex, drugs, or pregnancy**
- **Preventing transmission during home care**

HIV is a virus that infects white blood cells, primarily those called *CD4 cells* (also called *T4 cells* or *T-helper cells*). CD4 cells are found in several body fluids, but mainly in blood and in genital secretions. HIV is passed, or transmitted, when the CD4 cells from one person's blood or genital secretions get inside the body of another person. This method of transmission does not account for every case of HIV infection, but it does account for 97 percent of those people who have AIDS and would probably account for most of the remaining 3 percent if the necessary information could be reliably obtained.

The scientific evidence to support this method of transmission is compelling. What is known about the risk of transmitting HIV has come from two types of scientific studies: partly from studies of the virus, called *virology*; and principally from studies of the people who are infected with the virus, called *epidemiology*. The epidemiologic studies came first in time. In 1981, epidemiologists began tracking cases of pneumocystis pneumonia in gay men; by 1983, when HIV was finally discovered, epidemiologists knew most of what was necessary to know about the spread of the disease. They knew that the disease, whatever its cause, was transmitted by sexual intercourse and by blood and by passage from an infected mother to her unborn child. They knew that this sort of transmission suggested that a microbe was responsible (other microbes, including cytomegalovirus and hepatitis B virus, are transmitted in precisely the same ways). In 1983, a French researcher, Luc

Montagnier, reported the virology studies that described the virus that came to be called HIV.

But whether the scientific evidence is compelling or not, misunderstanding of how HIV is transmitted is widespread and causes people a lot of worry. The purpose of this chapter is to discuss, first, what is known and what is not known about the risk of transmitting HIV, and second, how to prevent transmission. In other words, it is about how not to give someone else HIV and about how not to get it yourself.

Most of the public's misconception is based on the belief that HIV is transmitted the way more common viruses, like the influenza virus, are transmitted. We think it is important to emphasize that viruses like the influenza virus and HIV are enormously different, not only in the way they are transmitted, but in the way they behave to cause disease.

Principles of Contagion

Preventing transmission begins with understanding the principles that govern how infections are transmitted. These principles are called the *principles of contagion.*

The terms *infectious diseases* and *contagious diseases* refer to different things. Infectious diseases are caused by *microbes*; microbes are viruses, bacteria, fungi, and parasites. Contagious diseases can be spread from person to person. Some diseases, like toxic shock syndrome or Legionnaires' disease, are infectious but not contagious. HIV infection, however, is both infectious (it is caused by a microbe) and contagious (with specific kinds of contact, it can be spread from one person to another). This chapter will begin by comparing HIV infection to another infectious and contagious disease most people know well from firsthand experience: influenza.

The microbe that causes influenza is a virus found in the nose, throat, and lungs of the person who is infected. Influenza is spread when secretions from the nose, throat, or lungs of the infected person are passed to another person. When an infected person coughs or sneezes on another person, or touches another person, these secretions and the virus they carry are transmitted.

People can be either susceptible or not susceptible to an influenza virus. If they have been infected with that particular virus or a closely related one before, or if they have been vaccinated against the virus, they already have antibodies against it, so they are not susceptible and will not get influenza. If they do not have these antibodies, they are susceptible and will get influenza.

Whether susceptible or not, the person will not become infected if the type of contact is wrong. Specific viruses can live only on specific tissues within the body. An influenza virus on the skin of your hand will not give you influenza; the same virus on the membranes of your nose, throat, or lungs will. If the virus is on your hand and you bring your hand to your mouth, however, you may get influenza.

Given susceptibility and the right type of contact, some viruses are more likely than others to be spread from person to person, that is, some viruses are transmitted with greater efficiency than others. Some viruses are difficult to spread; for others, like the influenza virus, even very brief contact with a person who is infected is likely to result in transmission. Highly efficient transmission accounts for the annual epidemics of influenza.

The efficiency with which a virus is transmitted also depends on the number of viruses a person is exposed to, or the *inoculum size*. Living with a person with influenza is obviously more likely to result in successful transmission than simply working with that person in the same office. And being sneezed upon poses a greater risk than passing someone in a hallway. In short, how efficiently a virus is transmitted depends both on the number of influenza viruses and the type of contact.

A person, once infected, may continue to feel well for a day or two but, during this time, can still pass the virus to others. This early period between infection and the beginning of symptoms is called the *incubation period.*

HIV, like influenza, follows the same general principles of contagion. An infected person is the source of HIV. HIV is contagious if a person is susceptible and the contact is of the kind necessary for transmission. And HIV has a certain efficiency of transmission and a certain incubation period. There the resemblance ends.

This point deserves emphasis. Much of the misunderstanding about AIDS is based on the assumption that HIV is transmitted like other common infectious diseases. It isn't. In brief, for HIV, the types of contact are very specific, transmission is inefficient, and HIV's incubation period is very long.

Sources of HIV

A person with HIV infection is almost the sole source of this infection. The only time a person is not directly the source is in the laboratory when a researcher has taken inadequate precautions and is infected while working with large numbers of the virus. Any person with HIV infection, regardless of symptoms, should be considered capable of transmitting the disease.

Types of Contact

The white blood cells that HIV infects, the CD4 cells, are found in differing numbers in different body fluids. As a result, the numbers of HIV also differ in different body fluids. The numbers of HIV are greatest in semen, breast milk, and blood, including menstrual blood. The numbers of HIV are fewer in women's genital secretions. HIV is unlikely to be in saliva or tears, though it has been found in these fluids in a minority of people, and then only in very low numbers. HIV has not been found in urine or feces. In order to cause infection, HIV must travel from the body fluids of an infected person into the bloodstream of an uninfected person. The skin that covers the outside of the body is a formidable barrier. If the skin is intact, simple contact between HIV and the skin will not transmit HIV. The mucous membranes that cover most of the insides of the mouth, vagina, and rectum are also a barrier to the virus. But we are less certain whether mucous membranes are as formidable a barrier as skin.

If the skin or a mucous membrane is broken—if it has cuts or sores— the virus can get into the bloodstream. Thus, infected blood, menstrual blood, vaginal fluids, or semen on intact skin is almost invariably safe. But on skin or mucous membranes that have an open sore or a cut, the same fluids can possibly transmit the virus. Injecting large amounts of infected blood into the body—like a transfusion of blood from an infected person—is the most efficient method of transmission.

We can provide absolute assurance that most types of common contact carry no risk of transmitting the virus. These include a variety of experiences often referred to as "casual contact": shaking hands, hugging, sharing a toilet, sharing eating utensils, closed-mouth kissing, being sneezed on, and so forth. Not only has infection through casual contact not happened, it is biologically unrealistic to suppose it might.

There are three primary types of contact that can result in transmission of HIV:

Sexual contact, that is, contact with infected genital secretions (semen, vaginal fluids, menstrual blood)

Injection of infected blood through transfusions or needle sharing

Pregnancy in an infected mother

Other kinds of contact more rarely result in transmission of HIV. These are:

Breast-feeding by an infected mother (transmission to baby)

Breast-feeding by an infected baby (transmission to mother)

Organ transplantation using organs from infected donors

Artificial insemination from infected sperm donors

Needlestick injuries in health care professionals caring for infected people

Dental care and possibly surgical procedures done by infected health care workers

Whether oral sex, either cunnilingus (oral sex performed on a woman) or fellatio (oral sex performed on a man), transmits HIV infection is controversial. There are stories about HIV being transmitted through oral sex, but in most cases, people who practice oral sex also practice other kinds of sex that definitely do transmit HIV. So no one knows for sure whether oral sex alone can transmit HIV. We do know that breast-feeding is a pretty high risk for transmission, and breast-feeding and oral sex may risk transmission in similar ways. Both breast milk and semen have lots of lymphocytes (lymphocytes carry HIV), and swallowed lymphocytes may be a substantive risk.

The combined total for these rarer types of contact accounts for about 0.1 percent of cases, actually amounting to only about 200 of the first 200,000 cases of AIDS reported to the Centers for Disease Control (CDC) (transfusions, now screened for HIV, are excluded from this number).

We are sure about what kinds of contact do and do not transmit the virus. Over 250,000 people with AIDS have been studied by the CDC. The types of contact listed above together account for 95 to 97 percent. When researchers went back and looked specifically at the remaining 3 to 5 percent of people not accounted for by these types of contact, they found that most were problematic: many people acknowledged risks when questioned by a more experienced interviewer, some people were so seriously ill at the time of reporting that no reliable medical history could be obtained, and some never had HIV infection to begin with. By the time researchers were done, the type of contact responsible for transmission remained ambiguous in less than 1 percent of the people. Given the likelihood that people will lie about such sensitive issues as homosexuality and the use of illegal drugs, 1 percent is an incredibly low figure.

At the same time, it must be acknowledged that other types of contact, though unlikely to transmit HIV, might transmit HIV, at least in theory. HIV has been found in low numbers in saliva and tears. HIV has not been found in feces or urine. Although transmission through these fluids is biologically possible, it doesn't seem to happen; the CDC, which tracks all cases of AIDS, has no case in which the only type of contact was clearly through saliva, feces, urine, or tears. Perhaps the inoculum size—the numbers of virus—in these fluids is simply too low. In any case, transmission of HIV through these types of contact is extremely inefficient and is not known to happen. Unfortunately, the CDC and other groups continue to talk about "body fluids" as the source of HIV infection. This gives the wrong impression that the source of infection is all body fluids. In fact, the only body fluids that are the source of infection are semen, vaginal fluids, breast milk, menstrual blood, and blood.

One type of contact that people worry about is mouth contact. HIV is found in low numbers in saliva, so deep kissing, mouth-to-mouth resuscitation, biting, being spat upon, and the like might potentially transmit the virus. It is noteworthy that HIV is actually found in saliva in only about 1 or 2 percent of people with HIV infection. Moreover, even in these people, the numbers of the virus are so low that researchers believe that transmission through saliva is biologically improbable and perhaps impossible. For this reason, the CDC has removed saliva as a potential source of infection for health care workers. The result is that a nurse who is spat upon or bitten by a patient with HIV infection is not considered to have been exposed to HIV. Nevertheless, we periodically hear of a case where saliva is a suggested type of contact. As a result, contact through saliva remains a theoretical concern that cannot be totally excluded.

Another type of contact people worry about is indirect: becoming infected by a virus on a surface outside the body. To repeat, no one (except the rare laboratory worker using high concentrations of the virus) has ever become infected by the virus living on a surface outside the body. The reason is that HIV cannot survive outside its host cells, and outside the body, cells die quickly. When host cells die, HIV dies with them. Although HIV can survive outside the body on a surface for up to fifteen days, the numbers of viruses on a surface fall rapidly to levels well below those necessary for infection.

A third possibility that people worry about, probably because the news media have paid a lot of attention to it, is that insects, particularly mosquitoes, could conceivably transmit the virus. The argument is that insects transmit other microbes in the blood, such as malaria. But even in Africa, where mosquito-borne diseases like malaria are common, scientists have not been able to find a clear case in which HIV has been transmitted by a mosquito. AIDS in Africa is a disease found almost exclusively in babies and sexually active adults, especially those in cities. Mosquitoes, however, do not select out babies and sexually active adults in cities to bite; mosquitoes are everywhere and bite everyone.

Epidemiological studies have been done specifically to study the possibility that HIV is spread by mosquitoes. These studies found that the areas in the United States with large populations of mosquitoes have no more cases of HIV infection than other areas; nor do they have more cases of HIV infection whose source of infection is unknown. Further studies in the laboratory show that mosquitoes cannot transmit HIV mechanically. The conclusion by most authorities in this field is that mosquitoes are not a source of HIV infection.

A fourth possibility is that a patient might get HIV infection from an infected health care worker, like a surgeon or dentist. The worry about this possibility followed the widely publicized case of the dentist in Florida who apparently infected five of his patients. An extensive investigation of this case by the CDC showed that the five patients appeared to get this infection from their dental care. Exactly how the dentist transmitted HIV infection has never been sorted out and never will be. This case raised a new possible mechanism of infection—acquisition from your dentist or possibly from your surgeon, presumably by mixing of blood. Ensuing studies seemed to show that this case was an isolated event. Testing of about 20,000 patients who had surgery or dental care from someone with HIV infection failed to turn up a single case of HIV transmission. Nevertheless, the possibility had been raised and required a response to a worried public. So the CDC then did some mathematical calculations with very limited data. It concluded that the risk of getting HIV infection from major surgery, called *exposure-prone invasive procedures*, by an infected surgeon was between 1 in 41,000 and 1 in 410,000. The same risk with an untested surgeon is about one hundred times less than being murdered and is about the same as the risk of being struck by lightning or the risk of dying from driving three miles. Despite such odds, the CDC has recommended voluntary HIV testing of surgeons and dentists. The CDC recommends limitations in the practice of those who are found to be infected.

Efficiency of Transmission

Because the types of contact are so specific and the numbers of the virus in some body fluids are so low, HIV is not transmitted efficiently. Certain kinds of contact transmit HIV more efficiently than others. This section will discuss efficiency of transmission in terms of the likelihood that a given type of contact will transmit HIV. The types of contact that transmit the virus most efficiently are those with the highest risk for infection.

There are four categories of risk for HIV infection, from the kinds of contact that are most likely to transmit the virus to the kinds that are least likely to do so.

1. Very likely risks. These are well-established, common ways to transmit the virus. They account for over 99 percent of cases. The order in which they are discussed below does not imply that there is a hierarchy of risk within this category. All these behaviors pose a very likely risk of infection.

The first very likely risk is nonsafe sex—that is, sex without condoms or spermicides or sex that involves exchange of body fluids—with people known to have HIV infection, or with people who have a high risk for HIV infection: The risk of getting HIV through nonsafe sex with an infected person is roughly estimated from studies done of spouses of people with HIV infection. For every five hundred to eight hundred episodes of nonsafe sex, the spouses had one chance of becoming infected.

How efficiently HIV is transmitted during sexual intercourse depends on a number of factors. One of the most important is whether the uninfected person has open sores on the genitals. The most common cause of genital sores are other sexually transmitted diseases such as herpes, syphilis, and chancroid. Open sores allow the virus to enter directly into the blood. The risk of transmission increases enormously when sores are present on the genitals.

Another factor is whether the person with the infection is a man or a woman. Most sexually transmitted diseases, like gonorrhea, syphilis, and herpes, are more easily transmitted from men to women. Women are also more likely to become infected with HIV than men, by about twenty to one. The study that produced these results looked at discordant couples, that is, couples in which one partner had HIV infection and the other didn't. An uninfected woman having regular intercourse with an infected man was twenty times more likely to become infected than an uninfected man having regular intercourse with an infected woman.

A third factor increasing the risk of transmission is the type of sexual practice. Virtually all sexual contact that has resulted in infection with HIV has been either anal or vaginal intercourse. Studies of transmission of HIV infection among gay men suggest that anal intercourse is an especially efficient means of transmission. During anal intercourse, the thin walls of the rectum are often cut or scraped, exposing blood vessels to infected semen. The vaginal wall is thicker and less likely to be cut, so transmission is less likely but still distinctly possible. Any sexual practice that exposes the blood of an uninfected person to the blood (including menstrual blood) or semen or vaginal fluid of an infected person will allow transmission of HIV.

A fourth factor is the numbers of HIV. The idea is that infection is simply more likely if there are more viruses. The numbers of viruses are different in different body fluids (see above). So semen, with higher numbers of viruses, is more likely to transmit HIV than vaginal fluid, with lower numbers of viruses. The numbers of viruses are also different at different stages of HIV infection. Both very early and relatively late in the course of the infection, the blood and presumably menstrual blood and all genital fluids have relatively high numbers of viruses. Early means the first several weeks or months of the infection, before the development of antibodies. Once the body forms antibodies, the numbers of viruses drop. In the late stages of the infection, when the person has relatively few CD4 cells, antibody levels decrease and the numbers of viruses increase again. So theoretically at least, people with HIV infection are more likely to transmit the virus early and late in the course of the infection.

A fifth factor that may influence the risk of transmission is the strain of the virus. HIV can change form within one person over the course of infection, and from one person to the next. Some forms of the virus may be more contagious than others. Or introducing new forms of the virus into your body may speed the course of infection. None of this is known for sure. But to be cautious, continue practicing safer sex even if both partners are infected.

A second very likely risk is sharing needles or works (spoons, cotton, needles, syringes) with a person who injects drugs, especially in cities with a high incidence of HIV infection among intravenous drug users. HIV can be transmitted by blood left on a contaminated needle, or by blood left in the syringe, or by blood on any other components of the works used to prepare the drug for injection. The risk of HIV transmission with needle sharing is not defined, but it apparently is very high: in 1989, children in Russian hospitals were infected by the tiny amount of blood left in a syringe when that single syringe was used for injecting many patients. Factors that influence the efficiency of transmission include the amount of blood, how long the blood has been outside the body before injection, whether the blood is dried, how many viruses are in the blood.

A third high-risk factor is pregnancy in a woman with HIV infection. An infected mother has a 30 to 35 percent chance of transmitting HIV to her unborn child. Exactly how or when transmission happens is unclear. Transmission might take place while the infant is still in the uterus, but it now appears that most of these transmissions occur when the baby passes through the birth canal and is in contact with the mother's genital secretions and blood.

2. *Likely risks.* This section discusses the ways in which HIV *may be* transmitted. The risks are scientifically established, though actual transmission in these ways is rare.

Safer sex (with condoms and with spermicide, or sexual contact that does not involve getting semen, blood, or vaginal fluid from one person's body into another's) with people known to have HIV infection or with people who have a high risk of HIV infection: Though safer sex is known to be safer, no one believes it is completely safe. Exactly how safe it is, no one knows.

Nonsafe heterosexual sex with multiple partners, especially if partners are anonymous, intravenous drug users, gay or bisexual men, or prostitutes in cities with high rates of HIV infection: No one knows exactly what the risk of nonsafe sex with multiple partners is; the risk depends entirely on whether your partners are likely to be infected. Other studies show that the risk of infection might be higher.

Breast-feeding: The risk of transmitting HIV with breast-feeding is hard to measure. Most children with HIV infection probably became infected before they were born, or while they were being born. The best studies on the risk of breast-feeding were done with women in Africa who became infected after their children were born and who were breast-feeding. Twenty-five to 50 percent of their babies became infected during breast-feeding. Furthermore, some babies also might infect their mothers during breast-feeding.

Needlestick injury, primarily for health care workers: One in 250 needlestick injuries has transmitted the virus to the person stuck. Of the four million health care workers, thirty-one to one hundred have become infected, almost all of them by "sharps injuries." A sharps injury is an injury with a sharp instrument like a needle or a scalpel during which the health care worker's blood mixes with the patient's blood. Of every 250 sharps injuries involving patients with HIV infection, one health care worker will become infected. If sharps injuries with all patients, infected and uninfected, are considered, the risk is 1 in 5,000. There are also about five health care workers who became infected when blood splashed into their eyes, mouth, or skin. This kind of transmission is rare, certainly less than 1 per 1,000 when the blood carries HIV. It appears that rare patients may acquire HIV infection from infected health care workers as well: We know of one dentist who transmitted HIV to five patients. Just how the transmission occurred, however, is unclear, and some feel it has no relevance to surgery.

Blood transfusion, artificial insemination, or organ transplantation from an infected donor: Between 1978, when HIV infection first appeared, and 1985, when the Red Cross began screening all blood for HIV, this was a high risk if the donated blood contained HIV. About 90 percent of the people who received HIV-contaminated blood became infected with HIV. Now the blood supply is almost, but not completely, clear of HIV: it is estimated that about 1 in 225 thousand units slips past the HIV screening process. The same scenario held for hemophiliacs, who are treated with a blood product called *clotting factor* that is pooled from the blood of several thousand donors. Between 1978 and 1985, 30 to 70 percent of hemophiliacs who were treated became infected with HIV. Currently, not only are all blood donors screened, but the clotting factor is treated so that any HIV that does slip through is destroyed before transfusion. Screening donors and treating blood works very well but not perfectly. Of the 6 million people who have received transfusions since screening began, 15 have become infected. During the first three years after screening began, about 18 hemophiliacs became infected from clotting factor; currently, the annual rate is less than 1 per 1,000. And there is one famous case of HIV being transmitted by organ transplantation. A man killed by gunshot donated various organs and tissues to 58 people. Though his blood test was negative, 7 of the recipients became infected. Probably the donor was tested in the "window" between infection and a positive blood test (see "Understanding Tests for HIV, beginning on page 299). Note that this is the only case of infection among the 60,000 organs and one million tissues transplanted since 1985. Finally, in the United States, one woman has become infected through artificial insemination, but the donor had not been screened for HIV.

Unprotected oral sex: No one knows just how much of a risk unprotected oral sex is. On one hand, there are a few stories about people becoming infected with HIV through oral sex. On the other hand, the researchers who gather statistics on risk can only occasionally find people who have oral sex exclusively (in other words, they never have anal or vaginal sex), so few studies confirm those stories. Certainly infected semen in the mouth could transmit the virus through any cuts or sores. Infected menstrual blood in the mouth could do the same. Infected vaginal fluids in the mouth are less likely to transmit HIV but are theoretically able to as well.

It is important to emphasize the infrequency of the transmission of HIV in this second category of "likely risks" compared to the first category of "very likely risks." If we add up all the documented cases since 1985, the total is less than 200; the total number of people with HIV infection in the United States is estimated to be one million. So those 200 cases account for about 0.02 percent, or 1 in 10,000.

3. Biologically plausible risks, but unlikely and unconfirmed. These types of contact might possibly transmit HIV, but are unlikely to. They are obviously controversial. If they do transmit HIV, they do so only rarely. As a matter of fact, there are no established cases in this category at all; these risks are totally theoretical. We include them to pacify the "what-if" crowd, the people who worry about risks that are biologically plausible but cannot be proved or disproved.

Sharing toothbrushes or razors with an infected person

Exposure to body fluids (tears, urine, feces, saliva, sweat) other than genital secretions or blood

Exchange of saliva with deep kissing

Caring for a person with HIV using proper precautions (excluding needlestick injuries)

Mosquito transmissions (according to studies, improbable and probably impossible; it is placed in this category simply to be conservative)

4. *Transmission that is not biologically possible.* Transmitting the virus through the following types of contact is inconceivable. The first lesson learned in medical school is "never to say never"; nevertheless, these types of contact not only lack precedent but also appear absurd on the basis of our current scientific knowledge of HIV infection.

Shaking hands

Sharing a toilet

Sharing eating utensils

Being sneezed upon

Living in the same household

Working in the same room or attending the same classroom

Sexual transmission by partners known to be monogamous and uninfected

Any contact with any pet

Closed-mouth kissing

Incubation Period

For most infectious diseases, the incubation period—the period from the time of infection until the person feels the first symptoms—is a few days or weeks. HIV infection is almost unique; its incubation period is five to eight years. This long incubation period accounts for the large reservoir of persons who are infected for years before they are aware of it.

Despite not having symptoms, the person infected with HIV is contagious to others throughout the incubation period.

Preventing Transmission through Sex, Drugs, or Pregnancy

Safer Sex

Methods to reduce sexual transmission of HIV are commonly referred to as "safe sex practices." Safe sex, to be absolutely safe, means no "exchange of body fluids"; that is, semen, blood, menstrual blood, or vaginal fluids must not pass from one person's body into another person's. Perhaps, taking human fallibility into account, the better term is "safer sex."

One good way to prevent transmission of HIV during sexual intercourse, either vaginal or anal intercourse, is to use a barrier against body fluids—that is, condoms. Testing of over one hundred thousand domestically produced latex condoms by the Food and Drug Administration showed HIV could permeate fewer than four condoms per thousand. The following suggestions should improve the safety of safer sex:

1. Use latex condoms. They are less porous—that is, they are less likely to have minute holes through which the virus can pass— than condoms made from animal skins. The latex variety are also substantially less expensive. Condoms manufactured by large companies—Ansell, Inc., Carter-Wallace, Circle Rubber Company, and Schmid Laboratories—are generally more reliable than those from small companies which are sold in novelty shops.

2. Reduce the risk of breakage by leaving the condom in the package until used. Condoms should be stored in a cool and dry place out of direct sunlight. With appropriate storage, most condoms retain their durability for up to three years. Condoms that are in damaged packages or show such signs of age as brittle texture, sticky surface, or discoloration should be discarded. Maintain an adequate supply of condoms.

3. Use water-based lubricants. Avoid oil-based lubricants, like petroleum jelly, cooking oils, lotions, and shortening. Oil-based lubricants weaken latex. The water-based lubricant usually advocated is

K-Y jelly, which is readily available in any drugstore. The lubricant should be placed on the outside of the condom and inside the partner.

4. The spermicide nonoxynol 9 rapidly kills both HIV and sperm. It also kills other microbes that cause sexually transmitted diseases like gonorrhea and chlamydia. Nonoxynol 9 is available as spermicidal creams, jellies, or contraceptive sponges. Most other spermicides are also effective. Condoms containing spermicides are available, but it is better to inject spermicides (using the syringes that are often packaged with spermicides) inside the partner as well.

Some women have an allergic reaction—vaginal irritation or ulceration—to spermicides such as nonoxynol 9. As a result, some authorities caution against using spermicides because any irritation or ulceration on the vaginal lining could conceivably permit transmission of HIV. Other authorities note that few women have these allergic reactions and advise using a spermicide unless the vaginal lining becomes irritated.

5. Spermicides are not substitutes for condoms. They should be used with condoms to provide additional protection.

6. The condom must be put on before any sexual contact, oral or genital.

7. Condoms should be used for fellatio (oral sex performed on a man). Rubber or latex dams placed over the woman's genitals should be used for cunnilingus (oral sex performed on a woman). Latex dental dams are available in dental supply stores.

8. Anyone who makes a mistake and has unprotected sex should use a vinegar douche as quickly as possible. Vinegar kills HIV in the test tube and so may kill HIV in the body as well. Vinegar douches are not a substitute for safer sex. How well they work has not been established. Do not rely on them.

9. Avoid contact with the menstrual blood of any person with HIV. Menstrual blood also contains HIV. Use a condom and spermicide.

Safer sex using condoms has two drawbacks. One is that condoms are not fail-safe. For birth control, condoms have failed for about 10 percent of the couples who use them. Reasons for the failure of condoms in birth control are probably improper usage and breakage. If condoms are not put on properly, they can come off during or just after intercourse. With vaginal intercourse, approximately one condom in one hundred will break. With anal intercourse, the breakage is probably ten times higher, or as many as ten broken condoms in one hundred. The most practical solution is to withdraw before ejaculation, so that the condom neither breaks nor comes off.

The other drawback condoms have is that all too often people simply do not use them. Surveys indicate that, among couples with one infected partner, only about one-half who continue having sexual intercourse actually use condoms on a regular basis. This is a disappointingly small number. Explanations for nonuse vary, but in most surveys the major reasons are that condoms seem to diminish the pleasure of sex, that many people find purchasing condoms embarrassing, and that many people find themselves without condoms at the moment when condoms are needed. Virtually all concerned persons can overcome these reasons for not using condoms. For the woman whose sex partner refuses, there is the female condom. This consists of two flexible rings. One is inserted in the vagina and the other hangs outside, covering the labia. This product appears to work well and is intended to empower women, although it is more expensive than the male condom and the initial tests showed concerns about aesthetics.

The alternative to condoms and spermicide is to have sexual contact that does not exchange body fluids at all. This kind of contact includes body-to-body rubbing, acting out sexual fantasies, or mutual masturbation using disposable latex gloves.

The basic principle of safer sex is to avoid getting the body fluids of a person with HIV infection into the body of another person. That can be accomplished by a barrier—condoms, latex dams, latex gloves—between the body fluids of the person with HIV infection and the other person, or by sexual contact or play that does not involve body fluids at all.

Avoid Intravenous Drug Use

The obvious way to avoid transmitting HIV during intravenous drug use is to stop using drugs that are injected. Many people who use drugs, however, are unable to curb this habit. Some people who would like to stop using drugs may have difficulty finding programs—such as methadone clinics or detoxification centers—that are available. Those who find it impossible to stop using drugs intravenously should avoid sharing needles, avoid sharing works, and, of course, practice safer sex.

Anyone who can't avoid sharing should clean the needle and works between use. Clean needles and syringes by flushing them with household bleach and then rinsing with water, as follows:

1. Use full strength household bleach.

2. Pour the bleach into a glass, immerse the needle and syringe to cover completely, and then draw the bleach up to fill the syringe. Bleach should probably be left in the syringe not less than two minutes. The two-minute period is absolutely critical.

3. Discharge the bleach and repeat the process.

4. Rinse the syringe by filling and discharging water twice.

5. Alcohol is an adequate substitute for bleach.

The drawback to these ways of preventing transmission of HIV is that using any drugs at all reduces a person's inhibitions. With reduced inhibitions, people are much less likely to practice safer sex and to avoid sharing needles and works, in spite of good intentions. Other substances that reduce inhibitions carry the same danger. This applies to mind-altering drugs that are not necessarily injected, such as alcohol, cocaine, crack, amyl nitrate (poppers), marijuana, barbiturates, and amphetamines (speed).

Avoid Pregnancy and Breast-Feeding

Women with HIV infection should probably avoid pregnancy. One reason is that the risk of transmission of HIV from an infected mother to her unborn child is 30 to 35 percent. A second reason is that children of women with HIV infection often end up requiring foster care. And a third reason is that HIV infection in children tends to progress rapidly. We therefore recommend that women with HIV infection use birth control and avoid pregnancy.

The most reliable method of birth control is tubal ligation, or having your tubes tied. The birth control pill is also extremely reliable, 98 percent effective. The rate of failure with condoms is 10 percent, so condoms are considered unreliable. To prevent transmission of HIV infection and other sexually transmitted diseases, use condoms. To prevent transmission and pregnancy, use condoms plus the pill.

One option for a pregnant woman who has HIV and is concerned about transmitting HIV to her baby is not to continue the pregnancy. Unfortunately, there is no method to determine before birth if the baby is infected, so that the decision to have an abortion must be made without knowing whether the baby has HIV or not. Whether or not the baby is infected, the mother will also have to consider in that decision who will care for the baby if her own health deteriorates.

If abortion is desired, it is best performed during the first fourteen weeks of pregnancy, when it is considered most safe. Abortions during the period of fourteen to twenty weeks are offered by some specialized clinics, but hospitalization is usually required and the risk to the mother is somewhat greater.

A woman who chooses to continue the pregnancy needs to tell her obstetrician about her HIV infection. Taking drugs against HIV during pregnancy might reduce the risk of transmitting HIV to the baby, though we do not know this for sure. Moreover, the safety of the drugs used for HIV is not well established. This means some doctors will not prescribe these drugs. Doctors who do prescribe the drugs will usually warn that the drugs may cause damage to the unborn child.

The woman who chooses to continue the pregnancy also needs to tell her pediatrician about her HIV infection. The pediatrician will then know what to look for during the child's medical evaluations, will increase the number of visits, will decide whether to change the schedule of childhood vaccinations, and may begin drug therapy with the child. Many pediatricians do not feel competent to care for children with HIV infection. Nor do many pediatricians know which tests for telling whether the child is infected are currently in vogue (the standard blood test for HIV infection will not give valid results until the child is fifteen months old). It might be best to ask your pediatrician to refer you to a pediatrician with a specific interest in HIV infection.

The woman who continues the pregnancy should also plan not to breast-feed her baby. HIV is found in breast milk, and the baby could also be infected by breast-feeding (see above, page 35).

Women who are already pregnant and who live in cities where the incidence of HIV infection is high, or who are in the high-risk categories, should take the test for HIV. The purpose of this testing is for the sake of both the mother and the child. Some obstetricians offer such tests to all pregnant women, some offer the test only to those considered at risk for HIV infection, and some do not think of HIV infection at all unless reminded.

Preventing Transmission during Home Care

Home care means living with or caring for someone with HIV infection. It does not include sexual contact. These guidelines are based on recommendations by the CDC and on extensive experience with home care and hospital care. You should know that these recommendations are intentionally overcautious.

Reality of the Risk

There is no risk associated with simply living in the same household or working in the same office with a person who has HIV infection. This generally involves the types of nonintimate contact previously referred to as "casual contact" (see above, under "Types of Contact").

The type of contact that might involve the risk of transmitting HIV nonsexually usually takes place during medical care in the more advanced stages of disease. Every health care worker who has acquired HIV infection nonsexually has been exposed to the blood or bloody fluids of a person with HIV infection; transmission usually occurs after health care workers inadvertently inject infected blood into themselves.

The type of contact involved in home care of a person with HIV infection carries, in CDC's extensive experience, almost no risk. Only two of the tens of thousands of people who provide home care for people with HIV infection have acquired HIV as a result of nonsexual contact. Many of the people who did not become infected provided complete care of people with HIV infection for many months or even years without the benefit of any special training and without any special precautions to prevent HIV infection. Nevertheless, we recommend that caregivers use some simple precautions to be extra safe.

The two exceptions: One was a woman in England who apparently acquired HIV infection while caring for a man from Africa who was dying and who did not know he had AIDS. The second exception is a woman in the United States who apparently acquired the infection while taking care of an infant with transfusion-acquired AIDS; this mother did the usual maternal chores of disposing of excretions and so forth with no precautions whatsoever. These two women appeared to have no other risk factors, and neither had used any special precautions at all.

How can we be sure these are the only two exceptions? We obviously cannot, although most physicians question people with HIV infection for type of contact, and any physician would promptly report contact through home care because of its importance as a public health issue. Testing the blood of people who are caregivers of people with HIV infection answers the question more formally: fourteen studies of well over one thousand caregivers have not identified any additional people who acquired HIV infection by nonsexual contact.

In short, for those who live in the same household and do things that are common for friends and relatives to do, the risk is nil. For those who care daily for people who are seriously ill, the risk is very low, but not zero.

Guidelines for Preventing Transmission of HIV during Home Care

People with HIV infection and those involved in their care will want to lower the already low risk of transmission. This is easily accomplished by using the basic and simple guidelines described below.

Handwashing. Handwashing is the most important way to prevent the spread of most infectious microbes, not just HIV.

The usual recommendation is to wash under hot running water. Apply soap or a germicide like alcohol, rub vigorously for at least ten seconds, rinse thoroughly, and then dry the hands.

Gloves. Wear gloves if your hands have any cuts, sores, or torn cuticles. Wear gloves to handle blood or feces or urine, or to clean open sores. Wear gloves for cleaning surfaces that have been soiled by blood or feces or urine. (Feces and urine are included in this guideline not because they might transmit HIV but because they can contain many other infectious microbes). The preferred gloves are latex. Latex gloves may be superior to vinyl; plastic and cloth gloves are not recommended. After they are used, gloves should be taken off or changed before going on to some other task. Following use, soiled gloves should be washed with soap and water, then dried, and then discarded in a plastic container such as a trash can lined with a plastic bag.

Disinfectants. These are chemicals that kill microbes. No one is known to have become infected from contacting HIV on a surface outside the body. Nevertheless, this virus has been shown to survive outside the body on a surface for several days (though in lower and lower numbers), and it is probably wise to clean up blood or other bodily secretions on clothing or hard surfaces. Studies show that HIV is killed by heat and by nearly all chemical disinfectants.

The most commonly used disinfectants include bleach and alcohol (70 percent isopropyl). Other disinfectants that are effective include hydrogen peroxide, iodophors, phenolics, and quaternary ammonium compounds. These disinfectants are readily available in pharmacies and grocery stores. They are registered with the Environmental Protection Agency (EPA) with direction for use and precautionary information.

Although each of these disinfectants kills HIV, they kill HIV at varying rates of speed, the effect they have on other microorganisms is variable, their effect on different materials differs, and they may be harmful if used inappropriately. Some disinfectants remove the color from fabrics, some corrode metal, some will etch glass, and some will stiffen plastic. All this information is included on the disinfectant's label.

The most common disinfectant used is sodium hypochlorite, commonly known as household bleach (the most common brand is Clorox). This is available as a 5.25 percent solution wherever household cleaning products are sold. Household bleach kills a broad range of microbes, including HIV. To clean surfaces contaminated by blood or secretions, use a 1:10 dilution. A 1:10 dilution contains one part of 5.25 percent household bleach and nine parts of tap water (for example, one-fourth cup bleach and two and one-fourth cups water). Leave the 1:10 dilution on the surface for ten minutes, then wipe it off.

If the surface is cleaned before using the bleach, a 1:100 dilution may be used. Some people find it convenient to use the 1:100 dilution of bleach in a spray bottle, to spray on surfaces after they have been wiped clean. Bleach may corrode metals. It may also damage electrical and electronic equipment. Undiluted, it can leave white spots on fabric or eat holes in fabric. Contact with the skin and especially the eyes should be avoided. Use gloves to protect the skin when cleaning and disinfecting with bleach. If bleach comes in contact with skin, eyes, or mouth, the area should be washed or rinsed thoroughly with water. This applies to undiluted bleach and to the 1:10 dilution. Inhaling bleach fumes should also be avoided.

Household bleach may be stored in the original container (or in any opaque container) in a cool area, for up to a year. Bleach in solution is unstable and loses potency when exposed to sunlight, heat, or metal. Diluted bleach solutions should be used within a day or discarded.

Seventy percent isopropyl alcohol is also a very effective disinfectant. One problem with its use on surfaces is that it evaporates quickly. It may also cause skin irritation. This is the usual disinfectant ingredient in waterless handwashing products that are marketed in sealed packets. Isopropyl alcohol need not be diluted before use. Undiluted isopropyl alcohol kills high concentrations of HIV in less than one minute.

Hydrogen peroxide is usually sold in a 3 percent solution, which is too weak to disinfect. Iodine is an adequate skin disinfectant, but it must be used carefully since it stains fabrics, corrodes metal, cracks plastics, and dissolves rubber.

In summary, the most practical disinfectant to keep on hand is household bleach. Bleach should be properly stored and clearly labeled to avoid misuse or accidental drinking. In addition, 70 percent isopropyl alcohol can be used to clean cuts or other open wounds.

Dishwashing. There is no reason to provide separate dishes, glasses, or silverware for people with HIV infection. Washing dishes in a standard dishwasher or in hot soapy water is adequate.

Laundry. Laundry should be washed with detergent, using the hot cycle. Adding one-third cup of household bleach per ten gallons of wash water will assure disinfection, although it is really not necessary and may damage some fabrics. Fabrics that are soaked with blood or other body secretions should be presoaked and then washed separately.

Dry cleaning will disinfect any fabric.

Cuts and other injuries. Any fresh bleeding cut or sore on the caregiver or the person with HIV infection should be wiped free of blood and washed with soap and water or with alcohol (70 percent isopropyl).

Blood spills. Blood, including menstrual blood, spilled on a surface should be cleaned by a person wearing disposable gloves and using disposable cleaning cloths. After wiping up the blood, clean the area with a disinfectant like household bleach in a 1:10 or 1:100 dilution. Sponges, mops, and fabrics that have blood or body fluids on them may be cleaned with soap and water or with bleach in a 1:10 dilution.

Disposal of waste. Liquid waste that may have HIV in it can be poured into the toilet or sink. This will not contaminate the sewer system: sewage is decontaminated using methods that are clearly adequate to kill HIV and virtually all other microbes as well.

Soiled materials such as bandages, sanitary napkins, disposable gloves, soiled cleaning cloths, and the like should be placed in plastic bags for disposal. This is important primarily when they are soiled with blood.

Sharp instruments such as needles, syringes, used razor blades, and broken glass should be placed in containers such as a metal coffee can for disposal. To be extra cautious, some health departments recommend also adding bleach to the container.

To summarize: Caregivers should be cautious and sensible but should not worry excessively. In ten years, of all the people who are and have been caregivers, only two are known to have become infected by nonsexual contact. Neither of these two persons used any precautions at all.

Preventing Transmission of Infections Other Than HIV

People with HIV infection are susceptible to infection by a multitude of other microbes. These microbes cause what are called *opportunistic infections*. The most common opportunistic infections are pneumocystis pneumonia, thrush, infection disseminated throughout the body caused by either cytomegalovirus or *Mycobacterium avium*, and a brain infection called toxoplasmosis. (These and other opportunistic infections are discussed at great length in Chapter 3 and Chapter 6.) People commonly want to know whether the caregiver can also be infected by these opportunistic infections. The short answer is: with rare exceptions, no.

Most of these opportunistic infections are caused by microbes that we all come in contact with every day. People with HIV infection usually do not develop opportunistic infections until relatively late in the disease after their immune systems have become profoundly impaired. The caregiver's immune system does not permit such organisms to flourish. In other words, none of these infections can be transmitted from the person to the caregiver either in the home or in the hospital.

Pregnant caregivers are sometimes worried about exposure to people with cytomegalovirus, but most authorities believe these concerns are unjustified (see section on cytomegalovirus in Chapter 3).

In fact, the person with HIV infection is not a significant source of opportunistic infections even for another person with HIV infection. The reason is that most of these microbes are and always have been everywhere around us, and everyone has been exposed to them for a long time.

Exceptions to the rule. Some infections *may be* transmitted to the caregiver, and to avoid these infections, the caregiver should use special precautions.

The most important exception is tuberculosis, which is caused by a bacterium called *Mycobacterium tuberculosis*. *Mycobacterium tuberculosis* is related to another bacterium that people with HIV infection are prone to, *Mycobacterium avium*, or MA, which causes infections throughout the body. MA is not contagious—that is, it cannot be spread from person to person. *Mycobacterium tuberculosis*, however, *is* contagious.

Tuberculosis has always been recognized as a contagious disease. Since 1985, the number of all cases of tuberculosis has been increasing every year. People with HIV infection are exceptionally vulnerable to infection with tuberculosis, and, once infected, they get the disease severely. Moreover, many of these people are infected with a strain of the TB bacterium called the "multiply drug-resistant strain," that is, a form of the TB bacterium that does not respond to the usual drugs. Most of the multiply resistant strains are found in New York City, but may easily be elsewhere.

All people in the same household as someone with tuberculosis are at special risk. The risk is highest during the period before diagnosis and treatment. This is equally true for people in the households of someone with tuberculosis and HIV infection. People not in the household—visitors, co-workers, casual friends, golf partners, and the like—are not usually considered to be at risk, but this depends to some extent on the type of contact. In any case, people usually become infected by inhaling the droplets in the air after the infected person has coughed.

Whenever a case of tuberculosis is detected, medical authorities evaluate others in the same household. The evaluation starts with a skin test.

Because the skin test can take three months to become positive, sometimes treatment is started immediately. And treatment is often started immediately for any children in the household. If the skin test for tuberculosis is positive, the evaluation proceeds to the next step, a chest x-ray. Once tuberculosis is treated with drugs, the infected person rapidly becomes noncontagious. For this reason, the main threat of tuberculosis comes from the person whose tuberculosis has not yet been detected or treated. People infected with the resistant strain of tuberculosis, which persists in spite of treatment, are an exception. These people require special care and may need to stay in the hospital for prolonged periods. And because the resistant strain of tuberculosis is a major threat to public health, people may even be kept in the hospital against their wishes.

Another infection that is an exception is hepatitis B. Most people with hepatitis B are not aware they have it; they develop antibodies to it and are subsequently protected from infection. However, about 5 or 10 percent of people with hepatitis B will develop a persistent infection, and therefore may infect others for many years. Some people with persistent hepatitis will develop a liver disease called *chronic active hepatitis* that may eventually result in cirrhosis.

The virus that causes hepatitis B is transmitted the same way HIV is: by sexual contact, by blood contact, or by passage from mother to infant. Therefore, the activities that carry a risk of infection with HIV also carry a risk of infection with the hepatitis B virus. People at greatest risk for hepatitis B are men who have homosexual sex, people who use drugs intravenously, and men who have hemophilia. Like HIV, hepatitis

B may be also transmitted to someone exposed to the blood of an infected person.

Hepatitis B has three features worth emphasizing:

1. Hepatitis B virus is transmitted much more efficiently than HIV. A needlestick injury with blood that contains the hepatitis B virus is twenty times more likely to transmit hepatitis B than a needlestick injury with blood that contains HIV is to transmit HIV infection.

2. The same guidelines for preventing transmission of HIV through blood and body fluids apply to preventing transmission of hepatitis B.

3. A vaccine can prevent infection by the hepatitis B virus. The hepatitis vaccine is readily available, though it is expensive.

Outside of tuberculosis and hepatitis, the infections that could conceivably be transmitted from the person with HIV to a caregiver are salmonellosis, herpes simplex infection, herpes zoster infection, and cryptosporidiosis. If the caregiver is otherwise healthy, these infections may cause a temporary disease that is not serious.

Salmonellosis is an infection of the intestine by bacteria called salmonella. The main symptom of salmonellosis is diarrhea. Salmonellosis is relatively unusual, and transmission to others is relatively infrequent.

Cryptosporidiosis is also an infection of the intestine, but is caused by a parasite. The main symptom of cryptosporidiosis is also diarrhea. It is transmitted by lapses in personal hygiene; that is, small amounts of feces on the hand carry the parasite to someone else's hand, and then to that second person's mouth.

Herpes simplex, usually known as "herpes," causes a blister on the skin, most commonly on the mouth or genitals, though people with advanced HIV infection can also have herpes over much of their bodies. The caregiver can get herpes by touching the blisters, and can avoid transmission easily by wearing gloves when touching the areas with sores until the sores are crusted over.

Herpes zoster, also called shingles, is caused by the virus that causes chickenpox. The virus is transmitted when people inhale it. However, most older children and adults have had chickenpox, even if they don't remember it, and thus are protected by antibodies against the virus. Those who are concerned about herpes zoster are urged to have a blood test to see if they have antibodies to herpes zoster; and to be safe, they should avoid going into the same room as the infected person until the sores are crusted over.

All these infections are discussed in greater detail in Chapter 3 and Chapter 6.

Preventing Transmission of Infections to the HIV-infected Person

Both health care workers and home caregivers are understandably worried that they might transmit infection to the person whose immune system has been damaged by HIV infection. Although this worry sounds rational, in reality it is not much of a problem.

The kinds of infections common in otherwise healthy individuals include upper respiratory tract infections like colds, sinusitis, and pharyngitis; influenza, or "flu"; gastroenteritis with diarrhea, vomiting, and fever; and skin infections. Some of these sound like infections, but in reality they are not. Some are infections that are not contagious and cannot be passed from one person to another. And some are contagious diseases in the usual sense. The latter category is the only important one. The most common examples are colds, bronchitis, influenza, and gastroenteritis. Most of these are caused by viruses.

However, people with HIV infection do not get these common contagious diseases any more frequently or any more severely than anyone else. The viruses that cause the common contagious diseases affect a person with HIV the same way they affect other people. The reason seems to be that the part of the immune system that HIV attacks is not the same as the part that defends against colds and flu.

People also worry whether pets can carry infections to people with HIV infection. The most common worry is about the *Toxoplasma gondii* parasite, which causes a brain infection called toxoplasma encephalitis. The parasite is commonly found in the stool of cats. This worry is probably not justified: *Toxoplasma gondii* is one of those microbes that 20–30 percent of all people have in their bodies, and the person with HIV infection who gets toxoplasmosis has probably had this microbe a long time.

If You Think You Have Been Exposed

Persons who think they have been exposed to HIV infection or any of the infections noted above should seek the care of a physician. The physician might recommend a blood test for antibodies to HIV to exclude the possibility of transmission. Because the body usually takes three months or so to form antibodies to HIV, blood tests for the antibodies are usually done at the time of exposure, and then again six, twelve, and twenty-six weeks later (see "Understanding Tests for HIV," beginning on page 299). Thus, a negative blood test three months after exposure gives over 95 percent assurance that the virus was not transmitted. During this interval, we recommend no sex or safer sex and other precautionary measures.

Table 1. Sources of HIV Infection in the Estimated 1–1.1 Million Americans Thought to Have This Disease

How Transmitted	Est. No. in U.S.	Body Fluid	Comments
Sexual contact	800,000	Genital secretion	Most are gay men, although heterosexual transmission accounts for an increasing portion of new cases
Injecting drugs	235,000	Blood on shared needles	95% are regular users (more than 1 time/wk); 5% are occasional users
Blood transfusions	40,000	Blood	Largely stopped in 1985 due to screening of blood donors; about 20 documented cases since 1985
Hemophiliacs	10,000	Blood products	As above; about 20 documented cases since 1985 (less than 1/1,000/year)
Infants	5,000	Mother to fetus	Projected annual increase, 1,000–2,000
Health care workers with exposures in the workplace	31	Blood	These are only the well-established cases; about 70 additional cases are less well established
Patients with exposures to health care workers	5	Blood	All 5 cases are patients of the Florida dentist
Organ transplant recipients	38	Blood or organ tissue from donor	This group largely stopped due to screening of donors; the exception is 7 cases from a single donor with a false negative screening test in 1985

Table 1. (*Continued*)

How Transmitted	Est. No. in U.S.	Body Fluid	Comments
Home providers of health care for people with AIDS	1	Not known	
Artificial insemination	1	Semen	Donor was not screened; there are 5 cases in other countries
Unknown	10,000	Not known	1% with no known risk; probably most have major risks listed above if properly queried

Note: Data are based in part on estimates by the U.S. Public Health Service for 1992. There are several references to cases reported since May 1985, the date when the blood test first became available for screening blood and organ donors.

53

Table 2. Common Infections in People with HIV Infection and Their Risk to Others in the Household

Microbe	Most Common Infection	Risk to Others
Candida albicans	Mouth (thrush) Esophagus Vagina	None: most healthy persons have this organism in their mouths or digestive systems
Cryptococcus neoformans	Meningitis Pneumonia	None
Cryptosporidium	Diarrhea	Minimal: may cause brief bout of diarrhea in healthy persons; transmission is by contact with stool
Cytomegalovirus	Infection through-out the body (lung, digestive system, eye, etc.)	None: most healthy persons have this organism, but it doesn't cause serious disease in otherwise healthy people
Hepatitis B virus	Liver	Transmitted by sexual contact and blood, especially IV drug use; blood donors screened for this virus
Hepatitis C virus	Liver	Transmitted by blood and especially by IV drug use; blood donors screened for this virus
Herpes simplex	Cold sores Genital ulcers Skin infections	Transmitted by contact with or without sores, primarily oral or genital contact by kissing or sexual contact; gloves should be worn when touching sores until sores are crusted over
Herpes zoster	Shingles	Same virus that causes chickenpox. Healthy persons who have had chickenpox are protected; persons who have not yet had chickenpox may get it from inhaling the virus

Table 2. (*Continued*)

Microbe	Most Common Infection	Risk to Others
		in the air and should avoid being in the same room until sores are crusted over
Mycobacterium avium	Infection through-out the body	None: everyone comes in contact with this organism; often it is in the drinking water
Mycobacterium tuberculosis	Tuberculosis of lung and other sites	Can be transmitted to healthy persons; people who are being treated are usually not contagious, but household contacts (people living in the same house) prior to treatment should be tested with the tuberculosis skin test
Nocardia	Lung	None: these bacteria cause infection only in people with weakened immune systems
Pneumocystis carinii	Lung	None: healthy persons cannot get this infection; most already have this microbe dormant in their lungs
Streptococcus pneumoniae	Pneumonia	None
Taxoplasma gondii	Brain	None: about 20–30% of healthy adults have this microbe in a dormant state; usual source is cat dung or eating uncooked meat
Salmonella	Diarrhea	May be transmitted to others, including healthy people, by contact with stool; most healthy people with this infection have no symptoms or only mild symptoms

Chapter 3

HIV Infection and
Its Effects on the Body

- Transmission of HIV
- Acute infection
- Seroconversion
- Asymptomatic period
- Early symptomatic HIV infection
- Late symptomatic HIV infection, or AIDS

The effects of HIV infection on the body have been studied thoroughly. Many studies have followed people who engage in high-risk behaviors, from before they were infected, through the entire course of the infection, to the final stage of AIDS. We now know the usual course of HIV infection with considerable precision.

In most people, HIV infection follows a clear course: transmission of the virus is followed by an acute infection that clears up spontaneously; then there is a prolonged period during which the person feels good and has no symptoms of infection, that is, is asymptomatic; the person gradually develops the symptoms that are called either AIDS-related complex (ARC) or early symptomatic infection; eventually, the person develops the disease referred to as acquired immune deficiency syndrome (AIDS) or late symptomatic infection, which is defined by a blood test showing low numbers of the immune cells infected by HIV, or the presence of a variety of other infections in many different parts of the body, the so-called opportunistic infections.

Based on extensive studies, researchers have determined the duration, on average, of each stage. Individual people, however, spend widely varying amounts of time in each stage. Some people with positive HIV blood tests have remained healthy for over ten years, though most have declining numbers of CD4 cells, suggesting some suppression of the immune system.

The course of HIV infection is *generally* as follows:

56

Transmission of HIV, usually by blood exposure or through sexual intercourse.

One to six weeks: Acute infection, meaning the development of an infectious mononucleosis-like illness from which people recover in one or two weeks. Some people do not even notice this stage.

Four to twelve weeks, sometimes longer: Seroconversion, that is, the body develops antibodies to HIV, and as a consequence, the results of the blood test for the presence of antibodies to HIV are positive.

Asymptomatic interlude, during which the person feels well and functions normally except for the psychological stress that accompanies knowledge of a positive test.

Five to eight years, with considerable individual variation: Early symptomatic HIV infection, that is, the first symptoms or conditions that indicate weakening of the immune system, or immunosuppression. These conditions were previously called AIDS-related complex, or ARC.

Eight to ten years: Late symptomatic HIV infection with severe opportunistic infections and tumors. These opportunistic infections and tumors (called AIDS-defining diagnoses) or a CD4 cell count below 200 are the criteria for AIDS.

This chapter, like Chapter 6, discusses the infections and conditions that accompany each phase of HIV infection. Chapter 6 offers practical information on the symptoms of each condition, and on how each condition is diagnosed and treated. This chapter offers background information: What causes the condition? How often does it occur? Is the condition different in people with HIV infection? Is it treatable? What does the condition imply about the progress of the infection?

Transmission of HIV

HIV is transmitted—that is, the virus enters the body—almost invariably by sexual contact, by blood-to-blood contact, or through pregnancy.

When HIV enters the body, it attaches itself only to certain sites on the walls of certain cells. The site on the cell wall is called the CD4 *receptor,* and the cell most commonly infected is called the CD4 *cell.* The CD4 cell is a white blood cell, or a *lymphocyte.* It belongs to a class of lymphocytes called T *cells,* which, along with B cells, are central parts of the immune system. (The CD4 cell is also called a *T4 cell* and a *T-helper cell*.) The CD4 cell's job is to help coordinate the immune system's defense against a variety of infectious diseases. HIV is carried by CD4 cells and other white blood cells to all parts of the body, including the brain. HIV also attaches itself to certain cells in the brain.

Once HIV attaches to a CD4 cell, it enters the cell. At this point, in a complicated series of events, the virus becomes part of the cell's genes. Genes are composed of DNA, a molecule which is responsible for directing the reproduction of the cell. HIV is a virus and has only RNA, a molecule which is actually the mirror image of DNA but which cannot produce new viruses. HIV, however, is a *retrovirus,* meaning that it has a protein called *reverse transcriptase.* Reverse transcriptase allows the viral RNA to turn into a mirror image of itself; that is, it allows viral RNA to turn into viral DNA. This DNA then directs the infected cell to produce, not new CD4 cells, but new HIVs instead. The virus eventually destroys the CD4 cell, and the new viruses that have been produced then infect other CD4 cells. As CD4 cells are infected and destroyed, the immune system functions less and less effectively.

Acute Infection

The first symptoms of HIV infection, sometimes called acute infection or primary HIV infection, occur early in the disease process. The interval between transmission of the virus and the first symptoms of acute infection lasts, on average, between one and six weeks. Probably 50 percent and possibly 90 percent of all people with HIV infection have the symptoms of acute HIV infection.

Many of the symptoms of acute infection are nonspecific; that is, they are also symptoms of many common viral infections. Symptoms include fever, sweats, malaise, fatigue, achiness, joint pain, headaches, a sore throat, trouble swallowing, and enlarged lymph glands. Some people have a rash consisting of red spots or splotches over the chest, back, and abdomen. Some have evidence of infection of the brain: severe headaches, mood changes, personality changes, irritability, and confusion. Occasionally, people lose the use of their arms or legs for a short time, then regain use again.

Because some of these symptoms resemble those of infectious mononucleosis, the acute infection stage is sometimes referred to as a mononucleosis-like syndrome. Mononucleosis, however, is caused by an entirely different virus, and with acute HIV infection the blood test for mononucleosis is negative.

Some people with HIV infection have no recollection of an acute infection stage, some mistake it for a common viral infection, and a minority of people feel sick enough to go to a physician. A physician will find enlarged lymph glands and an enlarged spleen. A blood count will show fewer white blood cells than normal—but then, a low white count accompanies most viral infections. Liver tests may show changes suggesting mild hepatitis, but many other conditions cause similar changes. A spinal tap to analyze cerebrospinal fluid, the fluid that bathes the brain and spinal cord, may show evidence of meningitis. The usual blood test for HIV, which detects antibodies to HIV, will be negative at this time, but will usually become positive within three to ten weeks. Blood tests for HIV instead of the antibody to HIV would be positive, but are not usually done: these tests are expensive and few laboratories offer them (see Chapter 14). When these tests are done, they show very high concentrations of HIV in the blood. The concentration of HIV decreases when the antibodies to HIV develop.

Acute HIV infection can last from a few days to three weeks; it usually lasts one or two weeks. Occasionally, people have excessive fatigue that may last weeks or months. Virtually all people recover from the stage of acute HIV infection. The immune system, after fighting off the acute infection, returns to normal.

Seroconversion

At the time of acute infection with HIV, the body has not yet made antibodies to HIV. Antibodies, proteins produced primarily by certain white blood cells called *B lymphocytes,* attack substances foreign to the body, including viruses. The fact that symptoms are present even though the blood test to detect antibodies to HIV is negative is not unusual. In most other infections, symptoms precede the body's production of antibodies, and the symptoms disappear once antibodies are produced.

The body usually takes several days or weeks to recognize a foreign substance like a virus, and then produces antibodies to attack it. Six to twelve weeks after HIV has entered the body, antibodies to HIV appear in the blood in sufficient concentration to give a positive blood test. Physicians call this appearance of antibodies *seroconversion.* That is, the result of a test for antibodies in the blood serum converts from negative to positive. Occasionally, seroconversion may take up to a year or longer. The reason for the delay in some people is not known. For some reason, the virus is dormant; that is, it is not actively reproducing, so the immune system is not manufacturing antibodies against it.

Antibodies against most viral infections, once they appear, eliminate the virus and then stay in the body to protect against future infections by the same virus. Virtually all people with HIV infection develop antibodies against HIV. These antibodies reduce the concentration of HIV but do not eliminate HIV. As a result, the person with HIV remains infected and capable of transmitting the virus for life.

Asymptomatic Period

For several years after seroconversion, people with HIV infection feel good. Because they have no symptoms of the infection, this period is called the *asymptomatic* (meaning "no symptoms") period. During this period the person will be unaware of the HIV infection unless a blood test shows antibodies to HIV. About 70–80 percent of the people who presently have HIV infection are in this asymptomatic period.

The length of time people remain in the asymptomatic period is highly variable. The average is five to eight years until the symptoms of HIV infection appear, and eight to ten years until AIDS is diagnosed. The shortest time, two years or less from infection until the development of AIDS, is highly unusual. Most people stay asymptomatic for five years or more. Based on four different studies (done before any effective treatment was available), the time lapse between transmission of HIV and AIDS is as follows: After 1 year, 0 percent of the people with HIV infection were diagnosed with AIDS; after 2 years, 0 percent; after 3 years, 3 percent; after 4 years, 6 percent; after 5 years, 12 percent; after 6 years, 20 percent; after 7 years, 27 percent; after 8 years, 36 percent; after 9 years, 45 percent; after 10 years, 53 percent.

The reasons for this great variation are unknown. We know that treatment makes a decisive difference in the rate of the infection's progression. We would like to think that "wellness"—a psychological sense of well-being, good nutrition, exercise programs, and other general health measures—increases the length of the asymptomatic period, although we don't know that.

Other factors may contribute to the length of the asymptomatic period but are beyond the control of the person with HIV infection. One of these factors is the inoculum size, or number of viruses when exposure took place: the lower the inoculum size, the less likely that the exposure will cause infection (people can be exposed to the virus without necessarily becoming infected). Another factor is the specific strain of the virus: some strains of HIV seem to cause the infection to progress faster. A third factor is the age of the person infected: the infection progresses much faster in children and somewhat faster in older people. The final factor is the genetic makeup of the person infected: some people seem to have genes that make them prone to faster progression of the infection.

The presumed reason for the long delay before symptoms appear is the body's enormous number of CD4 cells (the white blood cells that help the immune system and that the virus infects). At first, the virus infects only a relatively small number of CD4s, then more and more of them, but the process is slow. Several years go by before the body loses so many CD4s that the immune system cannot defend itself against other infections. Most people lose about 80 to 90 percent of their CD4s before AIDS develops.

Keeping Track of Asymptomatic HIV Infection

During the asymptomatic period, your physician will probably keep track of the progress of the infection by physical examinations and with two principal tests. One test is to count, at regular intervals, the number of CD4 cells in the blood. The normal count is between 700 and 1,300 CD4 cells per milliliter of blood (five milliliters is one teaspoon). The average person has a CD4 count of about 1,000. People's CD4 counts vary for several reasons. One reason is that different laboratories, counting CD4 cells in the same person or the same blood sample on the same day, can get counts that differ by as much as 20 percent. Another reason is that the CD4 count naturally varies in any one person over time, for reasons that are independent of HIV infection but are poorly understood. Consequently, a CD4 count of 500 one time may be 400 or 600 the next time; this is considered a normal variation. Because of this normal variability in the counts, a test showing a dramatic change in the count might need to be repeated.

Most people with HIV infection do not develop symptoms until their CD4 counts are below 300, and the average CD4 count for a person with a serious opportunistic infection or tumor is 50–100. In people with HIV infection, the CD4 count decreases, on average, by 50 to 80 cells per year. At this rate, the person who starts with a count of about 1,000 will develop symptoms after five to eight years, and will develop AIDS two or three years after that. The CD4 counts in some people fall more rapidly, while the CD4 counts in other people stabilize for several years. A recent study of over 1,000 gay men with HIV infection showed that 6 percent developed AIDS four years after seroconversion. Another 10 to 17 percent, however, have CD4 cell counts that remain steady, and it is predicted that these men will be AIDS-free twenty years after seroconversion. The CD4 count is the best measure of the progress of the infection. Physicians also use the CD4 count to determine what sorts of treatment will be helpful and to determine the benefit of the treatments used.

Blood counts are also important for keeping track of the course of

HIV infection. Blood counts are counts of the numbers of the different kinds of cells in the blood: red cells, white cells, and platelets. Red blood cells deliver oxygen to the rest of the body; without enough oxygen, the person loses energy, is tired much of the time. A low count of red blood cells is called *anemia*. White blood cells (the CD4 cell is only one kind of white blood cell) are part of the immune system's defense against certain types of infection. A low count of white blood cells is called *leukopenia*. Platelets are cells that are critical in the process of blood clotting; a low number of platelets may result in excessive bleeding. During the asymptomatic period, the blood counts, like the CD4 counts, may also fall. That means that the body has progressively fewer red blood cells, fewer white blood cells, and/or fewer platelets. The body, however, has a great reserve, a large overabundance, of all three kinds of blood cells. The blood count must be lowered severely before symptoms occur.

Other barometers also help keep track of HIV infection. Some, like the CD4 cell count, are measures of the status of the immune system: beta 2 microglobulin, neopterin, and p24 antibody tests. Others are measures of the amount of HIV: p24 antigen and quantitative PCR tests. All these tests can be used to supplement CD4 cell counts and are commonly used to study new therapies.

Persistent Generalized Lymphadenopathy

Medical evaluation during the asymptomatic period may also reveal a harmless condition called *persistent generalized lymphadenopathy*. Persistent generalized lymphadenopathy, or PGL, is a long name for persistently swollen lymph nodes, or glands. The lymphatic system is an extensive network of channels, like the blood circulation system, that carry lymph. Lymph is a clear fluid containing lymphocytes, or white blood cells (including CD4 cells), that are a part of the immune system. Lymph is absorbed from tissues by tiny capillaries and sent to the lymph glands, where it is filtered. Lymph glands are clumps of lymphatic tissue distributed widely throughout the body. Many lymph glands are near the skin surface and can be felt, even in healthy people, like marbles or bumps under the skin, at the back of the neck, along the jaw, at the front of the neck, and in the armpit and the groin. Lymph glands are also located deep within the chest and abdomen, where they can be seen only with x-rays or scans.

A swollen lymph gland usually means the immune system is fighting an infection. Many infections cause the lymph glands to swell. In certain infections, only the nearest lymph glands are swollen. Thus, an infection in the foot may be associated with swelling of the lymph gland in the groin of the same leg; a strep throat may be associated with swollen, tender lymph glands in the neck. Usually, swollen lymph glands recede several weeks after the infection begins.

Because HIV infection is distributed throughout the body, lymph glands all over the body might be swollen. The definition of PGL is swollen lymph glands in at least two different locations in the body that remain swollen for six months or longer, and for which there is no explanation other than HIV infection. (Swollen glands are so common in the groin that this site is not considered in the diagnosis of PGL.)

The lymph glands may be swollen to the extent that they are visible as bumps, and they may be painful or tender to the touch, especially in the neck. Lymph glands can also be swollen but neither visible nor painful, and the person is unaware of them.

Medical consultation is generally necessary to assess the significance of swollen lymph glands. In most cases, a physician can simply feel the glands and determine whether they are normal or enlarged. In some instances, the physician might recommend a lymph gland biopsy—minor surgery to obtain a small piece of tissue from the gland or to remove the whole gland and examine it under a microscope. On rare occasions, lymph gland enlargement can be caused by a cancer of the lymph system called *lymphoma* or by an opportunistic infection.

At one time, PGL was more or less seen as a sign that the HIV infection was progressing. Recent studies of people with HIV infection indicate that the lymph nodes are the sites of rapid growth of HIV. This is a time when the patient feels well but HIV is reproducing. As a symptom, PGL seems to be of little importance.

The Psychological Burden

People with asymptomatic HIV infection carry an enormous psychological burden (see Chapter 4). One aspect of this burden is that people are often sensitized to their health and have an understandable tendency to overreact. People with colds may conclude they have pneumonia, a forgotten appointment may be interpreted as dementia, and a newly discovered freckle raises fear of Kaposi's sarcoma. The fact is, most colds, forgotten appointments, and freckles are normal. People with HIV infection have the same trivial medical conditions as anyone else. The average person develops three colds and one case of infectious diarrhea a year; over 90 percent of the general population has occasional headaches. The great majority of these common medical conditions are of no importance to the person with HIV infection. Symptoms such as fluctuations in mood, aches and pains, and fatigue are common to everyone. For people with HIV infection, a certain amount of depression is also normal. Some people, however, become extremely depressed. Their psychological burden becomes incapacitating; some may even consider suicide. These people would do best to consult a psychologist or psychiatrist.

Except for the immensity of the psychological burden, people in the asymptomatic period feel well. They continue to work and participate in life's activities more or less as if they were not infected. Most will go along for several years without symptoms, and some will probably do so for decades. It also seems likely that new therapies may greatly prolong this asymptomatic interlude.

Early Symptomatic HIV Infection

Early symptomatic HIV infection is the stage at which the first symptoms or conditions of a weakened immune system occur. Early symptomatic infection is sometimes called AIDS-related complex, or ARC. The conditions are usually less severe than those used to define AIDS, but not always. In any case, the onset may or may not mean that the immune system is weakening.

The most common early conditions are thrush, oral hairy leukoplakia, shingles, idiopathic thrombocytopenic purpura, and constitutional symptoms, which include chronic fever, weight loss, and chronic diarrhea. Many of these complaints are experienced by people who do not have HIV; the biggest difference is that in someone with HIV infection, the symptoms tend to be chronic, that is, they persist for several weeks or months. Most people with these early symptoms have a relatively low CD4 cell count, usually less than 300; some have no symptoms until the CD4 cell count is less than 50.

Thrush

Thrush is a yeast infection of the mouth caused by the fungus *Candida albicans*. The symptoms are white patches in the mouth, along the gums, on the inside of the cheeks, or on the tongue. Thrush is a common medical condition that also occurs in people who do not have HIV infection, most frequently in people using antibiotics or cortisone, and in diabetics. Thrush virtually never occurs without some underlying medical problem. It is also one of the infections people with HIV infection most frequently develop: about 80 percent of those with HIV infection have thrush at some time.

Thrush is easily treated with a variety of medicines and is generally controlled after one or two weeks of treatment. It does, however, tend to recur when the drugs are stopped, so these drugs are often given in prolonged courses, initially to control the infection and then to prevent its recurrence. If any one of the drugs for thrush fails, another drug will usually control the infection.

Oral Hairy Leukoplakia

Oral hairy leukoplakia is an infection of the mouth which resembles thrush. Its cause is unknown, but it appears to be associated with the virus that causes infectious mononucleosis. Most infections by the infectious mononucleosis virus produce only trivial symptoms or no symptoms, but once the infection with mononucleosis virus occurs, the virus remains in the mouth for the duration of life. The person with oral hairy leukoplakia does not have the usual symptoms of infectious mononucleosis and does not transmit infectious mononucleosis to others. Oral hairy leukoplakia appears to be an unusual reaction to the common presence of this virus in the mouth.

As noted earlier, most of the conditions that occur in people with HIV infections also occur in the rest of the population. Oral hairy leukoplakia appears to be an exception: it occurs almost exclusively in people with HIV infection.

Unless the person is in pain, treatment is not warranted. Oral hairy leukoplakia does seem to indicate that the immune system is increasingly suppressed, and that the development of a severe opportunistic infection and AIDS is probable within the next few years.

Herpes Zoster, or Shingles

The symptom of herpes zoster, also called shingles, is bands of painful blisters called shingles. The virus that causes shingles is also responsible for chickenpox. Every adult who had chickenpox during childhood has the shingles virus living in his or her nerves for life. Usually the virus causes no problems. Sometimes, however, decades later it becomes active, causing not chickenpox, but shingles. It seems to become active at times of stress or in people with weakened immune systems, but sometimes it becomes active for no apparent reason. The assumption is that the virus is continually present but is held in check by the normal defense mechanisms. Shingles, then, often occurs when this balance is upset, which is the presumed explanation for the association with HIV infection.

Shingles is a relatively common condition that occurs sometimes in otherwise healthy people, especially older people. It is not life-threaten-

...g and inevitably cures itself, but can cause severe pain. Shingles may occur when the CD4 count is still relatively high and does not necessarily imply a weakening immune system.

Gynecological Problems

Women with HIV infection have gynecological problems frequently and at a relatively early stage of HIV infection. The major problems are vaginal yeast infections and cervical cancer. In fact, cervical cancer is now considered an AIDS-defining diagnosis. A less frequent problem during the early symptomatic stage is pelvic inflammatory disease. These are the same gynecological problems that all women have, but women with HIV infection have them more frequently and more severely.

Idiopathic Thrombocytopenic Purpura (ITP)

When a person has idiopathic thrombocytopenic purpura, or ITP, the body for some reason produces antibodies which attack the platelets that allow the blood to clot. Thus, the symptoms of ITP are excessive bruising and bleeding. ITP is a relatively unusual medical condition that can occur in people without HIV infection, but it is far more common in those with the infection. Most people are unaware of this condition; it is usually discovered with routine laboratory testing. Several forms of treatment are considered effective.

Whether ITP means that HIV infection is progressing is unclear. Many studies have shown that people with HIV-related ITP do not go on to get AIDS any faster than people with HIV infection who do not have ITP. Other studies have shown that people with HIV-related ITP develop AIDs more quickly than people who have HIV infection but do not have ITP.

Pneumococcal Pneumonia

Pneumonia is an infection of the lung. The bacterium, pneumococcus, is one of the most common causes of pneumonia in people with or without HIV infection. Pneumococcal pneumonia, because it occurs in people without HIV infection, is not really an opportunistic infection; people who get pneumococcal pneumonia do not necessarily have weakened immune defenses and are not uniquely susceptible. Nevertheless, people with HIV infection have pneumococcal pneumonia more severely and about one hundred times more frequently than people without HIV infection. Pneumococcal pneumonia can be sometimes prevented with pneumococcal vaccine, or it can be treated with antibiotics. When pneumococcal pneumonia recurs repeatedly, it is considered an AIDS-defining diagnosis.

Constitutional Symptoms

Constitutional symptoms are the vague, general symptoms that often accompany chronic illnesses. Included are weight loss, chronic weakness, diarrhea, fever, and fatigue. Any of these symptoms may also be caused by certain opportunistic infections. Because some of these opportunistic infections are treatable, when these symptoms develop, see a physician.

In people with HIV infection, the distinguishing feature of all of these constitutional symptoms is that they are chronic, that is, they don't go away. Fever, fatigue, achiness, malaise, and diarrhea are periodically experienced by everyone; when they are caused by an acute viral infection like influenza, they interfere with daily activities, but only for a few days. These symptoms can be considered the constitutional symptoms of early symptomatic HIV infection only when they have been present for at least one month. These symptoms usually occur only when the CD4 count is below 200.

Weight loss. Weight loss is a common symptom for people with HIV infection. One reason is that fever, any active opportunistic infection, and HIV infection itself can all increase the body's metabolic rate: the motor runs more quickly and calories are burned at a faster clip. People with increased metabolic rates may eat voraciously and still lose weight. Another reason for weight loss is starvation: people do not consume enough calories. The cause might be loss of appetite, depression, sores in the mouth, or loss of the sense of taste. Some people starve because of severe diarrhea. The food goes through the digestive system without being absorbed.

Diarrhea. Diarrhea is also common for people with both early symptomatic and late symptomatic HIV infection. Sometimes diarrhea is caused by an infectious microbe which laboratory tests can identify. For many people, however, diarrhea is irregular: on some days loose stools are frequent and on other days bowel habits are relatively normal. Such cases of diarrhea are not often caused by an infectious microbe. Instead, they are caused either by HIV infection itself or by some opportunistic infection produced by a microbe that cannot be detected.

Fever. Fever, like other constitutional symptoms, is common; it can be caused by an opportunistic infection, or it can simply be due to HIV.

The temperature we call a "normal body temperature" is actually different for different people; furthermore, a person's "normal" temperature usually varies during the course of a day. Usually a person's temperature is relatively low in the morning and has increased by about one or two degrees by the evening. This daily fluctuation in temperature is exaggerated during any illness. Though no single temperature is considered normal for everyone, temperatures above 99.6 degrees F (37.5 degrees C) are usually considered the upper limits of normal, especially if measured during the day (rather than at night). Most people with a fever are aware that they have a fever; nevertheless, the physician will want to know what the person's temperature is when measured by a thermometer. Rapid rises in temperature are commonly preceded by chills. Chills are an indication of the body's attempt to retain heat by constricting the blood vessels of the skin where heat is given off. Along with fever, some people also have "night sweats," sweating at night which can be severe enough to require changes in bed clothing. Night sweats are usually but not invariably accompanied by fever.

The combination of fever, chills, and night sweats is relatively common in the late stages of HIV disease. Often fevers, especially fevers over 101 degrees or those accompanied by shaking chills, indicate the presence of some infection other than HIV. If you have such a fever, see a physician; at least 80 percent of fevers in people with HIV infection occur with an infection that can be diagnosed and treated. The person with fever who does not have a specific treatable infection can obtain relief with aspirin, acetaminophen, or a variety of drugstore remedies that contain these agents. Acetaminophen carries on the label a warning that it causes liver or kidney damage; although the probability of this is low, it might be best to limit the amount of acetaminophen you take. The maximum adult dose is 0.6–0.9 mg (usually two or three pills) taken every four to six hours.

Fatigue.   Fatigue is an especially common constitutional symptom. Its severity is often profound and its causes are diverse. Likely causes are opportunistic infections, depression, anemia (low red blood cell count), and HIV-associated dementia. Many cases of fatigue, however, have no clear cause and can be blamed on HIV infection itself. This is true only when the CD4 cell count is low.

A medical evaluation can help sort out the cause of fatigue. A simple blood count will show if the cause is anemia. Such symptoms as fever, cough, and diarrhea often accompany an opportunistic infection. Most causes are treatable (unless fatigue is due to HIV itself).

Late Symptomatic HIV Infection, or AIDS

The late stage of HIV infection is severe immunosuppression, that is, severe weakening of the immune defenses of the body. This stage is called either late symptomatic HIV infection or AIDS. The exact definition of the stage, however, has been a moving target. The original definition in 1982 (which came before knowledge of HIV as the cause) was an opportunistic infection in a person who had no reason for it. In 1986, the definition changed to a specific list of opportunistic infections or tumors, called AIDS-defining diagnoses, that occur only in people with weakened immune defenses. In 1987, the list expanded.

The problem with this definition of AIDS is that some people go through the entire course of HIV infection and die without ever getting an AIDS-defining diagnosis. This is not a problem for medical care, but it *is* a problem for benefits like disability and eligibility for some social services. So now, as of January 1, 1993, the definition includes the same list of AIDS-defining diagnoses but adds some new conditions and a CD4 cell count below 200. (The number 200 was picked because at that point, people begin to be vulnerable to serious opportunistic infections or tumors.) Despite the advantages of the new definition, it has two problems. One problem with the proposed definition is that the Social Security Administration has refused to accept it as a criterion for disability. Another problem is that CD4 cell counts vary considerably: the counts on the same sample of blood can vary by 20 percent.

In this book, we refer to AIDS-defining diagnoses (or conditions) because the term is commonly used, because the opportunistic infections and tumors are the dominant medical problems of the late stage of HIV infection, and because they still constitute a diagnosis of AIDS.

The most common of the AIDS-defining conditions are opportunistic infections. Most opportunistic infections are caused by microbes to which everyone is exposed on a regular basis but which lack clout; usually a modest effort by the immune system is enough to defeat them. A suppressed immune system, however, is unable to fight off these infections. Opportunistic tumors, primarily Kaposi's sarcoma and certain lymphomas, are also AIDS-defining conditions. Most opportunistic infections and opportunistic tumors that occur with AIDS also occur in other medical conditions where the immune system is suppressed. The most common and important opportunistic infections and tumors are described below. *Pneumocystis carinii* pneumonia and Kaposi's sarcoma are the most common of the opportunistic infections and tumors, respectively; the others occur less frequently.

AIDS is the only stage of HIV infection which by federal law must be reported. As a result, AIDS is the only stage of disease for which we have reliable statistics and can make reliable predictions. Studies of people with HIV infection show that some people with AIDS lived five years or more after an AIDS-deficiency diagnosis, continuing for a long time to enjoy life and be productive members of society. Furthermore, these studies were conducted at a time before there was any effective treatment for AIDS. Advances in treatment, like AZT and the new drugs for opportunistic infections, allow such people to live even longer and healthier lives. Although AIDS is the stage of HIV infection at which the threshold of immune suppression is considered to have been crossed, people with AIDS should not think they will die any time soon.

Pneumocystis carinii Pneumonia

Pneumocystis carinii pneumonia (PCP) is an infection of the lung (pneumonia) caused by a parasite called *Pneumocystis carinii*. The parasite appears to be in the lungs of almost everyone, presumably acquired sometime early in life. (*Pneumocystis carinii* is found almost exclusively in the lungs, but like most facts in medicine, this is not an absolute, and pneumocystis infections have occasionally occurred in other parts of the body.) The parasite causes no problem unless the balance between the immune system and the microbial world is heavily tilted in favor of the microbe. As a result, physicians initially saw PCP mostly in malnourished children, in people with certain types of cancer, and in those who had received organ transplants. At present, over 95 percent of people with PCP have HIV infection.

The reason so many people with HIV infection get PCP is probably that the CD4 cell, which is infected by HIV, is also important in keeping *Pneumocystis carinii* in check. As the supply of CD4 cells decreases, *Pneumocystis carinii* is less constrained. In approximately 50 percent of the people with HIV infection, PCP is the first AIDS-defining diagnosis. Without preventive treatment, about 80 percent of all people with AIDS will develop PCP at some time during the course of the disease.

PCP in people with AIDS evolves slowly. In fact, most people have had the symptoms for weeks before they seek medical attention. The disease can be serious, and at first approximately 25 percent of people with PCP died. The prognosis is better now because of earlier medical intervention and improved treatments. PCP can usually be prevented. The preventive treatment is now considered an important part of the care of all people whose CD4 counts are less than 200.

Kaposi's Sarcoma

This is a curious and poorly understood tumor of the blood vessels that got its name from the person who first described it over a century ago, Moricz Kaposi, a Hungarian dermatologist. At that time KS was generally a tumor of the leg occurring in elderly men of Ashkenazi Jewish or Mediterranean desent. A KS tumor is purple or black in color and painless. Over years or decades, KS tumors in these men grew slowly in size and number, but seldom caused serious consequences. KS in people with HIV infection behaves differently: the tumors grow more rapidly and appear in parts of the body other than the legs, including the internal organs.

These tumors can appear any place on the skin. They can also occur in the gastrointestinal tract, where they cause abdominal pain or diarrhea; in the lymph glands, where they occasionally cause painful swelling in the neck, under the arms, or in the groin; in the lungs, where they cause shortness of breath, coughing up sputum, or collections of fluid that reduce breathing capacity; in the brain, where they cause seizures; and in the liver. KS may also occur on the roof of the mouth. KS is unusual in that the tumors grow simultaneously at different places both on the skin and within internal organs.

KS is second only to PCP as the initial AIDS-defining diagnosis in people with HIV infection. Although KS occurs without HIV infection, it is approximately twenty thousand times more frequent in people with HIV than in those without. Probably between 20 and 25 percent of all people with AIDS have KS, but the frequency is substantially greater in gay men than in other groups with HIV infection. KS was also more common in people with AIDS in the early stages of the epidemic than it is now, for reasons no one knows. Some feel that the epidemiology of KS suggests that it is a sexually transmitted disease and that the safer sex practices widely adopted by gay men in the early 1980s in response to the HIV epidemic account for the reduction in cases.

The prognosis is actually quite good, possibly because people with KS often have less severe immune suppression. Many people simply have tumors that persist or that increase in size and number. For this reason, treatment may not be necessary. Treatment is usually done for cosmetic reasons or for relief of any unpleasant symptoms. The most common symptom is fluid collection from blocked lymph drainage, causing swollen legs or a swollen face.

Tuberculosis

Tuberculosis, or TB, is caused by a bacterium called *Mycobacterium tuberculosis*. The bacterium causes an infection that is silent for years, and then, when the body's immune defenses are reduced, it causes disease. Unlike *Pneumocystis carinii*, which causes pneumonia only when immune defenses are weak, *Mycobacterium tuberculosis* causes tuberculosis when immune defenses are still relatively strong. As a result, tuberculosis often occurs relatively early in the course of HIV infection, when the CD4 cell count may be relatively high and the person otherwise comparatively healthy.

Tuberculosis was the major cause of death in the United States at the turn of the century. Since then, because of public health measures and antibiotic treatments, the number of cases has fallen steadily. That steady fall is one of medicine's greatest accomplishments; researchers thought the disease would disappear by the year 2000. But in 1985, the number of cases stopped falling, leveled off, and then started climbing. By 1993 there were forty thousand more cases than expected. The increase was attributed directly to tuberculosis in people with HIV infection. The connection between these two concurrent epidemics was logical. Many people are infected with tuberculosis bacteria but never get sick because their immune defenses hold the bacteria in check. People with HIV infection who are exposed to tuberculosis bacteria, however, are about fifty times more likely than someone without HIV infection to get infected. And once infected, they are also about fifty times more likely to get the active disease.

The problem of the connection between HIV infection and tuberculosis was further compounded by a particularly ugly strain of the tuberculosis bacterium. This strain, called multiply drug-resistant tuberculosis, does not respond to the standard tuberculosis drugs. The drug-resistant strain has been a particular problem for people with HIV infection and has caused several epidemics, primarily in New York City.

One result of all this is that health care workers are now especially aware of tuberculosis in people with HIV infection. Physicians are under appropriate pressure to pursue tuberculosis aggressively and to take precautions to prevent its spread. This means that everyone with HIV infection should have a tuberculosis skin test, and that everyone with tuberculosis should have an HIV blood test. A patient in a hospital who might have tuberculosis must be in a single room, and anyone entering the room must wear a mask. And someone who does have tuberculosis must take the full course of multiple standard drugs for at least nine months and do so under direct observation.

Mycobacterium avium Infections

Mycobacteria are special types of bacteria; the best known, *Mycobacterium tuberculosis,* causes tuberculosis. Though people with HIV infection do develop tuberculosis, they are far more likely to get an infection caused by a related bacterium, *Mycobacterium avium,* or MA. Some call this MAI, for *Mycobacterium avium intracellulare.*

MA in people with AIDS is distributed widely throughout the body. It can be found in the lungs, lymph glands, liver, spleen, blood, bone marrow, gastrointestinal tract (intestines), and in virtually any organ. In most instances, a person who has MA has it widely distributed in the body: 30 to 50 percent of the people with AIDS eventually develop MA infection, usually when the CD4 cell count is less than 100. The symptoms caused by MA depend to some extent on the organ involved. In the gastrointestinal tract, MA can cause diarrhea; in the bone marrow, it can cause a lowered blood count (further lowered from the effect of HIV); in the lung, it can cause pneumonia; in the lymph glands, it can cause enlargements; and in the liver, it can cause hepatitis. In many instances, the major symptoms are simply the constitutional symptoms reflecting the sum total of a widely distributed infection: fever, fatigue, and weight loss.

MA is easy to diagnose because it can be detected in the blood. It is somewhat difficult to treat, however, since many standard drugs don't work well and since, during the course of therapy, MA often becomes resistant. Physicians have two approaches to this infection. To prevent MA, many physicians will prescribe a drug when the CD4 count is very low. Once infection has taken place, the standard treatment is to give two or more drugs either to cure the infection or to reduce the numbers of mycobacteria.

It is important to note that MA is transmitted very differently from the mycobacterium that causes tuberculosis. MA is in soil and often in water supplies which are presumably the sources of infection. Unlike tuberculosis, MA is not transmitted from one person to another, and special precautions to prevent its spread are not necessary.

Another note: when various secretions and biopsies are sent to the laboratory to be tested for MA, the first test is a special stain to detect all mycobacteria. This stain will not distinguish *Mycobacterium tuberculosis* from MA. That distinction can be made only with a further test whose results are only available after several days or a few weeks. During this time, to be extra cautious, people may be advised to live as though they have tuberculosis. This means taking a brief course of drugs and using precautions against spreading infection until the lab sorts out the bacteriology.

Toxoplasma Encephalitis

Toxoplasma encephalitis is an infection of the brain that causes seizures and neurological impairment. Toxoplasma encephalitis is caused by a parasite, *Toxoplasma gondii*, which is commonly found in cat stool and in inadequately cooked meat. Whether cats and uncooked meat are the sources for the infection in any one person remains unclear. After infection, the parasite remains—generally dormant—in the human body for life.

Between 10 and 15 percent of all people with AIDS develop toxoplasma encephalitis.

About 30 percent of Americans have been infected with *Toxoplasma gondii*, though most people have no recollection of any disease associated with the infection. Like *Pneumocystis carinii* and other persistent microbes, *Toxoplasma gondii* has the opportunity to flourish when immune defenses are lowered. Thus, a person with AIDS who has *Toxoplasma gondii* dormant in his or her body might develop toxoplasma encephalitis if the parasite becomes active.

This is not an infection that can be passed from one person to another, and it poses essentially no threat to anyone who comes in contact with infected persons.

Toxoplasma encephalitis is one of the many infections in people with AIDS that responds well to antibiotics. It is likely to recur, however, when treatment is discontinued, so treatment is continued for extended periods. In many cases, the physician will find out who is vulnerable to toxoplasmosis by two criteria: (1) a low CD4 cell count and (2) evidence from a blood test showing prior infection with toxoplasmosis. People who meet both criteria are often treated with an antibiotic to prevent toxoplasmosis.

Cryptococcosis

Cryptococcosis is an infection caused by a fungus, *Cryptococcus neoformans*. The infection may develop in several different places in the body, including the lungs and the brain; it is most damaging and common in the brain. *Cryptococcus neoformans* is the most common cause of meningitis in people with AIDS. Between 8 percent and 10 percent of all people with AIDS develop cryptococcal meningitis.

Cryptococcus neoformans is widely distributed throughout the world, but the exact mechanism of transmission in unclear. It is clear, however, that *Cryptococcus neoformans* is not passed from one person to another. People with cryptococcal meningitis pose no threat to the caregiver, to people in the same household, or even to other people with AIDS.

The treatment for cryptococcal meningitis is effective, but it must be continued for life or the infection tends to recur. In many instances, cryptococcosis and other fungal infections can be prevented with new drugs called antifungal drugs, to be taken by mouth.

Cytomegalovirus Infection

Cytomegalovirus (CMV) is similar to microbes like *Pneumocystis carinii* and *Toxoplasma gondii*, which infect people and then remain dormant in the body. Most people have antibodies to CMV in their blood, meaning they have been infected and continue to harbor small numbers of the virus. The initial infection is usually associated with either trivial symptoms or no symptoms at all. For most people the presence of the virus in the body continues to cause no symptoms, but when the immune defenses are lowered, the virus proliferates.

Because CMV resides in blood cells, it is widely distributed throughout the body; in people with late symptomatic HIV infection, it causes infections in many different organs. In the lungs it can cause pneumonia, in the eyes it can cause inflammation in the retina (retinitis), in the gastrointestinal tract it can cause diarrhea, in the liver it causes hepatitis, and in the brain it causes encephalitis.

Probably 90 percent of people with AIDS develop CMV infection at some time during their illness. Retinitis occurs in 10 to 20 percent of people with AIDS, and gastrointestinal disease in about 10 percent. Many people simply have fever, and tests of the blood show the presence of CMV. For many, the only symptoms of CMV infection are fever, fatigue, and weight loss, that is, the constitutional symptoms described previously.

CMV is difficult to treat and impossible to cure. Antibiotics are at least partially effective against some forms of the disease. One treatable form is CMV retinitis, an inflammation of the eye which may progress to blindness in one or both eyes if it is not treated promptly and properly.

CMV can be transmitted through sexual contact. Like so many of the microbes previously discussed, CMV is not readily transmitted from one person to another. Even if it were transmitted, it is unlikely that it would be of any consequence for most people. Because CMV can cause serious disease in an unborn infant, there has been concern that pregnant women not take care of someone with CMV infection. However, careful studies indicate that people with CMV infection are unlikely to transmit the virus to caregivers, pregnant or not.

Herpes Simplex Infection

Herpes simplex infection takes two major forms, infection on the mouth and infection in the genital region, though it may spread to other places in the body. When the infection is on the mouth, transmission is usually through oral contact (like kissing) with a person who is infected with the virus and who may or may not have apparent sores on the mouth. When the infection is in the genitals, transmission is usually through sexual contact; the person who is the source of the infection may or may not have sores on the genitals.

With the first exposure, herpes simplex often causes water blisters, pain, and fever. This initial infection clears up, but the virus remains in the nerves nearby and is periodically reactivated. When the virus is reactivated on or in the mouth, it causes what people call cold sores. When the virus is reactivated on the genitals, it causes sores on the genitals or in the anal region. These reactivations are less severe than the initial infection. Cold sores on the mouth often occur predictably, at times of stress, with fever (causing what people call fever blisters), during menstrual periods, or with exposure to the sun.

Studies of blood tests show that 50 percent of people have had herpes simplex on the mouth and 20 percent have had herpes simplex on the genitals, even though many do not recall it. These people harbor the virus, but the virus remains dormant, that is, not actively reproducing.

In people with HIV infection, herpes infections lasting over a month are an AIDS-defining diagnosis. People with AIDS are subject to more frequent and more severe infections from herpes simplex. The presumed explanation is that the balance of immune defenses versus this virus becomes tipped in favor of the virus.

Treatment is generally successful in providing relief from an outbreak of sores. The relief is usually temporary; treatment does not eliminate the herpes virus, does not cure the infection, and does not prevent transmission. When the outbreaks recur frequently enough, treatment is given continuously.

Cryptosporidiosis

Cryptosporidiosis is caused by a parasite, *Cryptosporidium*. Its primary symptom is diarrhea. *Cryptosporidium* was originally described by veterinarians as a relatively common cause of diarrhea in animals, but it was not recognized as a cause of diarrhea in people until the 1970s. The parasite sometimes infects the gall bladder, where it occasionally causes gall bladder and liver disease.

Infection occurs when *Cryptosporidium* is ingested, by drinking contaminated water or by contact with animals or with infected people. In most instances, the source of the infection is not clear.

People with HIV infection are susceptible and account for the majority of cases, though they usually recover within one to two weeks. People with AIDS have the same symptoms as those without HIV infection, but the disease tends to be chronic and lasts several months or even years. The severe and prolonged diarrhea compounds the often already existing problem of weight loss and malnutrition. Probably between 5 and 10 percent of people with AIDS will develop this complication.

Cryptosporidiosis has no treatment that is especially effective.

The Tempo of AIDS

For about 50 percent of people with HIV infection, the first AIDS-defining diagnosis occurs within ten years of seroconversion; this is only an average. A very few people, less than 1 percent, progress rapidly from seroconversion to an AIDS-defining diagnosis within one year. At the other extreme are the people known as long-term survivors who remain well after having HIV infection for ten years or longer. Some of these long-term survivors have low CD4 cell counts that suggest complications in the near future. About 25 percent of them, however, have CD4 cell counts over 500. It is now estimated that 10 to 17 percent of people with HIV infection will remain well for at least twenty years without therapy; with therapy, the percentage should increase.

The course of HIV infection after an AIDS-defining diagnosis varies. Some people have repeated opportunistic infections or opportunistic tumors. Some people have general symptoms such as fever, fatigue, weight loss, and diarrhea that may be due to these opportunistic infections or to HIV itself. And some people are well for periods of a year or two or longer.

Much of this variation in the tempo of the disease is unexplained. One factor may be general wellness, that is, whether the person takes good care of his or her body and mind. Wellness is under the control of people with HIV infection (see Chapter 12).

In addition, the tempo of the disease may be slowed by treatments that prevent opportunistic infections, that fight HIV, and that stimulate the immune system. In particular, in 1986, AZT was found to prolong life in people with AIDS and advanced ARC. This was the first therapeutic breakthrough. Since that time substantial progress has been made in understanding, tracking, and treating HIV infection, and in treating and preventing opportunists. The present strategy to treat persons with HIV infection is a two-pronged attack: one, directed against HIV, is called *antiretroviral therapy* (because HIV is a retrovirus); the second attack is to prevent opportunistic infections by using antibiotics and vaccines. At the present time there is good scientific evidence that current treatments provide the following benefits:

1. Numbers of HIV in the body can be reduced.

2. Progressive decreases in CD4 counts can be stopped or at least slowed.

3. The time between HIV infection and development of an AIDS-defining condition can be prolonged.

4. Opportunistic infections can be prevented, and if they occur, can be controlled or at least slowed.

5. Life, including high-quality and productive life, can be prolonged.

The progress in treatments is obviously beneficial, but precisely how many years treatments add to a person's life is not yet known. Therapy has become a moving target, and recommended treatment changes quickly in response to research findings. It is gratifying to know that what is new and unusual this year is likely to be out of date next year because something better has been discovered.

Chapter 4

HIV Infection and Its Effects on the Emotions

- Anger and energy
- Depression and hope
- Fatigue and accommodation
- Fear and realism
- Guilt and self-worth

People's reactions to HIV infection differ widely, but nearly everyone shares to some extent feelings of anger, depression, fatigue, fear, and guilt. These feelings are not stages; they come in no order. Some people notice more of one feeling at certain times, more of another at other times. Some people have several or all of the feelings at once. All the feelings are part of human nature. They are all reasonable reactions to HIV infection. They are probably more or less unavoidable. This chapter describes the feelings, their causes, and the ways people have found to deal with them.

Anger and Energy

> *Lisa Pratt:* My husband had a lot of anger, which he first directed at me. He criticized, lashed out, once threatened to kill me. At first he refused to use a condom. He said, "Why did some jerk donate blood and now I have to use a condom?" He'd beat his fist on the table.

> *Alan Madison:* I am not particularly angry.

Some people, like Lisa Pratt's husband, easily admit and express anger. Others may feel anger but do not acknowledge it. And still others may not be angry at all. Whatever the case, anger is a perfectly reasonable response to HIV infection.

79

Reasons for Anger

One reason for anger is the unfairness of the situation. In the first place, being singled out by the virus at all is unfair. No one, regardless of how he or she became infected, asked for or deserved this infection. Steven Charles, who became infected through sexual intercourse, said: "Why me? I didn't do anything wrong, I never hurt anyone, I was doing what seemed right to me. I know people who are more promiscuous and they seem to be getting out without a scar." Helen Parks had found a good job in the post office of the small town in which she lives; she had stopped using drugs intravenously before she found out she was infected: "I hadn't been getting high any more. I was earning good money," she said. "Why bother to work hard and do good now?"

In the second place, being sick when you are young is unfair. "I won't get to fulfill my dreams," said Dean Lombard, who had always wanted to develop his singing talent. "The world owed me better than that. I didn't deserve that." Alan Madison became infected with HIV just as he was beginning to reach success and stability in his accounting business, and now he feels he should change his long-range goals. June's son, at age thirty-four, had just begun to practice medicine after long years of training and has had to discontinue his practice.

And finally, the social stigma, rejection, and even abandonment this particular virus seems to provoke are unfair. When Lisa Pratt's friends and priest could not respond to her request for help, she said she was hurt and angry. Dean says he feels like a leper: "And I'm not. I'm not unclean. I didn't ask for this virus."

Besides unfairness, another reason for anger is frustration at losing control over your life. "As my husband got sicker," said Lisa, "the more I did, the more he felt he was losing control. Sometimes he was grateful for help, sometimes he just screamed. He was so independent, and so full of life—he had no frame of reference for sickness and death." Dean had spells of being sick during which he had to be cared for by his long-time partner: "Once I messed the bed like a baby. I got so frustrated and angry at not being able to do what I want to do, I cried."

Expressing the Anger

Some people express anger directly and openly, usually in private, though Dean has cried in church. "Tremendous anger wells up in me," Dean says. "I cry during hymns, reading those words. At home alone, I lose my temper, bang doors, throw things, yell. It's important to me to release my anger, but I try to be careful not to hurt anything." Steven uses almost identical words: "I feel anger building up on a weekly basis. I want to run up and down the road and cry. When I'm really angry, I beat on the bed with a piece of hose, which is noisy and very satisfying. Or I go in the bedroom and jump up and down and yell."

Other people express anger more obliquely. "I'd cry every morning and night in the car on the way to and from work," said Helen. "Sometimes I'd have to pull over to the side. And I went through a period where I snapped at my customers in the post office. When they asked why, I'd say, 'Oh, the stupid Xerox machine won't work.'" In fact, people often express anger not at the true causes, at unfairness or at loss of control. Instead, like Helen and the Xerox machine, they get angriest at little things: "My husband expressed a lot of anger about things so small, they were all out of proportion to what he was angry about," said Lisa. "I'd fix him oatmeal, and it was not what he'd wanted, or it wasn't hot enough."

People also get angry at whatever is nearest. Sometimes, like Lisa's husband, they get angry at their caregivers. Some people turn their anger toward the medical system. They say that government medical assistance requires that you first become impoverished before you can get help, and that you fill out an amount of paperwork equaled only by the IRS. They say that hospital clinics make you wait for hours, that the clinic doctor you felt you had rapport with last time has been replaced by someone else, and the clinic clerks are rude. The drugs have unpleasant side effects, tests are painful and invasive, and so are the procedures. Hospitals do not allow a sense of control and privacy. Doctors seem impersonal and inattentive, nurses too slow. The rooms are too hot or too cold. And, Steven said to his doctor angrily, "Why are they taking so long to find a cure?"

Some people say they are not particularly angry, and they truly are not. Other people truly *are* angry but say they are not because they are uncomfortable expressing an emotion which is, after all, overwhelming. They worry that giving in to anger means losing face or losing self-control. Their anger at unfairness and loss of control, however, often has not disappeared. Instead of getting angry at co-workers or the medical system, these people turn their anger on themselves. They feel depressed or guilty or they dislike themselves: Alan felt hopeless and stopped seeing his friends. Some eat too much: Lisa gained twenty pounds after her husband's diagnosis. Others rely too heavily on alcohol or drugs. Some continue the behavior that put them at risk for the infection in the first place: for a while, though she denied doing it, Helen went back to injecting drugs intravenously. In general, when people are depressed, they quit taking care of themselves.

Dealing with Anger

Anger is a natural and justifiable response to this infection. People need to be allowed to be angry. People also need to learn how to express anger appropriately. Directing anger at the wrong target—like Helen at the Xerox machine or like Lisa's husband at Lisa or like Alan at himself—is at best ineffectual and at worst harmful.

Anger turned on yourself is recognized as a form of depression. Those who feel hopeless or isolate themselves or eat or drink too much or continue the behavior that put them at risk for the infection are hurting themselves. Usually people realize they are treating themselves badly, and before too long, they stop of their own accord. Sometimes a friend or relative notices that the person is drinking a lot or seems unhappy and recommends getting help. If you do not seem to be stopping on your own, get help from a psychiatrist, psychologist, or social worker. These mental health professionals will help you identify and understand the anger and will help the anger find its proper target. If necessary, they can also recommend alcohol- or drug-treatment programs.

Even anger turned outward can be overwhelming. Certain actions and attitudes help people deal with anger. First, separate the anger from its target. Lisa's husband, after talking to a psychiatrist, understood he was angry at the circumstances, not at Lisa for serving him oatmeal. Steven, who had been furious at the doctors he saw in the clinic, was able to say, "The doctors aren't the people I'm mad at. I can identify the feeling now and separate it out." Alan came to see he was depressed because he was turning his anger at the disease on himself and punishing himself with hopelessness and feelings of isolation.

Second, find mechanisms that discharge anger. These will be different for different people. Helen screams, hits the bed until she is tired, and takes long walks through the fields around her small town. Steven jogs and works out in a gym. Dean tires too easily for regular physical exercise; instead he yells, writes out his anger in a journal, and talks to his partner, parents, and relatives. Alan, though he remains somewhat depressed, finds he feels calm and relaxed after he meditates.

If You're a Caregiver

If you are taking care of someone with the virus, understand that the disease is the target and you are not. The person you're caring for is feeling anger, not hatred; they do not blame you. Lisa said, "The anger and rage my husband felt were his issues and not in my control. I knew it was just his guilt for bringing the virus into our lives. It's easier to deal with his annoyance over something understandable than it is to deal with the feeling of being unloved."

Allow the person with HIV infection to express the anger, though that can be difficult when, as Lisa said, "they're shouting at you." Dean did a certain amount of yelling in the presence of his partner; his partner told him, "Go ahead and get it over with. Get it out of your system. It's understandable." Try not to judge the person or to confront him or her: judgment and confrontation will only further misdirect the anger toward you.

Acknowledge the struggle the person is having. Try saying, "I know it is hard for you. Cold oatmeal really does not taste good, and I'll heat it up again." This may help the angry person dissipate the anger and understand its true target.

Still, you need not try to achieve sainthood during your lifetime. No caregiver is neutral; often caregivers have long histories with the people they are caring for, and many old sources of anger get confused with the new ones. Nor is letting them talk about their anger the same as letting them take it out on you. Remind them that their anger is difficult for you to hear, and difficult to separate out from old problems. Dean's partner not only told him to get it over with, but also said, "Thank goodness you don't go blowing up all the time." When Dean's partner felt he had taken too much abuse, he would pull away. Dean said he noticed this, calmed down, and worked to recover his perspective.

Directing Anger

Finally, anger holds a lot of energy. Directing the energy of anger at its appropriate target has accomplished wonders.

Lisa was angry at the social stigma her husband's illness had brought her. After her husband died, she began a newsletter for people in her city with HIV infection, so that others would feel less isolation than she had felt. Steven, who was angry at the medical profession for not finding a cure, volunteered for a research study to test drugs. June, who was angry about the financial problems of her son and his friends, formed an organization that raised money to help local people with HIV infection pay for their rent, medicines, and food.

Lisa, Steven, and June are not exceptions. All over the country, people affected by HIV have used the energy from their anger to found buddy systems, political action groups, telephone hotlines, newsletters, fund-raising groups, and newspapers. Directing anger puts that frightening energy where it will do the most good; it returns to you a sense of control over your own life. Sometimes it accomplishes near-miracles.

Depression and Hope

Helen Parks: Sometimes I'm in my room, in my chair, and I think about the people in all the stages of this disease and the people who have left the world with this disease. And I wonder what I'm going to do when I get sicker. I get confused. I get drastic thoughts. I sit in my chair and cry. I get real depressed.

Steven Charles: I think, maybe they'll come up with something that will help, but I don't think so. You start to wonder why you're going to the doctor, why take the medication, why fight for another month, another year, just to be sick longer.

What Depression Feels Like

Depression is one of the most painful feelings a person can have. People say they feel alone and helpless in an indifferent world. They say they lose interest in things, have no energy, feel generally tired. They feel empty and uninterested in things they are normally interested in. They feel lonely and alienated from their friends, relatives, neighbors, co-workers. They doubt themselves or blame themselves or feel they have failed. Like Helen, they have "drastic thoughts": they think about dying, sometimes about killing themselves. Sometimes depression affects not only the mind, but also the body. Some people report they cannot think as clearly or quickly as they used to. Some stop eating, others eat too much. Some cannot sleep, others sleep too often. The inability to sleep in the morning is especially characteristic. In general, people dealing with depression say they are mostly sad and lonely, and they often cry a lot: "For a while, I cried all the time," said Lisa Pratt. "I didn't want to cry in front of my family. I cried when I was alone—in the car, in the shower."

At bottom, depression seems to be the absence of hope. Hope is the sense that life is good, that it holds comforts and delights, that what you do makes a difference, that one way or another things will be all right. Sometimes, for a while, this sense of hope fails you. "What good are all my comforts, my things?" said Alan Madison, who for a long time had spent his extra money on collecting art from the 1920s. "I've always worked for comfort in my old age. Now maybe I'm not going to be old. I've always thought, next year it'll be different. I'll get a new haircut, be more outgoing. Now maybe I have no next year."

Faced with hopelessness, people feel helpless. They feel they have no alternative but to continue feeling depressed. They feel they no longer have the power to change how they act or how they feel. Some people, especially early in the course of the infection, consider suicide.

Depression varies in intensity and duration. Sometimes it is a mild feeling of being "down," or sad, or demoralized. Sometimes it is severe, and feels like despair, deep apathy, or true hopelessness. For most people, depression comes and goes: "I get bouts of these depressions," says Steven. The bouts can last a few hours, a few weeks, a few months.

Causes of Depression

One cause of depression is a sense of being stuck in a frustrating, disheartening situation. Such situations are everywhere in life. Most people at one time or another must face something which they cannot fix, to which they can only adjust. HIV infection is certainly reason for depression: "One of the worst things about this virus," said June, "is that you never know what's coming next. I'm beginning to feel over my head. That's pretty depressing." For people facing HIV infection, depression, like anger, is a reasonable response.

Another cause of depression is predisposition: people who have been depressed before their diagnosis might be more likely to be depressed afterward. Another cause is medications. Many of the medications used to treat opportunistic infections and HIV itself can sometimes cause depression.

Alcohol, which is a depressant, is a particularly treacherous cause of depression because it can start a cycle. To feel better about their depression, people drink, which makes them feel depressed and out of control. So to feel better, they drink some more, get more depressed, and so on and on.

Occasionally, depression may be caused by the virus itself. That is, depression can be a symptom of dementia, a condition that results when the virus enters the brain (see Chapter 7).

Frequently, depression is caused by unexpressed anger. Anger is hard to express, especially if it is directed at something as vague as fate, or something as personal as your own body or your behavior. People who do not express such anger either consciously restrain it or unconsciously ignore it. In either case, they unknowingly turn their anger inward on themselves and become depressed.

What to Do about Mild Depression

Depression that is unexpressed anger will disappear if the anger is recognized and dealt with. Depression that is basically sadness, loneliness, and hopelessness almost always runs its course within days or weeks, and then goes away. For some people, this happens without their intervention. Others need to be more active in dispelling depression. One way to lessen or end depression is with physical activity: get outside, go for walks, cook a wonderful meal, go boating or driving or fishing or bowling, go shopping and buy yourself a little treat. Try to accomplish something you want done. A sense of accomplishment can come from doing something small, like cleaning out a closet, writing a letter, or polishing your shoes. No matter how small, a sense of accomplishment is a great weapon against depression.

Another way to lessen or end depression is with mental activity: read novels or biographies or science or philosophy or poetry; go to the movies or the theater or the opera or an art gallery; talk to your neighbors or friends or family; play a musical instrument or draw a picture or take some photographs or write a poem. The possibilities of undemanding and pleasurable activities are endless. "I'm not one of those people who immerse themselves in the sickness," said Steven, who is a technician in a scientific laboratory. He takes in stray dogs, operates a ham radio, and reads up on scientific discoveries in all fields. "I keep my regular life going, keep on working," he says.

When Helen gets depressed, she has a list of things she does: "I usually notice depression when I hit the house after work. Then I find things to do, to keep my mind relaxed. I dig in the dirt. I walk, anything physical. Clean the closet, walk through the mall and window shop. I take a bubble bath. Read the Bible, help someone else." Lisa Pratt's husband did the same: "For months," said Lisa, "my husband sat in a chair and stared. Nothing interested him. Then he got into his workshop and started making crafts, carving wooden ducks." Dean gardens; he says it takes little energy and gives him a great sense of peace and beauty. June finds that her son is less depressed after he goes out for a walk around their neighborhood: "I nag at him. I tell him, 'You can't sit there and watch TV. I want you up, dressed for the weather and outside, and I don't want to see you for 25 minutes.'"

These and other activities will not make your life wonderful again, but they do seem to dissolve depression, at least temporarily. Sometimes, during a walk, the balance between hope and hopelessness seems to shift back toward hope, and you feel more yourself again. And when the next bout of depression moves in, you, like Helen, will have your list of activities and distractions and small pleasures handy.

What to Do about Severe Depression

Sometimes, for some people, depression is too severe or it lasts too long. They feel alienated from everyone, deeply apathetic, profoundly hopeless. Severe, persistent depression is often best treated with medication. Talk to a doctor. If medication taken for another condition is causing depression, the doctor can change the drug or lower the dose. If the depression is part of dementia, the doctor will prescribe medications that ease the symptoms. Most of the persistent depression in people with HIV infection, however, is simply the natural reaction to knowledge of a devastating disease. Like the depression that accompanies the loss of a loved one or a diagnosis of cancer, it can be successfully treated with appropriate support and medications. In this case, the doctor will recommend a psychiatrist, who can prescribe medication that restores sleep, appetite, and mood. The drugs currently used for severe depression are nearly miraculous. They do for depression what penicillin does for pneumonia: about 80 percent of severely depressed people with HIV infection respond, and about 50 percent are cured. For most people, treatment of depression is temporary but critical.

Either the doctor or the psychiatrist might recommend professional psychological help (see section on mental health professionals in Chapter 12). Psychiatrists, psychologists, and social workers can help you talk through whatever is blocking the healing process, though only psychiatrists are trained medically and can prescribe medications. Psychotherapy may concentrate on the overwhelming problems people must face and feel they cannot solve: How can I face rejection? How can I deal with anger? How can I feel less guilty? How can I have sex without hurting myself or anyone else? Why me? Why now? What will I do with the rest of my life? What will happen to my kids? My parents? The people I love? Will I die? How will I die? Am I a good person? By helping you confront problems you feel are unsolvable and find new perspectives on those problems, a psychotherapist will help you take control of your life. He or she will help you deny, not the fact of your infection, but your own helplessness and hopelessness in the face of it.

Thoughts of suicide are usually only temporary: the suicide rate among people with HIV infection is low. Researchers say that people seem to consider suicide mostly as a means of regaining a feeling of control over their lives. And that makes sense—it is as though people were saying, "This disease does not control whether I live or die, I do." Nevertheless, if thoughts about suicide persist, and if thoughts of taking pills become plans to collect specific pills, and if these persistent, concrete thoughts are coupled with an increase in guilt and sense of punishment, then get help. Call your doctor or psychotherapist.

Fatigue and Accommodation

The Causes of Fatigue

Fatigue often accompanies depression: people dealing with depression lose not only a sense of hope but also their physical energy. They are tired, sometimes exhausted, sometimes apathetic.

Fatigue is also an indirect result of HIV infection. In this case, it is usually accompanied by weight loss, fever, and night sweats. These symptoms are most likely to occur relatively late in the course of the infection when the CD4 count is low, usually well below 300 (see chapters 3 and 6).

HIV infection causes fatigue by depriving the body of some of its sources of energy. People with HIV infection often have anemia, or lower numbers of red blood cells. Red blood cells, among other things, carry oxygen; oxygen supplies the muscles with energy. People with fewer red blood cells therefore have less energy and tire easily, though the anemia must be severe before people notice symptoms.

In addition, people with HIV infection sometimes have diarrhea. With diarrhea, food is eliminated from the body before being absorbed, so food is also unavailable as a source of energy. Again, the diarrhea must be severe or last for several weeks to cause the fatigue that accompanies malnutrition.

For some people, fatigue is caused by opportunistic infections like MA or CMV.

Medications can also cause fatigue or sleepiness, which is often interpreted as fatigue. These medications include, among others, narcotics, antihistamines, and antidepressants.

The Effects of Fatigue

Although the causes of fatigue may be physical, the effects are psychological. In fact, depression not only causes fatigue but is also caused by it. Dean said he has had good days and bad days. On the good days, he has more energy. After a rough night and diarrhea, he will be tired the next day: he said, "Those are the crying days." "Fatigue is my son's biggest obstacle," said June. "He sleeps 18 hours. By ten in the morning, he's done. He says to me, 'Why aren't I beating this?' I don't think he could get through a work day. He loses motivation and courage. Sometimes he stops caring for himself, stops eating. He's too tired to eat."

Another psychological effect of fatigue is irritation. Lisa Pratt's husband "had always been a go-getter," she said, and resented his fatigue. "For my husband," Lisa said, "AIDS was a series of little deaths. He had to give up little things he liked because he had no stamina. For years, he had been an actor in our local community theater. After he got AIDS, he couldn't keep up with the rehearsal schedule and thought he was going to have to quit. It hurt to not go. And it made him mad to give in." Dean said that until he learned to pace himself, he regularly worked fourteen hours a day running a small newspaper, came home angry, then "got the blues."

Accommodating to Fatigue

Fatigue is an integral part of this infection. Whether its cause is psychological or physical, fatigue cannot be ignored. First, talk to your doctor: some medications can counter fatigue. The best way to deal with fatigue may be to accept it and go on from there. Decide what you want to do most, be sure it is possible, plan it out, and pace yourself. When Dean wants to go to a concert on Thursday, he begins resting on Tuesday and takes off Friday and Saturday. Lisa's husband stayed in the community theater but tried out only for small roles. Steven gets up late, goes to work late, and goes home early. Dean kept his job but cut back his hours and tried to have meetings in his office rather than in offices across town.

Try to plan things that can, if necessary, be changed or postponed. Dean's long-time partner helps him in this: "We deal from day to day. We don't look ahead because the illness is so powerful and changes at any time. Plans for one day can easily be impossible, so we just do what we had planned a few days later." June's son had planned a trip to Europe in great detail: reservations for travel and for hotels, sites to visit, places to eat, tickets for everything. When he realized he was too easily fatigued to go, he planned another trip, in the same detail, to a part of the United States he had always wanted to see.

Know what times of the day you have most energy, and plan accordingly. If possible, cook and eat at those times when you have energy: food is the body's best source of energy. Otherwise, use those times of the day for things you want to get done, things that will give you a sense of accomplishment. Alan schedules appointments for late morning or over lunch. Lisa's husband asked the community theater to change rehearsal times to early evenings, when he had most energy; the theater was happy to accommodate him.

In general, try to find ways to accomplish what you want with less energy. Lisa's husband's fatigue also affected their social life: "Socially, we didn't go out as much. But then we redefined 'socially.' Instead of going out drinking and dancing, we entertained at home. Our social life didn't disappear." People who find driving tiring can often take public transportation. Or they consolidate several trips into one, or ask their friends to drive them. When they want to buy clothes or household supplies or presents, they order from catalogs. Catalogs from large department stores have enormous selections of everything from shampoo to shirts to lamps to sheets. To buy groceries, they find a store that delivers, or ask their friends. They get their medication from pharmacies that deliver.

If cooking is tiring, buy foods that are prepared or that can be microwaved. Try cooking a large amount of food and freezing what you don't eat. Spaghetti sauce, chili, pot roasts, stews, and soups all taste good made in large amounts and reheated, and they freeze well. If eating is tiring, use nutritional supplements that come as powders and are mixed with milk. Or make a nutritional supplement out of milk, ice cream, and fruit mixed in a food processor. Alan used to do all the cooking, and he still does most of it, but when he is tired, Alan says, "My partner offers to do parts of the meals. He makes great desserts." Helen does the dishes immediately after eating; she finds that less tiring that letting them stack up and doing several meals' worth at once. She keeps a chair in the kitchen for when she needs to rest. Dean keeps a chair in the shower, and sometimes he showers sitting down.

Cleaning services may not be prohibitively expensive; friends might help with cleaning too. To minimize what must be cleaned, try consolidating your living into one area or one floor. Make a bedroom on the first floor, or turn the bedroom into a living area. Consolidating your living also saves steps. Put a dorm-sized refrigerator next to your bed for juice or fruit. Keep the phone near your bed.

Wear clothes that are easy to wear and to care for: jeans, knitted shirts and pants, sweatsuits, clothes with elastic waists and no buttons, clothes that can be washed and dried easily and do not need ironing. Alan used to do the laundry alone; now he and his partner do it together. "I don't get as tired," Alan says, "and it's more fun that way."

If several friends or relatives have offered help, do not be shy about accepting it. After all, you need the help, and if circumstances were reversed, you would want them to accept your help. Try making lists of things you would like help with. Perhaps one friend would not mind regularly watering plants, another might feed your cat, another might help with the laundry.

Fatigue often makes paying bills particularly onerous. Friends can help with regular bills; they can write the checks for the mortgage, rent, utilities, taxes. Some banks will deduct payments for monthly bills directly from your banking account.

Do what you can; don't give up before you need to. June worries that people give in too soon to their fatigue, and then they miss doing what they are capable of doing. When June is not at home caring for her son, she visits other people with AIDS. "Some are tired and giving up," she said. "I say to them, 'Don't tell me you can't go out next Wednesday. This is only Sunday. How do you know how you'll feel on Wednesday? If you think tired, you'll *be* tired.'" Steven says, "I keep pushing myself. I do wake up tired and don't like that. I make myself get up. I get out of that bed." Alan agrees: "The main thing is that I not feel like an invalid. I still cook, even though my partner helps out a lot now. But I still cook."

If you know you've done your best, then relax and rest. Try not to let fatigue affect your good opinion of yourself. You've done what you could.

Fear and Realism

> *Alan Madison:* I'm scared as hell at different periods. I have little sores on my skin, and my leg tingles. I'm going to be crazy until I see the doctor. I wake up at night and cry a little.

People fear what they do not understand and cannot control. Like Alan, they worry about symptoms that may or may not be serious. They fear being a patient in a hospital, or undergoing painful medical tests and procedures. They fear dependency: "My husband had a tremendous fear of being bedridden and me caring for him," said Lisa. They fear rejection: Alan was afraid that people would treat him as though he had leprosy; Helen said she was fearful of telling her sons. People with HIV infection are afraid they will give someone else the virus. Caregivers fear contagion.

People with HIV fear what the infection might do to them: they fear becoming blind, or losing their cognitive abilities. They fear dying. They say they fear not death, but the way death comes. "I could handle dying," said Alan, "if I knew how I might die. My biggest fear is what the end will be like." When June goes with her son to the hospital, she feels fear: "It is hard for me to see his friends who are also in the hospital. I think, what's the last time going to be like for him? It's so frightening. You can drive yourself crazy thinking these things. And you're also crazy if you don't think these things. You are faced with that ultimate fear all the time." People fear the future. All these fears are realistic responses to a situation that in fact includes the possibility of sickness, pain, dependency, rejection, and death.

Sometimes these fears can actually be useful. Fearing contagion can be a useful way to avoid transmitting or becoming infected with the virus. Fearing dependency can be a good way of remaining independent as long as possible. The point is not to live without fear, only to live without being unduly troubled or hindered by fear. Sometimes what people feel is not fear but anxiety. That is, they have feelings of fear that are unrealistic. People who are anxious say they feel as if something terrible were about to happen. They cannot say what exactly they fear, only that they have a sense of underlying uneasiness. They feel restless and uncomfortable wherever they are. They are irritable, tense, and preoccupied with their bodies. They have trouble breathing, are nauseated, break out into cold sweats, have racing pulses. Some have periods of feeling panicky.

People whose feelings of anxiety persist too long or are too severe should see a mental health professional or a doctor who might in turn recommend a visit to a psychiatrist. Persistent anxiety takes a tremendous amount of energy, and it is often curable. Psychiatrists can prescribe medication to relieve anxiety. Mental health professionals can teach techniques that help you relax. Physical relaxation usually makes people feel calmer and more themselves again.

Dissipating Fear with Information

Many fears do not hold up in the cold light of reality.

If you fear sickness, find out which symptoms you should see your doctor about and which you should ignore (see Chapter 6). "I found out what's what," said Alan, "and now I don't worry about every little cough."

If you fear medications, tests, and procedures, educate yourself about them. Read what you can find, ask your doctor, ask people who have had the experience. Learn about drugs like AZT and their side effects. Talk to someone who's had a bronchoscopy, who's gone through a scanner, who's had a lumbar puncture. The fear of such things is often much worse than the things themselves.

If you fear dying, talk to a therapist or pastor or other people in your situation or someone you love. Death, whether your own or that of someone you are caring for, seems like a dark thing we cannot talk about. Talking makes the unknown much less frightening. Talk as openly as you can.

If you fear rejection and desertion, find out if those you love will in fact stand by you. Try saying, "This is what will happen to me. Can you deal with that?" As it turns out, people are rarely completely abandoned by the people they love. "I know," said Dean, "that given my resources in life, which are my relatives, I will always have a roof. That's helped me with anxiety." Steven said that he quit being afraid when his cousin said she'd come stay with him. Sometimes those people you love cannot offer unqualified support. In that case, you and they will need to negotiate what they feel able to give. People usually know and can be specific about what they can and cannot provide.

If you fear what the disease might do to you, ask your doctor, hospital mental health professional, or other people with HIV infection. During a stay at the hospital, Dean roomed with a man who was dying and, like June, Dean was full of fears for the future. "My roommate in the hospital was dying. I asked him lots of specific questions. I asked him, Could he care for himself? He told me that when he got too tired to follow a routine, he didn't. I wondered, Was he lucid? I found out that things didn't get bad for him until right before. He was religious—so am I—and that was reassuring to me. His lover was very attentive, and that was reassuring, too."

If you are a caregiver afraid of contagion, inform yourself about how to take the precautions that avoid infection—June said she had "learned to be precautious" (see Chapter 2). While you are doing this, try not to communicate your fear to the person you are caring for. Make that person feel you are comfortable being around him or her.

Put the fear into perspective. Alan said, "I went to a therapist for a while. Then I had a big gigantic turning point. I was taking a shower and realized that all my problems were coming from the fear itself. Fear was creating all the problems, even the fear. Realizing that made the fear dissipate in a gush. Of course, it came back again, but it kept going away again too."

Guilt and Self-Worth

What People Feel Guilty About

One of the many peculiarities of HIV is the amount of guilt it seems to inspire. People feel guilty for having become infected. They feel they are somehow to blame for having gotten the virus, that they brought it on themselves. "I feel a little guilt," said Steven. "I should have known to practice safer sex, even though at the time I got infected, no one even knew the virus was around. I know how stupid that sounds, but I feel guilty anyway." They feel guilty about bringing HIV infection into the lives of other people: about putting their partners or spouses at risk, about having those closest to them go through the trauma of caregiving, about telling their children they have HIV infection, about distressing their parents, their families, and their friends.

Many people also feel guilt about the behavior that put them at risk in the first place. The behaviors that exposed most people to the virus—

gay lovemaking and intravenous drug use—are behaviors of which society often disapproves. For many people, social disapproval is distressing, and they feel isolated and punished. Sometimes they unconsciously take social disapproval on themselves as guilt. "A lot of us took society's view," said Dean, "and felt guilty about being gay." The same is generally true for IV drug users: "I was real upset with myself," said Helen. "This disease makes me feel like I've been a dirty person, and I'm not. I'm a clean person."

Even those whose exposure to the virus came through conditions society does not disapprove of—blood transfusions, hemophilia—still feel guilty. They feel they are to blame for involving their families in a disease that is socially isolating, and for putting their spouses at risk. Lisa said her husband had been afraid their daughters would say, "What did you do to our family?"

Even caregivers feel guilty. Steven's mother feels that if she had been a better mother, Steven would not have been gay and come in contact with the virus. June feels guilty that she will probably survive her son.

Causes of Guilt

Guilt does not necessarily have a cause. Guilt, like fear, is a feeling that may or may not have anything to do with the facts. Some people truly did something they should not have done. Perhaps they knew they ran a risk when they became infected. Others are accepting blame for something over which they had no control. Perhaps they knew nothing about the virus or they thought they were taking appropriate steps to avoid infection or they unknowingly received infected blood. Guilt, like all other reactions to this infection, is a natural human feeling. Sooner or later in their lives, most people feel guilty about something, sometimes justifiably, sometimes not. Alan, for instance, remembers stealing a plastic toy from a dime store when he was seven years old, and though he does not feel like a criminal, he does feel a vague sense of shame and is not able to forget the incident.

Perhaps guilt comes from a sense that good behavior deserves reward and bad behavior deserves punishment. Perhaps people feel that since the virus feels like a punishment, they must have behaved badly. Perhaps social disapproval operates the same way: people feel isolated and punished, so they feel they must have done something wrong to deserve it. Both of these possibilities are built on bad logic and are just plain wrong.

What to Do about Guilt

First, separate the virus from a sense of punishment. Lisa states: "What I say is, it's a virus, not a punishment. I didn't get the virus and my husband did. Does that make me good and him bad? That's ridiculous. Everyone got this virus like my husband did: being in the wrong place at the wrong time."

The virus does not set out to "get" anyone. It has no brain, no judgment, no ability to pick out who is worthy and who is not. The virus has nothing whatever to do with punishment. Nor does anyone set out to get infected with the virus. The behaviors that put most people at risk for the virus may well be behaviors that are directed by biology, and in any case, are not the result of a conscious intention. No one makes a conscious, informed decision that they will become gay or will use drugs.

Understand that guilt, except when it keeps you from repeating mistakes, is a remarkably useless emotion. Feeling guilty means worrying about something you cannot change. Whether people knowingly ran a risk or not, the past is beyond anyone's power to change. Guilt keeps people captured in the past and prohibits them from doing what they can to improve the present. Guilt uses emotional energy that would be better used on the real problems of life.

Balance guilt by understanding your own worth. Ask yourself, outside my worries, who am I? A pastor who has had experience with people with HIV infection asks people, "What else besides the things you feel guilty about are you? What do your friends like about you? They tell me 'That I helped them move the piano, that I had some good kids, that I was a good friend.'" Sometimes the pastor had to remind his parishioners what is good about them: "One man with HIV was having trouble with guilt and thought he was all bad. I had to remind him he was our church organist, and when he played, he would rock the timbers of the church with music."

In the process of focusing on your own worth, guilt usually fades away. People come to like themselves for who they are. Some people speed up the process by getting help from a therapist. During therapy, they deal with the attitudes and behavior, often left over from childhood, that make them feel guilty. They learn to feel comfortable with themselves and free themselves of their old, useless burden of guilt.

Chapter 5

HIV Infection and Its Effects on Interpersonal Relations

- Sympathy and worry
- Helplessness, dependency, and control
- Feelings about sex
- Relationships with your children
- Relationships with drug users

Sympathy and Worry

By the imagination we place ourselves in [their] situations, we conceive ourselves enduring all the same torments, we enter as it were into [their] bodies, and become in some measure the same person with [them]. . . . [We] not only feel a sorrow of the same kind with that which they feel, but as if [we] had derived a part of it to [ourselves]; what [we] feel seems to alleviate the weight of what they feel. . . . The sweetness of [our] sympathy more than compensates the bitterness of that sorrow.

(Adam Smith, *Theory of Moral Sentiments,* 1892)

People are built to feel connections to one another. The word *sympathy* comes from a Greek word that means "feeling with," or more literally, "co-suffering." When we see someone in pain, we feel pain too. It is as if, as Adam Smith said, we become in some measure the same person. When someone sympathizes with us, our pain is relieved. It is as if we could split the same packet of pain between us.

For caregivers, feeling sympathy means being intensely involved with those being cared for. "I want to be a part of taking care of Dean," Dean Lombard's partner says. "If God wants him back to where he was, I want to be a part of that, of getting him to walk out the door." For people with HIV infection, sympathy amounts to a cure. It provides comfort, sustenance, healing; it is an antidote to pain, loneliness, and loss. June Monroe's son says, "My mother has the ability to keep me alive."

As in all human relations, what sometimes is an alliance is at other times a source of conflict. People with HIV infection sometimes feel their caretakers' sympathy and involvement as a burden, a responsibility: "It gets to be hard," Steven Charles said about all his worried relatives, "making myself comfortable and everyone else too." And as in many conflicts, both sides are right.

One Side: People Who Take Care of Those with HIV Infection Are Worried

"My son had pneumocystis pneumonia, then neuropathy," said June. "He was very sick. It worried me so much, I didn't even want to leave him alone at night." Lisa, remembering the care of her husband, said, "It was such torture and grief, I wonder how I did it. I went out of town one weekend to visit friends. But I spent the whole time worrying how things were going, and finally cut the weekend short. I had to come home. I couldn't stay away." June's and Lisa's inability to leave their relatives is a measure of how connected they felt, of how little they could separate themselves.

Caregiver's feelings are varied and confused. They feel sympathy, they are co-suffering. They don't know where the boundaries are between themselves and those they care for. They expect themselves to somehow *know* what the sick person feels and wants. Then they expect they should be able to supply it. They also understand, however, that no one really knows what someone else feels. They see the problems the sick person is having, and they try to figure out all the solutions. They feel guilty that they weren't the ones struck by illness. They worry that at some critical moment—during a seizure, for instance—they will not know what to do, and the result of their not knowing will be a catastrophe. So they worry, they have an intense desire to know what is going on. "What do I expect myself to do?" said June. "Everything. I think, I will find out what's wrong with my son. I will get him cured. Once I was even going to carry him the 60 steps down from his third-floor apartment. I am going to do it all."

Needless to say, no one, no matter how strong and determined, can do everything. Caregivers who try to do everything inevitably have periods when they burn out. They feel depressed, hostile, impatient, agitated; they think they can't cope, and they lose their sense of humor. They have trouble concentrating and sleeping, and sometimes they overeat or drink too much or rely on drugs. They get sick and feel distant from other people.

The Other Side: People with HIV Infection Sometimes Feel Unable to Reassure the Caregivers

"The people who are my support," said Alan Madison, "also upset me most. My partner, when I came home from work early, gave that look of, 'Oh God, he's sick, he's probably dying.' " Caregivers' worries about people who are sick occasionally seem to be requests for reassurance, as though the caregivers want the sick person to say, "No, I'm not sick at all. Nothing to worry about." When people are tired and not feeling well and a little worried themselves, reassuring others is trying. Steven's caregiver is his cousin: "My cousin gets too doting. She gives me her entire schedule and wants to know mine. But I can't feel accountable to her—we're both full grown—in spite of her good intentions."

People with HIV infection are extremely aware that they are affecting the lives of their caregivers. They worry that they are causing trouble and suffering, and they feel responsible for that. Perhaps they also occasionally feel some guilt for inflicting trouble on their caregivers. As a result, people with HIV infection protect their caregivers. Sometimes they keep worrisome information to themselves, or they minimize symptoms and pains. They say they don't want to make the caregivers' burdens any heavier. They worry that the caregivers will burn out and be unable to help them in times of urgent need. They also worry that no one is caring for the caregivers: "My cousin hasn't had an easy life," says Steven. "She lost her father, and now she's losing me. She's having a hard time and somebody should be watching out for her."

People with HIV infection are sometimes bothered by reassuring caregivers because they want not to be reminded of sickness, but to concentrate on getting well. Both people with HIV infection and their caregivers have times when they confront sickness and times when they enjoy being alive. Occasionally they are simply not thinking about the same things at the same time. They are not disagreeing on what is important; they are only out of sync.

Too often, what the caregiver expresses as sympathy sounds to the receiver like pity. The sick person sometimes hears the caregiver saying, "It must be awful to be you." "That kind of sympathy," says Steven, "makes me very uneasy."

Resolving the Conflict

Balancing sympathy and intrusion is difficult. For people dealing with HIV infection, sympathy, both as a blessing and a burden, is as much a fact of life as the infection is. At times, people make each other feel comforted and reassured. Other times, people's feelings are so overwhelming that they need to protect themselves from the pain, and just cannot help another person. When this happens, the person with HIV infection and the caregiver might want to take a break from each other. They might find other, temporary supports. Family members, friends, nurses, mental health professionals, support groups, buddies, home health aides, clergy—all can take some of the heat off, give both people some time out.

Caregivers especially need to take breaks. They often feel guilty about this, but breaks are essential to good caregiving. Without breaks, caregivers start burning out. June, who had expected herself to do everything, even carry her son down three flights of steps, said, "But I can't do everything. I need to enlist people. I have a friend who's a nurse. She can help my son some afternoons—she'll give me a breath of air."

Resolving the conflicts among people affected by HIV infection is a matter of managing these difficult facts of life, of balancing the blessings against the burden. No one resolution of the conflict will last forever. Nor will a single solution apply to all problems. Instead, people solve different problems, some small, some large, one after another. Those who do this best have learned to focus on the blessings and to negotiate the burdens. They appreciate the virtues in the relationship. They are willing to acknowledge another person's needs and to be flexible about their own. They are willing to lose something less important in order to gain something more important.

People who solve problems well often negotiate by talking. They acknowledge the other person's point of view, then state their own. Alan could say to his partner, "I know you're worried that I'm dying. I'm not dying. I'm just tired and have come home early. I know you love me and you're always worried. I wish you didn't have reason to worry." Alan's partner could say back, "I worry because I love you. I wish you didn't have the problem and I didn't have the worry." This way, what began as a source of tension ends as a source of comfort.

Caregivers can avoid asking for reassurance that creates a burden or that cannot be given. They can respect the abilities of the person with HIV infection to find his or her own solutions. They can understand that some things cannot be fixed. They will allow the person to talk freely and openly and without interruption or fear of judgment. They can listen, though they find it hard. They can let the person cry, and not try to make him or her stop. They can also allow the person to be alone, and not talk. They can understand that talking about depression, fear, anger, or guilt sometimes seems to undercut the positive attitude that is important to people with HIV infection. Caregivers can learn to accept their own helplessness, to give up trying to make everything right again. At the same time, they can learn not to run away. Lisa understood that her husband had all the burdens he could handle: "He needed me to keep talking, to reminisce about good things, to bring up happy memories, to touch him." People with HIV infection can see worry as love. Dean understood that his mother needed to ask him questions, and they worked out times when she could. "My mother has felt so helpless with this disease. Everyone does. But she talked only when I wanted to. She'd say, "Do you want to talk about this now?"

Helplessness, Dependency, and Control

> *Alan Madison:* One of the worst thoughts for me is, I don't want people taking care of me. No one wants to give up that control. I come from proud people. I've always felt the need to do it on my own.

No One Wants to Give up Control

Like Alan, all people want to "do it on their own." By that, they usually mean that they do not want to rely on other people; they want to rely only on themselves. They take care of their own needs. They want to do their fair share in a relationship, not only taking advice and help, but also giving it. When something goes wrong, they fix it; when someone has a problem, they solve it. They can do what they set out to do. In short, they have the sense that they are in control of their own lives.

HIV infection seriously undermines a person's sense of control. People with HIV infection have intervals of illness during which they depend on others for things they normally provide for themselves. Their dependency ranges from needing someone to shop, clean, and cook for them to needing someone to dress, bathe, and feed them. They dislike this dependency. They say that being dependent is hard on their self-esteem, their sense of self-worth. They don't feel like normal adults any more; they feel like babies.

Their caregivers have a different problem with the sense of control. Instead of feeling dependent on someone else, they feel helpless to change things. The person they love is sick and in emotional pain, and they can do nothing to fix that. They can fix problems that are physical—they can shop, clean, cook, give medications, talk to doctors, dress and bathe and feed the person they love. But problems that are emotional—anger, depression, fear, guilt—are often unfixable, or at least not fixable in the same way. Caregivers still want to fix them, to correct them, to make them disappear. Faced with an inescapable virus and inevitable emotions, caregivers feel helpless and stupid.

Different aspects of loss of control bother different people. Some dislike what seems like a reversion to childhood: at times, they need to be changed, bathed, dressed, groomed, fed, driven. Helen Parks, who has lived alone all her adult life, says she worries "about moving in with my parents and not having time to myself and having to have my dinner fixed and my clothes washed. I won't have my mother drive me or change me." June's son, who had been a doctor, now lives with her: "It was hard for my son to come home at age thirty-four and have his mom care for him," she said. "How much he can do for himself depends on how he's feeling. He always wants to do as much as he can for himself." Lisa said her husband "had a tremendous fear of being bedridden and me caring for him." Adults who must accept being cared for like a child feel they are a burden. Because their bodies must be cared for by others, they feel they have lost their dignity.

Some young people with HIV infection are upset that they may be unable to take care of their parents. They see this as losing control. They had expected, as they became adults, to care more and more for their parents, and they dislike the reversal in roles. Steven has two aging great-aunts and a grandfather he feels responsible for: "I should be taking care of them. I should see that they're getting their medication or their new glasses. People shouldn't be doing these things for me."

Other people hate giving up their roles with their partners. Lisa said that the more she took out the garbage, paid the bills, and mowed the lawn, the more her husband felt he was losing control, and the unhappier he became: "Sometimes he was grateful," she said, "and sometimes he just screamed." Dean said, "My partner used to be a cook, it's okay with me that he does most of the cooking. I had always done the heavy work, and sometimes still do. But sometimes I can make no contributions. The days I can't contribute are awful, just awful."

Others worry about financial dependency on their parents or on the welfare system: Helen says, "I'm surely not one for welfare." As people get sicker, they depend more and more on the social service and medical systems. Both systems require people to give up control, one system over their personal resources, the other over their bodies. The requirements, though necessary, are distressing. People who give over control of their resources and their bodies feel they have little left of their own. They feel powerless, ineffective, and incompetent.

Coming to Terms with Loss of Control

The trick is to balance acceptance of help with preservation of control. First, don't give up independence too easily. "I have a friend with AIDS," says Steven, "who sometimes asks me to bring stuff down from his attic or install his screen windows—things I know he can do for himself. I say no. I know, because I have other friends with AIDS, that he has to take some responsibility. Lots of people give up, but mental and physical health go hand in hand." People feel better about accepting help if they think they've done their best to accomplish the task on their own first.

Next, accept the fact that having some help is going to be necessary. Certainly such physical limitations as fatigue require that you accept help. Helen, who had worried about depending on her parents or on welfare, made her peace with getting help. "I know I'm not going to be able to count on myself for everything," she finally said. "I'm not going to be afraid of becoming dependent, of saying I need help. My father and stepmother have been very supportive. My church will always help." Some people feel they need help so badly they have no choice but to accept it. Some people feel they can accept help because they have helped others: what goes around comes around, they say. Some can accept help because they understand that their caregivers need to be involved with them. Some know that if circumstances were reversed and their caregivers were sick, they would help their caregivers. Some feel they have led good enough lives that they are worthy recipients of care.

Control What You Can

Finally, after you accept what you must, control whatever else you can. A friend of Steven's felt he was being a burden to his parents and moved into a private home for people with AIDS; he liked the home particularly because he felt needed by other people there. Another friend of Steven's had wanted to be sick at home, but after he had diarrhea and his sister had to change his sheets and wash him, he decided to go to the hospital instead.

If you cannot control your life in big ways, control it in small: you never lose control over everything. Lisa would ask her husband, "Do you want the water glass here or there? Do you want to wear your blue shirt or your white one? Do you want cocoa or coffee?" When Dean needs to go to the hospital, he routinely takes along his own lamp and radio. You can always affect the course or quality of your life somehow.

This strategy of controlling what you can extends to the social service and medical systems. For more on dealing with the social services, see Chapter 10; for more on dealing with the medical system, see Chapter 8.

Control and the Caregiver

For caregivers, problems with control are different. Caregivers need to balance several things at once. They need to deal with their own sense of helplessness, to allow the people they're caring for to maintain a sense of control, and to care for them, all at the same time. Maintaining this balance is tricky and confusing. "My son is so much in control and I always push that," June said. "But it backfires. When he really needs help, like with getting meals when he's sick, he doesn't ask. Sometimes I help him anyway. I also wish I could help him with the emotional things too, by just sitting and talking. But I'm afraid of smothering him. I just don't know where the line is."

On the whole, caregivers should probably try to let the people they care for determine where the line is. The problems and feelings that people with HIV infection face can be resolved only by them. In fact, for people with HIV infection, being told solutions to problems they know are insoluble, or whose solutions only they can find, is annoying and intrusive. The best help caregivers can give is listening. Caregivers find it hard just to listen; they feel passive and helpless. Nevertheless listening, as Dean said, "really helps."

Listening means being quiet, not interrupting, not judging, not giving advice, not trying to fix what's wrong. It means paying sympathetic attention, drawing the person out. Try saying, "I'm interested in that if you want to tell me." Or, "That sounds hard. How are you handling it?" If the person is crying, don't interrupt or make him or her stop. If you want to know why he or she is crying, wait until the crying is over to ask. Let the person cry it out—some things deserve tears. Listening also means picking up cues: perhaps the person does not want to talk, or wants to talk but is afraid of being a burden, or does not want help, or wants help but does not want to ask. The cues will help the caregiver decide how to act.

Sometimes giving this much control to someone else annoys the caregiver. Caregivers occasionally feel as though they are looking after a demanding and self-centered child. They feel manipulated and demeaned, as though they are being servants. Sometimes, the people they are caring for want things that seem unreasonable: to go on a long trip, to spend money a certain way. Lisa's husband inherited some money from his uncle and wanted to spend it all on a pickup truck. Lisa thought he was rapidly getting too sick to get much use out of a truck, but after she gave him the reasons against it, she thought, "Why shouldn't he have what he wants? It was his uncle and it's his money. He needs to control what's left of his life." Like Lisa, caregivers need to remember that people with HIV infection are in positions of dependency and need to feel as effective and competent and in control as possible.

Likewise, people who are being cared for need to remember they are placing unusual demands on the caregiver. They need to share control whenever they can. A caregiver could say, "I know how much you dislike feeling helpless, but I'm feeling bossed around. I'd like to decide what to fix for supper tonight." The person being cared for could say, "I wouldn't like taking orders either, and I appreciate your fixing supper. Whatever you make, could you make it spicy?"

What You Cannot Control, Relabel

Some people maintain control by what mental health professionals call *reframing* or *relabeling*. Relabeling means looking at situations in such a way that they seem benign or comforting or controllable. Try paying attention not to where your family or friends fail you, but to where they help. Try calling something a challenge rather than a struggle, a preference rather than a need. If the disadvantages of a situation are undeniable, so are the advantages.

When June's son had to quit driving, he said that although he felt frustrated at being unable to drive, he also now had extra money to spend on things he enjoyed. Dean was pleased that doctors caught an infection of cryptococcal meningitis early before he began getting the headaches he'd seen his friends endure. Dean also said that now that his partner has had to take over more of his care, they spend more time together and have become closer: "My being sick has made us closer, made us cherish our time together. It's not depending, it's mutual caring." People with HIV infection who have to quit work say they are happy to have more time to spend on gardening, developing photographs, working on old cars, or anything else they enjoy. They say repeatedly that they are happy to have more time to spend with the people they love.

Relabeling can be done only by the person with the problem, not by anyone else, no matter how well-meaning the other person is. If June had told her son that being unable to drive means having more money to spend, he would have felt she was making light of his problem. Having your problems relabeled by someone else is usually annoying.

Feelings about Sex

People's feelings about sex are varied. At different times and to different people, sex is a joy, a comfort, a distraction, a release, intimacy, reassurance, bonding. To some extent, people's feelings about sex depend on feeling healthy, enjoying life, liking themselves, trusting others, feeling relaxed, having the freedom to be spontaneous. HIV infection changes much of this. Everyone knows these facts: the virus occurs in great numbers in blood and semen, and in smaller numbers in vaginal fluid and menstrual blood. So while making love, people with HIV infection can unthinkingly transmit the virus. Even when both partners are infected, they can communicate variants of the virus to each other. To avoid this, people have no alternative but to have no sex at all or to practice safer sex. But both safer sex and the fact that sex can communicate the virus create emotional problems for people.

Problems with Feelings about Sex

Probably the most difficult problem is that some people equate making love with getting sick. They worry about getting sicker themselves, they worry about making other people sick. They feel guilty having sex. They mourn the loss of the sexual life they once had. They feel violated by the virus; the virus invaded their bodies when they were doing something enjoyable and natural. And all these feelings come at a time when people intensely need the closeness that sexual intimacy brings. "We've seen couples pull apart," said Dean. "We need closeness a lot more now."

Another problem for some people is that they feel safer sex is no fun. Safer sex seems to detract from spontaneity and a feeling of relaxation. It sometimes seems to add a barrier of constraint or artificiality between partners.

In addition, some people not in long-term sexual relationships fear that if they meet someone they like, they will have to begin the relationship by telling that person something unpleasant to hear. Perhaps that person will respond by rejecting them. Perhaps that person will spread the information about their diagnosis.

Solving the Problems

Some people react to these feelings, as Alan did for a while, by becoming celibate, not having sex at all. Celibacy is one solution. If you are uncomfortable having sex, or if you feel no desire to, don't bother with it. Many find sexual release in masturbation.

After a while, many people adjust to safer sex. "The way I've adjusted to safer sex," says Alan, "is by psyching myself into thinking I prefer it. It wasn't easy, but I did it, and now I can't *not* practice safer sex, even if my partner wants to do it differently. I can't ejaculate inside someone any more."

Lisa and her husband also worked out a mutually satisfying solution. "The virus was pretty hard on our sexual relationship. Oral sex had been an important part of our lives. I tried oral sex with him while he was wearing a condom, but it tasted too bad. We ended up having sex with him wearing a condom, and with mutual masturbation. It was satisfying enough."

Some people set limits on sex. Dean and his partner had sex less often. That made Dean feel guilty, but his partner said, "I can handle that better than he can. I look at him and he looks so tired." Some couples have sex quickly, and say that is better than nothing. Some couples in which only one person is infected give control to the unifected person to determine how often they make love and what happens during lovemaking.

One good solution is to accept the necessary changes in sexual practices, and where those changes are less than satisfying find other ways to accomplish the same intimacy, reassurance, comfort, and bonding. "Sex always created a bonding between me and my husband," Lisa said. "Safer sex could do that too. But I also tried to re-create that bond by doing more things together and having more communication." Dean said the same thing: "We gave up having sex and make love now." All kinds of physical intimacies that are not sexual can also create bonding: holding hands, touching, giving baths, giving massages, combing hair, napping together, taking showers together, playing card games, lying in bed together, sitting together to read the morning paper or to watch TV or to listen to music; sitting together and reading aloud to each other. Lisa found that her husband responded as she had hoped: "My husband had always had a fear of intimacy. I saw that dissolve. He told me things he never had before. It took time and love to overcome the fear and guilt."

Relationships with Your Children

Many of the problems people with HIV infection have with their children are, on the surface, the same problems they have with any other relative: how to tell them about the infection, how to deal with their worries, how not to be a burden on them. Under the surface, however, the problems are complicated by the uniqueness of the parent-child relationship. Parents and children are not equal partners in a relationship. Parents take care of children, not the reverse. Young children truly are helpless and cannot care for their parents. Older children may be unable emotionally to care for their parents, or the parents may be unable to accept care.

Problems with Telling

In many ways, telling your children about HIV infection is different from telling most other relatives. People feel responsible for their children; they want to protect them against fear and worry and life's hard facts. They think of themselves as their children's safe haven, and they want to avoid bringing uncertainty into their lives. As a result, many people decide to put off telling their children until they have to. They will have to tell, they say, if they get an AIDS-defining diagnosis. "With this virus," said Helen, "you don't know anything definite about the future. I have two kids, aged sixteen and seventeen, who live with their father. I will only tell them if I start getting really sick. They would be anxious, a little for themselves even, though they would believe I wouldn't hurt them. They'd be anxious about my dying." Dean also has a child by an earlier marriage: "I have a son, who's pretty well grown now. He knows about me. I told him only when I hit the AIDS stage."

Sometimes, in spite of their plans, people find that they must tell their children even before the first AIDS-defining diagnosis. People in the earlier stages of HIV infection are often fatigued and bothered with many minor illnesses. The children, who always see more than they seem to, sense that their parents are unwell and preoccupied. The children worry. Sometimes they suspect the truth; sometimes they come to entirely wrong conclusions.

One mother had two children she wasn't telling about her diagnosis. The children noticed her frequent sicknesses and doctor appointments, talked to each other about it, and decided she was dying of cancer. The children were upset: one child became a workaholic, going to school and then working into the night until early the next morning; the other got into trouble at school. When their mother finally told them she was infected with HIV and wasn't dying any time soon, they were almost relieved. At the least, they no longer had to deal with uncertainty.

Telling your children you have HIV infection usually also means telling them how you got the virus. People want their children to respect and look up to them. They don't want to look vulnerable or fallible. Most people, however, get infected in ways that society judges harshly: through using drugs intravenously or through gay sexual relations. Often people have hidden these behaviors from their children. People worry their children will make the same judgment society makes, and reject them. Drug users especially worry that they have set a bad example. Helen is proud that her children do not use drugs and have never seen her use drugs: "I'd rather die than lose my kids' respect," she said. One couple with two children told them that the father (who had HIV infection) had cancer. Several years before, the father had experimented with bisexuality and had become infected. Both parents were ashamed of this. The mother said she didn't want them to see her as a secret-keeper, but she couldn't tell them their father is bisexual.

Dean and his eighteen-year-old son managed to resolve the issue of homosexuality the way Dean and his parents resolved it. He talked openly and lovingly about his life and his son's place in it, and his son's relation to his partner. "Now my son just accepts it," Dean said. "He says, 'Dad is gay and has AIDS.' He brings his friends to our house. When the kids are around, my partner and I hold back our normal affections and don't use terms of endearment with each other." Sometimes children have more trouble with the situation than Dean's son, and are upset at their father's bisexuality. Sometimes they dislike their father's partner.

In general, people find telling the truth works out best. They naturally feel sadness and guilt and regret about the truth, and those feelings will complicate how they talk to their children. They find that the simplest truth works; they say things like, "You know I used to have a drug problem. At that time, I did things I wasn't proud of, and I got AIDS." Children in their teens understand this sort of information best.

Children's Worries

Children fear abandonment. Even young children seem to understand that they cannot feed and house themselves on their own, that they need parents to provide for them. Younger children, when faced with a parent's illness, will ask directly, "If you get sick, who is going to take care of me? Who will live with me if you go to the hospital?" Older children, though they are bothered by the same questions, try to tough it out, and often they will not ask.

Some children worry that their parents are not caring for themselves well enough. Helen's son, though he does not know she has HIV infection, sees that she occasionally loses weight and asks her, "You aren't getting high, are you? You're eating, aren't you? You're taking care of yourself, aren't you?" Other children worry not only about their parent's health, but about everything else the parent is normally responsible for: bills, rent, mortgage, car, groceries. These children are beginning to see themselves as their parent's caregivers, and they are trying to take on the role of a responsible adult.

Children often do not express their worries directly. Instead, they act their worries out; their worries are evident only in their behavior. Some children get depressed, some become withdrawn and stop talking, some become unusually aggressive. Parents who see this happening can try to encourage the child to express his or her worries directly. They can also get help from mental health professionals, especially those who deal specifically with families or children.

The Parent's Worries

A parent's worst worry is whether he or she has unknowingly infected a child. Fathers worry that they have infected their children through casual contact; mothers worry that they have infected their children during the birth process. If the child was born before the mother became infected, the child is almost certainly uninfected. If the child was born after the parent became infected, the child has a 30 to 35 percent chance of also having the virus. Parents do not always know exactly when they were infected, and do not know if they have passed the virus on to their children. The only way to find this out is to have the child tested. To decide whether to do this, ask, What would be gained by testing? What would be lost? Parents often decide to have their children tested. If you are worried about this, or if you are about to become a parent, get help with this decision from a mental health professional.

Parents also worry that they haven't yet done enough parenting. Some try to accelerate the child's social development, to help the child grow up, and become mature, responsible, and settled in life. Some parents want to teach their children everything immediately, whether the children are of the age to learn or not. Dean had a friend with a young child, and Dean's friend solved this problem by writing letters for the child to open as she grew up.

Parents with older children worry about being a burden on the children. "My son worries about who will take care of me," said Dean. "He's feeling the responsibility." People can often accept that a friend or relative worries about them, but they are unhappy to think that their children worry about them. The reversal of the normal role of parents and children makes parents uncomfortable; they feel intensely responsible for their children and hate the idea of being a burden on them. The children often understand this without being told, and do what they feel they can do. Some children are less worried about this than their parents are. "I've spent more time with my son," said Dean. "I'm very close to him. But now I'm worried that I don't want to become a burden on my son. When I tell him that, he just says, 'We'll cross that bridge when we come to it.'"

Parents with younger children—or with children of any age—worry about who will take care of the children. They worry that their own health may prevent them from caring for their young children, and they feel a moral obligation to provide for that possibility. They are intensely worried, and they are often more distressed about this than about their own health.

Deciding Who Will Take Care of the Children

To decide who should look after the children, parents need to consider a number of questions. Who wants the child? Who does the child like? Who is fit enough? Who is trustworthy? Who is emotionally capable of caring for a child? Who will think of the child first, will protect the child? Whose house is suitable? Who has enough room for a child? Who feeds their own children well? Who will pay attention to education, to developing the child's talents? Who values what you do? Who has the money to take on a child? Who has the physical energy? Who has a stable home life, is in a stable long-term relationship, has stable relationships with other relatives? Who holds a job? Who is not drinking or using drugs?

Needless to say, no one is saint enough to meet all these qualifications. For many parents, deciding who should look after their children comes down to two questions: Who among my friends and relatives do I love the most? Who loves me the most?

Some parents have several children and need to consider whether to try to keep them together or to place them in separate surrogate families. Social workers generally advise keeping brothers and sisters under one roof: they say siblings do best together.

But keeping the children together is not always possible. If not, perhaps their surrogate families will take on the responsibility of keeping brothers and sisters in touch with each other. Perhaps, if everyone agrees, this can be made part of a legal agreement.

Some parents have raised children alone. They need to consider a further question of whether they want the child's other parent to have custody of the child. In all states, at the death of one parent, custody of the child will normally be assigned to the remaining parent. If you do not want the child's other parent to have custody, see a lawyer. Sometimes the other parent will legally sign off his or her parental rights. Sometimes another person—an especially close relative or friend—can be given legal custody instead. In any case, your state's Department of Social Services or Friend of the Court can advise you on this decision, and help you find the attorney to make the necessary arrangements.

Once parents have made these decisions, they discuss the decisions with everyone concerned. When talking to their children, they often do not discuss their decisions outright. Instead, they tell the children gradually. They say, "What do you think it would be like living with your aunt?" Or they say, "If anything ever happened to me, your grandmother will look after you." Or, "If I should get sick, your cousin will care for you for a while." Whether people discuss this decision with their children gradually or outright, one way or another, they do let the children know who will take care of them. Children need this reassurance.

When talking to their relatives, they must be more forthright. This is not always easy: sometimes the people not chosen, especially relatives, are upset at the decision. Helen, though her sons are nearly grown, asked her father and stepmother to watch out for the boys and take them in when necessary. They all agreed. Helen also has a sister she did not choose, in truth because she trusted her father and stepmother more. But she did not want to hurt her sister, and so she gave her sister what she thought was a palatable reason for the decision: that the father and stepmother had more money, and that taking on two young men would thus be less of an imposition on them than on her.

In general, people find reasons for explaining their decisions that are not personal but are external to the person. In other words, they did not choose a certain person because he or she is more trustworthy, or has a better marriage, or a better temper, but because she or he has a better income, or better benefits, or a bigger house, or no other children, or children the same age.

When deciding what sort of legal arrangements to make between your children and their surrogate parents, get advice. The three options are custody, guardianship, or adoption. Custody means the person you choose has temporary responsibility for the child. A guardian has certain but not all parental rights. And adoption is the legal equivalent of biological parenthood.

You can choose an option and make the necessary arrangements at any time. Helen has a friend who has her second opportunistic illness and who arranged for her mother to legally adopt her young child; the mother is now that child's legal parent. Many agencies offer advice on this subject: the state Department of Social Services, social workers, and such private social services as Catholic Charities, Jewish Family and Children's Services, and Lutheran Social Services can help. In any case, to guard your rights as a parent, make any such arrangements only with the advice of your own lawyer.

Relationships with Drug Users

Resolving relationships between drug users and their caregivers is not always possible. Relationships between drug users and their parents and partners were often difficult even before an HIV diagnosis. Sometimes addiction is a family illness and everyone is participating in the addiction process: parents or partners pay bills, make excuses, solve problems, make problems bearable. Sometimes everyone in the family is a user of some sort and dependent on alcohol or drugs. Sometimes relationships cannot bear the strain of addiction, and families have already drifted apart. Sometimes, as with gayness, families have known all along. A friend of Helen's called a hospital social worker and said, "My brother is in the hospital, probably with AIDS, probably from using drugs. He won't tell me, and I don't want to ask. Can you help me talk to him?" The social worker agreed to say only that the sister had expressed concerns, and set up a visit. When they got together, he told her his life was changing and he was going to need her support. "Finally," said the sister, "we really got together. We had a wonderful time."

Some families simply accept the addiction. Helen's family says, "This is the way Helen is. We do what we can. We just keep going." Other families try to fight the drug problem by withholding care until the user is off drugs. When a friend of Helen's told his mother he became infected with HIV from injecting drugs, his mother took off her shoe, hit him with it, and said she'd take care of his infection but not his drug problem, so if he wanted help he'd better get off drugs. Like Helen's friend's mother, caregivers often insist on detoxification as a condition for care.

The decision of whether to fight the addiction or accept it is extraordinarily painful. Do you insist on detoxification and risk letting people be sick without your care and support? Or do you accept them as they are and risk letting them continue to hurt themselves? Get help with the decision from mental health professionals—psychiatrists, psychologists, social workers—or from the professional drug counselors. Professional drug counselors can be found in drug rehabilitation programs and programs in psychiatric hospitals, regular hospitals, Veterans Administration hospitals, or family and children's social service agencies.

This is not to say that the relationships between drug users and their caregivers are always unstable. If the relationship was stable before HIV infection entered their lives, it will be stable afterward. Caregivers of drug users, however, often need help from mental health professionals.

Chapter 6

What to Do When: Guidelines for Medical Care

- What to do when you feel well
- What to do when you feel sick
- Lung problems
- Skin problems
- Mouth problems
- Problems of the digestive system
- Gynecological problems
- Eye problems
- Head and nerve problems
- Problems affecting the whole body

HIV infection affects virtually every part of the body. The virus's effect is either direct or indirect, through opportunistic infections. Moreover, its effects, both direct and indirect, resemble symptoms of other diseases. As a result, people easily become confused and worried: Which symptoms should I see the doctor about? Which should I ignore? Which result from HIV infection and which are the normal flus and headaches everyone has? How are the conditions diagnosed? What are the usual treatments? What are the side effects of the treatments? For those who feel well, there is a separate question. What can I do to maintain good health?

This chapter, like Chapter 3, describes the different conditions that accompany HIV infection. Unlike the earlier chapter, the purpose of this chapter is to provide guidelines for the medical care of a person with HIV infection. The chapter is divided into two parts. The first part discusses what to do to maintain good health when you feel well. The second part discusses the medical complications of HIV infection: the symptoms for which people should see a physician, the most likely diagnosis of those symptoms, the tests that establish the diagnosis, and the best treatment. The second part of the chapter is organized first by which parts of the body the particular condition affects, then by what symptoms people notice. So someone worried about a red rash needs to go to the section on skin problems, and look up red rashes.

What to Do When You Feel Well

Most opportunistic infections occur only after you have had HIV infection for many years. The reason is that most opportunistic infections happen only when the cells responsible for defending us against certain microbes (the CD4 cells) are depleted. The depletion takes years because the body has an abundant supply of CD4 cells to begin with, and it loses them very gradually. The average person starts with about 1,000 CD4 cells per milliliter of blood, and the person infected with HIV loses about 30 to 80 CD4 cells each year. When the CD4 cell count is less than 200 per milliliter, opportunistic infections begin to occur. But these numbers are only averages: some people lose CD4 cells much faster and have opportunistic infections within a year of being infected. Other people remain relatively well for twelve years or longer. The average time from the time of getting infected to the time of having an opportunistic infection is eight to ten years. Why do some people lose cells quickly and others remain well for years? We know that treatment directed against HIV increases CD4 cell counts and slows the progress of the infection. In addition, what can people do to slow the progression of HIV infection?

This part of the chapter discusses the issues of wellness and how to stay well. Traditionally, medical science has defined wellness as the prevention or treatment of disease by drugs. This time-honored definition has proven successful: most of the serious epidemics of infectious diseases have been stamped out during the twentieth century. Wellness now has a second definition: maintaining physical health through adequate nutrition, adequate exercise, and good mental health. This second definition is attractive and, for some diseases, has established merit. For HIV infection, the merit of this second definition of wellness has not yet been convincingly established by the proper studies. But regardless of the lack of proof, most physicians believe that nutrition, exercise, and mental health certainly contribute to the quality of life, and probably contribute to longevity.

Get Regular Medical Care

All people with HIV infection should have regular medical care. Options for medical care will depend to some extent on the resources available (see Chapter 8; options for financing this care are discussed in Chapter 10).

For the person with HIV infection who feels well, regular medical care usually includes between two and four visits to a physician per year. During the visits, your previous medical problems should be reviewed, and any symptoms or conditions that may or may not be related to HIV infection should be discussed. During the visits, you should also have a physical examination and any necessary laboratory tests. Your physician should then candidly discuss your health status with you, and should recommend subsequent medical care. The laboratory tests and the drugs that may be prescribed are discussed below.

Laboratory tests. The laboratory tests to expect are those ordinarily done during a medical evaluation, plus those done to keep track of the status of HIV infection. The main blood test used to evaluate the status of the immune system and the status of HIV infection is the CD4 cell count. Other tests, used for the same purpose but less frequently, include the erythrocyte sedimentation rate, beta-2 microglobulin, the levels of antibody to reverse transcriptase, neopterin levels, and counts of lymphocytes other than CD4 cells. Other tests done to evaluate a person's general health include tests of kidney and liver function, a blood test for syphilis, and a complete blood count. Occasionally a chest x-ray or a test for the hepatitis virus will also be done.

Two tests are worth explaining in more detail. One is the test called a *complete blood count,* or CBC. The CBC is a standard laboratory test done during the medical evaluation of almost any condition. Few tests reveal more information for the price (usually $8 to $15 per test). CBCs count the number of red blood cells, white blood cells, and platelets. Any one or all three of these counts can be lowered by HIV infection, by opportunistic infections, or by various drugs. Red blood cells carry oxygen to all parts of the body; low red blood cell counts, or "anemia," can cause fatigue. White blood cells, which include lymphocytes and neutrophils, are the cells of the immune system; low lymphocyte counts are to be expected with HIV infection, and low neutrophil counts, or neutropenia, can predispose people to bacterial infections. Platelets (also called thrombocytes) are responsible for the clotting of blood, so low platelet counts, or thrombocytopenia, can cause a tendency to bleed excessively from minor cuts or injuries.

The second test worthy of special note is the CD4 cell count, a test regularly done with people with HIV infection to evaluate the status of the immune system. CD4 cells are those cells of the immune system that HIV infects. The CD4 cell count is therefore a reasonably good indicator of the strength of the immune system, of the stage of HIV infection, of the need for certain medicines, and of the potential importance of some of the symptoms described below. The cost of the test is usually $50 to $150, and no one seems to know why the charge varies so enormously.

Despite the importance of the CD4 cell count, a word of caution is necessary. The CD4 count varies significantly. The count can vary with the time of day and with medical conditions other than HIV—colds, drugs, and even emotional state. It can also vary depending on the laboratory technician who does the test and on the method used to do the test. The same laboratory technician doing the same test twice on the same blood sample can show counts that differ by as much as 20 percent. That means that a count of 500, if repeated, might be 400 or 600. When possible, it is desirable to have sequential tests done in the same laboratory and at the same time of day to avoid the variations.

The CD4 cell count considered normal has a large range. For most labs, the range is about 550 to 1,450, which is considered normal; 95 percent of people without HIV infection have counts in the same range. When major decisions about treatment depend on the CD4 count, as they sometimes do, the usual recommendation is to repeat the count a week later, to insure that the decisions are not being based on an erroneous test. Almost everyone with HIV infection knows his or her CD4 counts and has them measured at periodic intervals, usually every three to six months. This knowledge is good. Unfortunately, many people also have unrealistic expectations of the test and become alarmed when the count decreases slightly. But the CD4 cell count is not particularly fine-tuned, and modest decreases from one test to the next may or may not mean anything. Repeated tests showing trends over long periods are far more reliable than any isolated sampling.

The tests discussed above are done during the first medical evaluation of someone with HIV infection and are, at that time, called screening tests. Results of the tests will be discussed either by telephone or during a subsequent office visit.

Many of the same tests, especially the CBC and the CD4 count, are also done periodically throughout the course of the infection. Which tests are selected depends on the symptoms, on the presence of any other medical problems, and on the idiosyncrasies of the physician. The frequency of tests and which tests are selected also depend on which drugs are being taken, since these tests often reveal adverse reactions that are important to know about. For example, people taking AZT should have a CBC at regular intervals, because the main adverse reactions are anemia and neutropenia.

Drugs. We have mentioned that 50 percent of the people with HIV infection will develop serious complications within eight to ten years.

This percentage has changed, though no one yet knows by how much. The change is the result of the discovery of drugs directed against the virus: we now know that drugs will delay the loss of CD4 cells and the opportunistic infections that accompany HIV infection.

Drugs directed against HIV are called *antiviral* or *antiretroviral* drugs. The first antiviral drug against HIV was AZT: it was found in 1986 to prolong the lives of those with AIDS, and in 1990, to delay the progression of HIV infection to AIDS. Drugs that are chemical relatives of AZT, called ddI and ddC, were also found to be effective against HIV; ddI became available in 1991 and ddC in 1992. Many other drugs are being tested. So many are being tested and the field is moving so fast that at this point, making any recommendations about these drugs would be like trying to hit a rapidly moving target. Questions also remain about when during the course of the infection to begin taking drugs, which drugs to take, and which drugs are best taken in combination with other drugs. We do know, however, that taking antiviral drugs is critically important during the later stages of HIV infection.

Other drugs will prevent certain opportunistic infections from occurring. Vaccines prevent influenza, pneumococcal pneumonia, and hepatitis B. Antibiotics can be given to prevent pneumocystis pneumonia and other opportunists. Anyone with a skin test positive for tuberculosis, and who has no symptoms, should take a drug called isoniazid (INH) to prevent tuberculosis from becoming active.

Even though HIV infection cannot now be cured and no drug now eliminates HIV from the body, the progress of the infection through the body can be slowed down. As a result, we can now look at HIV infection in much the same way we look at other chronic medical conditions like diabetes and high blood pressure. We cannot cure these conditions, but we can manage them. And along with proper medical management comes some assurance of a long and productive life (see also Chapter 9).

Get Dental Care

The dental problems common to all adults—diseases of the teeth and of the supporting structures of the teeth—seem to occur more frequently and more severely in people with HIV infection. See your dentist regularly. Floss and brush your teeth assiduously. Tell your dentist about your HIV infection: people who are prone to dental problems should probably see the dentist more frequently, and the dentist may change some of his or her normal recommendations.

Unfortunately, dental care has some problems. One is that dental care is not always easily available to people with HIV infection. Some dentists are unrealistically afraid of catching HIV during dental care and will refuse to treat someone with HIV infection. If you have been an established patient with a dentist, such a refusal is unethical. (See Chapter 10, under "Legal Rights and Obligations.") Another problem is that medical assistance will pay only for emergency dental care and not for routine dental care. AIDS advocacy agencies in most cities have lists of dentists willing to treat people with HIV infection, including people on medical assistance.

Follow a Nutritious Diet

Nutrition is important for virtually all people with HIV infection for two reasons. The first is that weight loss is a common symptom of this infection, and during the later stages, many people lose weight excessively. Paying attention to nutrition early in the course of the infection might delay weight loss. The second reason is that good nutrition seems to help maintain a strong immune system, even apart from HIV infection. It is well established that the immune system functions less well in people who are malnourished, though malnutrition must be severe before immune defects become noticeable.

Malnutrition is more exactly called protein-caloric malnutrition. Calories come from most food, particularly fats. Proteins come from meat, milk products, poultry, eggs, fish, and dried beans and rice. People need diets that are a balance of calories, protein, and the necessary vitamins. The usual American diet provides an ample supply of vitamins, though some people with HIV infection might wish to take supplemental vitamins. If supplemental vitamins are taken, the usual recommendation is to take no more than the Recommended Dietary Allowances (RDA), the amount recommended by nutrition experts. The RDA is listed on the labels of all supplemental vitamins. In general, excessive doses of vitamins, along with macrobiotic diets and other fad diets, should either be avoided or be undertaken only with the advice of a certified dietitian.

Some people believe that progressive HIV infection is associated with deficiencies in what they call *micronutrients*—selenium, iron, zinc—and advocate taking supplements to correct the deficiency. The role of these micronutrients, however, has not been established scientifically, especially for the person with HIV infection who feels well. The bottom line is that a balanced diet makes sense. Fad diets, megavitamins, and supplemental micronutrients have no clearly established role in therapy.

Get Exercise

Aerobic exercise programs are widely advocated as a way of staying healthy and of preventing cardiovascular disease. Whether exercise is similarly helpful to people with HIV infection is unknown. Most people who exercise regularly, however, feel better both physically and emotionally. There is no reason for a person with HIV infection to avoid regular exercise as long as fatigue or other symptoms do not prevent it.

Keep Working

People with HIV infection should work as long as they possibly can. Work contributes to people's sense of self-worth, to their knowledge that they are contributing members of society. HIV infection should not keep people from working unless fatigue or other symptoms make it impossible.

Occasionally employers have used the fact of HIV infection to limit someone's employment or to change their job assignments. The employee has considerable legal recourse as a result of the Rehabilitation Act of 1973, which became law in the United States in July 1992. This protects every citizen against unfair discrimination based on sex, race, or handicap. Under this law, HIV infection is a handicap, and those who have HIV infection are legally protected. The employer must provide the employee with continued employment in the same job as long as she or he is capable of performing the job. This issue is discussed in more detail in Chapter 10.

Maintain Mental Health

HIV infection carries an enormous psychological burden, both because of the nature of the disease and because of society's reaction to it. It is critically important for a person with HIV infection to deal with the psychological impact of the disease. Mental health may even affect the state of the immune system. Methods of maintaining mental health will differ with different people. Resources available include mental health professionals (psychiatrists, psychologists, and social workers), support groups, and AIDS-advocacy organizations. Mental health and the methods of maintaining it are discussed in Chapter 4 and in Chapter 12.

What to Do When You Feel Sick

The rest of this chapter discusses the medical complications of HIV infection. Our purpose is to provide information on specific symptoms, their likely diagnoses, and their treatments. The chapter is organized by anatomy: lungs, skin, mouth, digestive system, eyes, and head and nerves, and concludes with a segment on the constitutional symptoms—like fever and fatigue—that affect the whole body. Each part of the anatomy is organized according to symptom, and then according to diagnosis. Thus, someone worried about a red rash would look up skin problems, find the symptom of red rash, and read which diagnoses are possible. The intent of this section is not to provide a substitute for medical care, but to list the symptoms that deserve attention and to inform the person with HIV infection of likely diagnostic tests and treatments. Nevertheless, both diagnostic tests and treatments are subject to rapidly changing guidelines, and some of this information can quickly become antiquated.

Overview

HIV affects the body in two different ways. The first way it affects the body is directly, causing an early mononucleosis-like disease or a late dementia called HIV-associated dementia. These are complications caused by the virus directly. The second way HIV affects the body is indirectly, specifically by infecting the CD4 cell (see Chapter 3). Most of the symptoms that people with HIV infection have are a result of opportunistic infections and tumors that would not happen with the usual number of CD4 cells. As noted previously, the usual CD4 cell count is about 1,000; a person with HIV infection loses, on average, about 30–80 CD4s each year, so that after seven or eight years the count is down to 200–300. Different people lose CD4 cells at different rates, but the CD4 count at which complications occur is less than 200, and often substantially lower. Some opportunistic infections and tumors are exceptions because they do not depend quite so much on CD4 cell counts. Those include Kaposi's sarcoma, lymphomas, idiopathic thrombocytopenic purpura, bacterial pneumonias (but usually not pneumocystis pneumonia), *Candida* vaginitis, salmonellosis, herpes zoster or shingles, and tuberculosis.

Most of the common and serious opportunistic infections occur when the CD4 count is below 200 per milliliter, and many people have few medical problems until the CD4 count is consistently below 50. These include pneumocystis pneumonia, disseminated (widespread) cytomegalovirus infection, disseminated (widespread) *Mycobacterium avium* infection, cryptosporidiosis, toxoplasmosis, cryptococcal meningitis, and HIV-associated dementia.

Lung Problems

Most infections of the lung, or pneumonias, regardless of their cause, have the same symptoms: cough, shortness of breath, and fever. In some lung infections, the cough is productive—that is, the cough produces sputum; in other lung infections, the cough is dry. Cough and shortness of breath may be accompanied by chest pain. The person with HIV infection should watch out for these symptoms and should seek prompt medical attention for them. They can be symptoms of complications that almost invariably respond to antibiotics if given early enough.

Cough and shortness of breath are relatively common symptoms of other medical conditions as well. Causes of these symptoms include asthma, bronchitis, and chronic lung diseases like those brought on by long-term smoking. When these symptoms occur in someone who has not previously had lung problems, when they are more severe than usual, or when they are accompanied by fever, the cause could be pneumonia. People with HIV infection get different kinds of pneumonias, but the most important are pneumocystis pneumonia, tuberculosis, and certain common bacterial pneumonias.

The standard diagnostic tests for these symptoms include a blood count, a chest x-ray, and culture of the sputum. Additional diagnostic tests will largely depend on the specific symptoms and on the results of the first set of tests.

Dry Cough, Shortness of Breath, and Fever

Symptoms that include a dry cough, shortness of breath, and fever when the CD4 count is below 200 are most likely to be *Pneumocystis carinii* pneumonia (PCP). The most characteristic symptom of PCP, compared to other pneumonias, is a dry cough that does not produce sputum and that begins subtly and progresses slowly. People with PCP first notice shortness of breath only with exercise, then begin to notice it with minimal activity; eventually, they notice it even when they are at rest. Fever is variable, but nearly all people with PCP have a temperature of at least 100 degrees F at some point during the day, usually in the late afternoon or evening. These symptoms of PCP usually come on over a period of many days or several weeks. By contrast, most other forms of pneumonia become serious much more quickly.

Because PCP usually (though not always) evolves slowly, people often put off going to the doctor. If PCP is left untreated, it is usually fatal. If PCP is caught early, it can be treated with pills rather than intravenous drugs that require hospitalization. PCP is relatively common late in the course of HIV infection: of the first 100,000 people who had AIDS in the United States, 80 percent had PCP sometime during the course of the infection, and 60 percent had PCP as their first major opportunistic infection. This percentage is now decreasing because drugs are given to prevent PCP in people with CD4 counts below 200.

PCP is caused by a parasite called *Pneumocystis carinii*. People acquire this parasite early in life, but it remains inactive or dormant in the lungs and causes no trouble until the immune system is weakened. Because virtually everyone already harbors *Pneumocystis carinii*, PCP is not considered a contagious disease. This means that people caring for a person with PCP need not worry about catching it.

The initial test for PCP will probably be a chest x-ray. In about 10 to 15 percent of people with PCP, however, the chest x-ray will be normal. Additional tests must then be done to show whether the lungs are affected: blood gases demonstrate whether oxygen supply is adequate, or a test on a breathing machine shows how well the lungs function.

The test that diagnoses PCP most specifically is one that shows the parasite in lung secretions. The problem with this test is that getting a sample of lung secretions is difficult: people with PCP, in contrast to people with other pneumonias, have great difficulty in coughing up sputum. As a result, sputum must be induced. Inducing sputum requires a trained technologist who uses specialized techniques to coax sputum up from the lung; alternatively, a specialist in lung diseases uses a bronchoscope, an instrument passed through the bronchial tubes into the lungs.

The tests to diagnose PCP can be tedious, expensive (especially bronchoscopy), and unpleasant. People often ask if the testing process can be simplified, and indeed, the person's symptoms and chest x-ray results are occasionally compelling enough to diagnose PCP without looking for the parasite. This approach, though simple and efficient, can occasionally lead to an inaccurate diagnosis; that is, the person is assumed to have PCP, and an alternate and treatable infection may be overlooked. Similarly, a delay in treating PCP may allow it to progress to the point that it is difficult to reverse. For these reasons, most physicians experienced in caring for people with AIDS will treat PCP aggressively when symptoms suggest it.

A variety of drugs can be used to treat PCP. The two most common are antibiotics: trimethoprim-sulfamethoxazole (the trade names are Bactrim and Septra) and pentamidine. The side effects of trimethoprim-sulfamethoxazole include nausea, vomiting, stomach pain, hepatitis, fever, a lowered white blood count, and a rash that may be serious. These side effects can occur at any time during treatment, but they are most common at the end of the first week and the beginning of the second week of treatment. Trimethoprim-sulfamethoxazole can be taken by mouth, but large doses are required. For severe cases, trimethoprim-sulfamethoxazole can be given intravenously, that is, by vein; when there is improvement, the treatment may be changed to pills. As many as half the people with HIV infection taking trimethoprim-sulfamethoxazole develop side effects, and the side effects are sometimes serious enough that treatment has to be changed.

People who cannot take trimethoprim-sulfamethoxazole can usually take dapsone-trimethoprim, which can also be taken by mouth, causes fewer side effects, and is sometimes preferred for persons with PCP who are not too ill. The other drug commonly used is pentamidine, which must be given intravenously. Serious side effects with intravenous pentamidine include nausea, vomiting, low blood pressure, low blood counts, low blood glucose, kidney failure, and hepatitis. You should promptly report dizziness or a feeling of faintness. Any of these three drugs should be continued for three weeks.

The side effects associated with any of these treatments are often serious enough that people cannot finish the entire three weeks. However, a variety of alternative treatments with different drugs or different doses of standard drugs have been developed to handle the situation.

Most people respond well to treatment. But those who recover are likely to develop PCP again; in fact, the recurrence rate is about 70 percent within one year. The drugs that prevent the recurrence of PCP include pentamidine given by aerosol; trimethoprim-sulfamethoxazole given by mouth; or dapsone given by mouth. People who are candidates for preventive treatment include not only anyone with HIV infection who has previously had PCP, but also people with HIV infection who have not had PCP but whose CD4 counts are less than 200. The best preventive treatment is trimethoprim-sulfamethoxazole: it works the best, it prevents many infections besides PCP, and it is dirt cheap. Many people can't take it because of reactions, so they get a reduced dose or one of the other drugs.

Productive Cough, Shortness of Breath, Fever

Productive cough, shortness of breath, and fever are symptoms of tuberculosis and pneumonia caused by certain types of bacteria; these symptoms may also be caused by PCP, certain viruses, Kaposi's sarcoma in the lung, and several other unusual conditions.

Tuberculosis (TB). The most common symptoms of TB are cough, bloody sputum, shortness of breath, fever, weight loss, chest pain with breathing, and night sweats. As with PCP, the tempo of tuberculosis is generally slow, usually progressing over a period of weeks or months. During this time the person is usually fatigued, has night sweats, and loses weight. TB can occur in the lung, but it can spread to almost any part of the body. TB, either in the lung or outside the lung, is now considered an AIDS-defining diagnosis. People with HIV infection often have TB relatively early in the course of the infection, when the CD4 count is fairly high: TB apparently has enough clout that it does not require a severely weakened immune system to cause disease.

TB, which is caused by a bacterium called *Mycobacterium tuberculosis,* can be active or inactive. When it is active, the bacterium is reproducing and the person has symptoms of TB. When it is inactive, *Mycobacterium tuberculosis* is dormant in the lung, much the way *Pneumocystis carinii* is dormant in the lung. People with inactive TB have no symptoms, and all cultures for *Mycobacterium tuberculosis* are negative.

The only way to find out whether a person has been infected with *Mycobacterium tuberculosis* is the skin test most people are familiar with, done on the forearm. The skin test is a shallow injection of a protein called a purified protein derivative, or PPD, made from *Mycobacterium tuberculosis.* If the area around the injection becomes red and thickened two or three days later, the person's immune system has responded to the bacterium, meaning that *Mycobacterium tuberculosis* is in the body. The person has TB, either active or inactive. The only other evidence of infection might be a chest x-ray showing the scars of previous infections with TB that the person may be unaware of. Most, though not all, people with active TB have had inactive TB for several years previously.

If the skin test is positive, it is followed by sputum tests for TB and x-rays. If the sputum test is also positive, if symptoms are ascribed to TB, or if the x-ray shows new changes, the person has active TB. Otherwise, the TB is inactive.

It is especially important for people with HIV infection to have a skin test. Inactive TB can be treated with a drug, isoniazid (INH), that will prevent active TB. Active TB is treated more aggressively, with three or more drugs.

Medical researchers have been greatly concerned about TB in people with HIV infection for several reasons. First, in 1985 the number of active cases of TB in the United States, after decreasing every year for eighty-five years, began to increase. The increase was largely attributed to the increase of TB in people with HIV infection. Second, TB in people with HIV infection often fails to obey the usual rules: the skin test is often falsely negative and the chest x-ray, though abnormal, does not show the changes usual in TB. Both these findings make detecting TB in people with HIV infection more difficult. Third, and most disturbing, is that a "new strain" of TB bacteria is resistant to standard TB drugs. Such resistant strains are usually caused by people failing to finish the full course of standard drugs. As a result, the drug barely taps the TB bacterium and doesn't destroy it, giving the bacterium a convenient training period during which to make the genetic changes that allow it to resist the drugs. The person with a resistant TB bacterium not only is hard to treat but may transmit this trained TB bacterium to others. The result is several large epidemics in some areas. For all these reasons, health care workers worry about this resistant bacterium and not only preach compliance with treatment but may insist on observing it.

Mycobacterium tuberculosis must be distinguished from a related microbe called *Mycobacterium avium,* or MA. MA causes infections in many organs throughout the body (see Chapter 3). This distinction between *Mycobacterium tuberculosis* and MA is important, not only for deciding what the treatment should be, but also for preventing transmission. *Mycobacterium tuberculosis,* the only contagious mycobacterial infection, can be transmitted from one person to another by close contact over a period of several months. For this reason, the people most likely to be infected are those who live with the infected person. But an infected person who has been treated with drugs against TB for several days is unlikely to transmit the infection to others. This means that once treatment has started, the likelihood that it will be spread to others is reduced or nil. The standard recommendation for testing those people who have been exposed to TB for long periods is to do the skin test, and if it is positive, to follow it with chest x-rays.

Bacterial pneumonias. Bacteria have always been a major cause of serious pneumonias. Before penicillin became available in the 1940s, bacterial pneumonias were the most common cause of death in the United States. Bacterial pneumonia, recurring repeatedly, is considered an AIDS-defining diagnosis.

The symptoms of bacterial pneumonias are fever, shortness of breath, and a cough that produces thick yellow or green sputum. For some people, the major symptom is chest pain, especially when they breathe. Unlike PCP and TB, bacterial pneumonias usually begin rather abruptly, and people see physicians within days rather than weeks or months.

Bacterial pneumonias can occur relatively early in the course of HIV infection. Unlike PCP, bacterial pneumonias do not necessarily indicate a severely weakened immune system. One common bacterial pneumonia is caused by a microbe called *pneumococcus;* people with HIV infection seem especially prone to pneumococcal pneumonia.

The diagnosis of bacterial pneumonias is usually established with a chest x-ray and sputum tests. Treatment with antibiotics is highly effective when begun early in the infection. Trimethoprim-sulfamethoxazole, which prevents PCP, will prevent pneumococcal pneumonia as well. Pneumonococcal vaccine also prevents pneumococcal pneumonia and is advocated for people with HIV infection. Bacteria other than pneumococcus cause pneumonias as well, but the symptoms, diagnostic tests, and treatment are all similar.

Viral pneumonias. The virus that most commonly causes pneumonia in people with HIV infection is cytomegalovirus, or CMV, which rarely causes disease until the CD4 count is less than 100. CMV can infect not only the lungs, but virtually all parts of the body. A test of respiratory secretions will show CMV in the respiratory system, but it is difficult to know whether CMV is causing the pneumonia, because when CMV is present, other microbes like *Pneumocystis carinii* are usually present as well. There are some drugs that can be used to treat CMV pneumonia, although proof that they work in most cases is not well established.

Influenza virus is like many viruses that attack the respiratory system. It is common in people without HIV infection, but there is no evidence that it is more common or severe in those with HIV infection, even those in advanced stages of HIV infection. The apparent reason is that influenza triggers immune defense mechanisms different from those triggered by HIV. Nevertheless, influenza vaccine is sometimes advised for people with HIV infection. The reason is that influenza symptoms may cause undue concern about PCP and other lung problems. In addition, we're not sure that influenza is totally safe in people with HIV infection, and the vaccine usually works well.

Miscellaneous infections. Other causes of lung problems in people with HIV infection are less common than those above. *Mycobacterium avium* (MA), though it usually infects other parts of the body, sometimes infects the lungs. Kaposi's sarcoma may be found in the lungs, where it causes cough and shortness of breath. People with Kaposi's sarcoma in the lungs will probably have changes on a chest x-ray or on special scans of the lungs, and Kaposi's sarcoma also on the skin. Occasionally, people with HIV infection will have a pneumonia called lymphocytic interstitial pneumonia, which appears to be due to HIV itself. Diagnosis of lymphocytic interstitial pneumonia requires a biopsy of the lungs using a bronchoscope. It often responds to treatment with corticosteroids.

Skin Problems

The skin is commonly affected in people with HIV infection. The conditions affecting the skin include a diverse array of infections and an unusual tumor called Kaposi's sarcoma. Other skin conditions—psoriasis, seborrhea, molluscum, fungal infections, and allergic rashes—are also common in people without HIV infection, but they are more common and more severe in people with HIV infection. Since most of these conditions are treatable, people should see their physicians, especially if the skin problem is painful, disfiguring, or accompanied by a fever.

As expected, the diagnosis of a skin condition is largely dictated by its appearance. In many cases, a diagnosis can be established simply by observation, but occasionally diagnosis will require a biopsy.

Purple or Black Spots

Purple or black spots on the skin are characteristic of Kaposi's sarcoma (KS), a tumor of the cells of the blood vessels. In most cases, there are several tumors, each approximately a quarter of an inch to an inch in diameter. They can usually be felt as a nodule or a fleshy collection of tissue. They can—but do not usually—cause pain. In light-skinned people, the tumors are usually purple; and in dark-skinned people, they are very dark brown or black. The tumors are not like freckles, either in color or to the touch.

KS tumors can appear any place on the skin, including the face, scalp, back, chest, abdomen, arms, legs, or inside the mouth. They appear most commonly on the tip of the nose, around the eyes, on the ears, behind the ears, and on the arms, the legs, the chest, and the genitals. Usually there are several tumors in different places. At times the tumors occur symmetrically, appearing in almost identical places on both arms, on both sides of the face, or on both feet.

Kaposi's sarcoma is a relatively common complication; it is found in about 20 percent of HIV-infected persons at some stage of the disease. KS can occur when the CD4 cell count is relatively high, though sometimes KS does not occur until late in the infection, after PCP or another AIDS-defining diagnosis.

Some have argued that KS is a sexually transmitted disease because it is extremely common in gay men with HIV infection and is quite unusual in hemophiliacs, children, or those who became infected through transfusions. If KS is sexually transmitted, the safer sex practices that prevent transmission of HIV also seem to prevent transmission of KS: among gay men with HIV infection, KS is disappearing.

KS on the skin is suspected based on its appearance and is diagnosed with a biopsy of the tumor. This is a simple outpatient procedure; Novocain is injected into the skin to make the procedure painless.

The treatment of KS is controversial. Many people do not have serious problems with the disease. Most people simply have KS on the skin, and though they may also have KS on their internal organs, it usually causes no problems. Moreover, many of the treatments for KS are either ineffective or have serious side effects. Cosmetic problems can often simply be covered with opaque makeup. Treatment can be considered necessary under several circumstances: if people have KS tumors on the face or other exposed areas of the body that they feel are unsightly or carry the stigma of AIDS; if the tumors are obstructing lymph channels and causing swelling of the legs, abdomen or face; if KS is causing pain, most commonly on the bottoms of the feet or roof of the mouth; if KS has spread to internal organs and is causing disabling or serious symptoms, like pneumonia or problems of the gastrointestinal tract; or if KS is causing fever, fatigue, weight loss, and similar symptoms.

The usual treatment of skin tumors is radiation, freezing, laser treatment, or injection of a drug called vinblastine. If KS has spread to internal organs, the treatment consists of taking the same drugs used to treat other cancers, or "cancer chemotherapy." A drug called interferon, taken by injection, is effective in some cases, but it generally works best when the CD4 count is above 400, and it has serious side effects.

The best advice about treating Kaposi's sarcoma will come from any physician with extensive experience in this area, particularly from an AIDS physician (see Chapter 8), from a dermatologist, or from a cancer specialist (an oncologist). Which physician does the treatment will depend on which therapy is used: radiation treatment will require referral to a radiation therapist, cancer chemotherapy will require referral to an oncologist, and interferon will require referral either to a dermatologist, an oncologist, or a specialist in AIDS or infectious diseases. The person contemplating interferon treatment for KS should be forewarned that interferon is the substance produced by the body during flu that causes the aches of influenza. The same achiness is a common side effect of interferon treatment.

Red Rash

A rash is usually either diffusely red all over or red only in spots or blotches. It usually appears on the chest, back, arms, face, and legs. Rashes can be accompanied by other symptoms, including fever, swelling of the face, giant welts, or itching.

The most common cause of a red rash covering large areas of the body in people with HIV infection is an adverse reaction to a drug. The most common offending drug is a sulfa drug—especially trimethoprim-sulfamethoxazole (Bactrim, Septra), the drug usually given for the treatment or prevention of *Pneumocystis carinii* pneumonia. Sulfa drugs are also treatments for many other infectious diseases in people with and without AIDS. Rashes that are a reaction to sulfa drugs are especially common in people with HIV infection: 30 percent to 50 percent of people with HIV infection have these rashes. In addition to rashes, many people also have fever, low white blood cell counts, or tests showing hepatitis. All these symptoms disappear when the sulfa drug is stopped.

Other drugs can also cause rashes; rashes simply seem to be especially common with the sulfa drugs. One of the problems with identifying the cause of rashes is that they can occur with almost any drug, and many people with HIV infection are taking many drugs. To find out which drug is causing the rash, the physician may stop one drug at a time every two or three days, beginning with the drug most likely to be responsible. Or the physician may suggest a drug holiday: all drugs are stopped, then only those that are necessary are started again.

When the rash occurs, talk to a physician. This consultation is especially important if the drugs causing the rash are also causing such symptoms as swelling of the face, difficulty breathing, large and itching welts, fever, or dizziness when standing (suggesting low blood pressure).

In addition to stopping the drug, the rashes are often treated with antihistamines like Dramamine which can be purchased without a prescription, or with prescription drugs that are sometimes more effective. More serious reactions may require treatment with corticosteroids.

Blistering Rash

Blisters are small, fluid-filled bubbles that often break, becoming open sores filled with clear fluid or pus. Blisters can occur in groups in one specific area of the skin, or they can be distributed all over the skin.

Like red rashes, blistering rashes can be caused by adverse reactions to drugs. The most common causes of blistering rash in people with HIV infection, however, are two related viruses, herpes simplex and herpes zoster.

Herpes simplex infection. Infection by the herpes simplex virus is extremely common in healthy people. There are actually two different types of herpes simplex viruses: Type I and Type II. Type I most frequently causes the infection of the mouth called cold sores. Type II most frequently causes sores on the genitals and the anal region and is regarded as a sexually transmitted disease. Herpes simplex hides in nerve cells and periodically becomes active, causing recurrent blistering rashes. In people with weakened immune systems, herpes simplex can also affect skin on other parts of the body, and can even affect the internal organs.

Blood tests show that 20 percent to 50 percent of otherwise healthy people have one or both types of herpes simplex. Most of these people have either no problems or rare outbreaks; some have attacks more frequently, but these are brief, not severe, and restricted to the lips or genitals. By contrast, people with advanced HIV infection can have herpes simplex infections that cover a larger area of the skin, can be more painful, can last longer, and are often difficult to treat.

Treatment with an antiviral drug called acyclovir (commercial name, Zovirax) usually controls symptoms. Acyclovir is available as pills and as ointment to be applied directly to the sores; when infection is severe, acyclovir can be taken intravenously. Treatment does not eliminate the virus. As a result, the infection can recur; recurrence can often be prevented or at least reduced in frequency by taking acyclovir pills. For people who do not respond to the usual doses of acyclovir, the options are to use high doses by vein or to use alternative drugs like foscarnet.

Herpes zoster, or shingles. Herpes zoster is caused by the same virus that causes chickenpox. Like herpes simplex, the herpes zoster virus stays dormant in the nerve cells. The virus recurs many years or decades after the original bout with chickenpox, causing a disease called shingles. Shingles is common not only in people with HIV infection, but in the elderly and in others as well.

The symptoms of shingles are blisters that are identical to those seen with chickenpox. The blisters are small and filled with a watery fluid; later, the blisters break, the fluid becomes pus, scabs form, and the skin heals. Unlike the blisters of chickenpox, however, the blisters of shingles are often extremely painful. In addition, they are not spread all over the body, but instead are distributed in bands or lines on the chest, the abdomen, down the leg, on the arm, or on the face. In most cases, the blisters occur on only one side of the body and stop abruptly at the middle of the body. The blisters follow this pattern because they are following the path of the nerve in which the virus is living, and each nerve serves only one side of the body.

The worst complication of this infection is pain. The pain may come before the blisters appear, or it may accompany the blisters. The pain may also occur once the blisters are gone and the skin is healed; this pain is called post-herpetic neuralgia. Fortunately, people with HIV infection who get shingles simply do not often develop post-herpetic neuralgia. This complication is most common in elderly persons with or without HIV infection.

A note about transmission: the blisters contain the virus that causes herpes zoster. Adults who have had chickenpox already have this virus, have antibodies to it, and are not susceptible when exposed to someone with chickenpox or shingles. However, young children and the rare adult who has escaped chickenpox could become infected with the virus that causes herpes zoster. These people may acquire chickenpox by contact with the blisters or by inhaling the virus. To prevent transmission, people who have not had chickenpox should carefully avoid contact and should even avoid being present in the same room. People who are hospitalized should expect strict isolation precautions—gloves, masks, and gowns—to be taken, to prevent transmission to the health care workers.

Shingles is not life-threatening and inevitably cures itself. But it can be especially severe in people with HIV, so treatment is generally recommended. Shingles can be treated with acyclovir, and other drugs such as nortriptyline may be given to control the pain. Acyclovir may be given by mouth, but the doses required are unusually large, and hospitalization for intravenous treatment is sometimes advocated. Foscarnet and ganciclovir are usually effective as well.

Thick, Discolored Nails; Red, Flaking Circles

Thick, discolored toenails or fingernails are usually caused by a fungus. Patches of red, flaking skin, on the feet or in the groin area, are called athlete's foot or jock itch. When the patches of red, flaking skin are in circular patterns on the scalp or the skin, they are called ringworm. Athlete's foot, jock itch, and ringworm are caused by fungi. These fungi cause infections of the skin and nails but are not capable of causing much else.

Treatment of ringworm with antibiotic ointments—clotrimazole (commercial name, Lotrimin) or miconazole—applied on top of the involved area is usually effective. Most of these ointments are available without prescription. When the nails are involved, when large areas of the skin are affected, or when ointments do not work, other antibiotics, like ketoconazole or griseofulvin, can be taken as pills and are usually effective.

Small, Colorless Bumps

A crop of small, colorless bumps is usually caused by a virus called *Molluscum contagiosum*. Each of the bumps often has a central indentation. The most common location is on the face, especially around the mouth, and in the genital region. *Molluscum contagiosum* seems to be especially common in people with HIV infection.

The major problem is cosmetic. No antibiotics are successful, but a dermatologist can remove the bumps by freezing.

Flaking, Scaling Rash in Patches

Red, scaling patches, most frequently on the scalp, face, ears, chest, and genitals, are symptoms of seborrhea. Some people have the patches symmetrically on both cheeks, in what is called a "butterfly" distribution. Many people simply have seborrhea on the scalp, where it is referred to as dandruff.

Seborrhea appears to be caused by a fungus, generally involves only the skin, and, at least when severe, is usually cared for by dermatologists. Seborrhea occurs in 50 percent to 80 percent of people with HIV infection. As the infection progresses, seborrhea is more frequent and more severe.

The treatment of seborrhea of the scalp is to use shampoos containing coal tar, available without prescription at drugstores. Seborrhea on the rest of the skin can be treated with ointments containing cortisone or ketoconazole. Cortisone ointments are available without prescription, but severe or persistent cases of seborrhea are best treated with stronger concentrations of cortisone, which require a prescription.

Excessive Bleeding

Excessive bleeding from nosebleeds, cuts, and injuries may be a symptom of idiopathic thrombocytopenic purpura (ITP). Other symptoms are easy bruising and bloody or tarry stools that result from intestinal bleeding. Some people will have many small red dots about the size of a pinhead on the lower legs and feet, called *petechiae,* that are tiny hemorrhages. Others have larger hemorrhages into the skin, called *purpura.* Unlike other red rashes, these hemorrhages do not disappear when pressure is applied to them. In other words, if you push on the red spot, the spot does not clear for several seconds but remains red.

Idiopathic thrombocytopenic purpura means low numbers (penia) of blood platelets (thrombocytes) that promote blood clotting, causing bruises or hemorrhages in the skin (purpura) for reasons that are unexplained (idiopathic). The cause of ITP is unknown: for some reason, the body produces antibodies that attack blood platelets. ITP can occur in people who do not have HIV infection. It can occur in people with HIV infection either when the CD4 count is high or when it is low. Most people who have ITP are unaware of it; ITP is usually discovered with routine laboratory testing when a complete blood count (CBC) shows that the number of blood platelets is low. The usual count in healthy persons is 150,000 to 300,000 platelets per milliliter of blood. People with HIV infection often have slightly lower counts—80,000 to 120,000 platelets per milliliter—though these counts cause no problem. People with ITP often have counts that are lower yet—5,000 to 30,000 platelets per milliliter.

Treatment of ITP may consist of drugs like corticosteroids that suppress the antibodies attacking the platelets. Other treatments include AZT, interferon, or gamma globulin given intravenously. Occasionally, people have surgery to remove the spleen. All these treatments seem to be beneficial, but not always so. Some people respond to one treatment but not another, some don't seem to respond to anything, and many who respond to one treatment will eventually have recurrent symptoms. Other people do well with no specific treatment, despite the low platelet count. The worry with ITP is the possibility of internal bleeding, during which large amounts of blood could be lost, or vital organs like the brain or lungs could be damaged. Obviously, the person with extremely low platelet counts should be extremely careful to avoid cuts and injuries.

Mouth Problems

Many of the complications of HIV infection involve the mouth. Because of this, it is important for all people with HIV infection to inspect their mouths regularly, pay careful attention to oral hygiene, and get regular dental care. Though most complications occur in the later stages of the disease, some occur early.

Pain in the Mouth

The most common causes of pain in the mouth include thrush, oral hairy leukoplakia, herpes simplex, aphthous ulcers, and Kaposi's sarcoma. All of these are described below. Most of them can be diagnosed largely on the basis of their appearance. The biggest problem with pain in the mouth is adequate nutrition. It obviously makes sense to avoid foods that cause pain: foods that are highly seasoned, for instance, or citrus fruits or certain vegetables that are highly acidic. Also avoid foods that are very hot or very cold. Instead, eat bland foods, foods that are soft, and nutritious liquids like milkshakes. Exactly what you eat should suit your own preference, as long as it is nutritious. (See the following section, "Problems of the Digestive System.")

White Patches in the Mouth

White patches in the mouth, sometimes painful, often painless, are most commonly symptoms of thrush, and less commonly symptoms of oral hairy leukoplakia.

Thrush. Thrush is a common infection of the mouth caused by the fungus *Candida albicans. Candida albicans* is found in the mouths of most people; thrush occurs only when the fungus begins growing out of control. Symptoms include white or grayish-white patches that look a little like cottage cheese along the gums, along the inside of the cheeks, or on the tongue. Thrush can be unnoticeable, or it can cause pain severe enough to interfere with chewing or swallowing. Thrush does not cause fever, malaise, fatigue, tooth loss, or headache. Since most people have the fungus in their mouths, thrush is not considered contagious.

What appear to be patches of thrush can also simply be food particles in the mouth. The distinction is easily made by rinsing the mouth to remove food particles. Thrush cannot be removed without direct scraping, and scraping will leave an inflamed spot where the white patch was. A physician can usually verify the diagnosis by simply inspecting the mouth. Microscopic examination of the patch to identify the fungus can be done but is usually not necessary.

Thrush can result from taking antibiotics, which inhibit the bacteria in the mouth that seem to control the growth of *Candida albicans.* People with HIV infection are therefore more prone to thrush when taking trimethoprim-sulfamethoxazole, tetracycline, ampicillin, amoxicillin, erythromycin, ciprofloxacin, or other antibiotics.

Thrush is commonly viewed more as a nuisance than as a serious problem. Symptoms are often trivial, and even when severe, they are easily corrected with medication. Thrush becomes more serious when it extends to the back of the throat to the esophagus: the pain from swallowing might cause people to stop eating, and the treatment given may be somewhat different than for thrush that is restricted to the mouth. The diagnosis of thrush in the esophagus can be made only with an endoscope, which is a tube put through the mouth by a medical specialist (gastroenterologist), or with an x-ray called a barium swallow. In many cases, these diagnostic procedures are unnecessary: the existence of thrush in the mouth, accompanied by painful swallowing, is enough to make the diagnosis.

Nearly all people with HIV infection eventually develop thrush; it is often the first condition indicating that the immune system is weakening. The CD4 count is usually around 100 to 400.

Common treatments for thrush include gargling with and then swallowing nystatin solution; sucking clotrimazole troches; or taking such pills as ketoconazole (Nizoral) or fluconazole (Diflucan). All of these are prescription drugs. If any of the drugs fail, another will usually work. Thrush is generally controlled after one or two weeks of treatment.

Occasionally people do not do well with any of these treatments, either because the diagnosis was wrong to begin with or because the infection has extended to the esophagus. In the latter cases, treatment with such drugs as amphotericin B, given intravenously, may be required for a few days.

In people with HIV infection, thrush tends to recur once treatment is discontinued. As a result, it is common practice to give these drugs for a long time, initially to control the infection and then to prevent its recurrence. Or people keep on hand the drugs prescribed for their original infection and use them intermittently whenever symptoms recur.

Oral hairy leukoplakia (OHL). White patches along the side of the tongue and occasionally in adjacent areas in the mouth are symptoms not only of thrush, but also of oral hairy leukoplakia (OHL). Oral hairy leukoplakia is named for its location in the mouth (oral), and its appearance as white patches (leukoplakia) with microscopic hairlike protrusions (hairy) from the tongue's surface. The patches can be a fraction of an inch in diameter or they can coat most of the tongue. Some people with oral hairy leukoplakia have a sore mouth and occasionally have voice changes.

The symptoms of OHL resemble the symptoms of thrush, though OHL is somewhat less common. Sometimes the first clue to a diagnosis of OHL is that the person does not respond to treatment for thrush. The best way to distinguish clearly between thrush and OHL is to look at tissue taken by biopsy under the microscope. Often the patch itself is sufficiently distinctive in appearance to make a biopsy unnecessary. Most people discover the patches themselves, when they examine their mouths.

Oral hairy leukoplakia is a rather unusual condition. Its cause is unknown, but may have something to do with the Epstein-Barr virus, the virus responsible for infectious mononucleosis. Whatever the association with the Epstein-Barr virus, OHL is not considered contagious. It is found only in people with HIV infection and no one else gets it.

There is little need for treatment except for pain, for interference with nutrition, or for voice changes. The usual treatment is an antiviral drug, acyclovir, taken by mouth. Occasionally other antiviral drugs like ganciclovir are also successful. The patches disappear within two or three weeks when treated, but like thrush, they recur when the medicine is discontinued.

Sores, Blisters, or Ulcers on the Lips or Mouth

Sores or blisters on the lips or mouth or in the throat are usually caused by one of two conditions. One is an infection by the virus herpes simplex; the other is a condition called aphthous ulcers, whose cause is unknown.

Herpes simplex. The sores in the mouth called cold sores or fever blisters can be an infection caused by the herpes simplex virus. The sores usually start as an area of irritation or pain that becomes inflamed, then forms a watery blister that breaks and forms an open sore with pus, and finally scabs over and heals. The sores occur on the lips, in the mouth along the cheeks, on the roof of the mouth or palate, or on the back of the mouth. These sores are usually round or oval, measure about a quarter of an inch or less in diameter, and can have a characteristic white raised border. The sores of herpes can be very painful and often interfere with chewing; when in the back of the mouth or esophagus, the sores can interfere with swallowing.

Herpes simplex remains in the nerves serving the area of the mouth for the remainder of the person's life; it can be reactivated and cause new sores. The interval between outbreaks is unpredictable, but outbreaks are frequently associated with stress, exposure to sunlight, surgery, colds, menstrual periods, fever, and pneumonia. These associations explain the common name of these sores: cold sores or fever blisters.

Infections of the mouth from herpes simplex are extremely common: probably 50 percent of healthy Americans have had this infection at some time. Herpes simplex infections of the mouth are more frequent, more severe, and last for longer periods in people with HIV infection. This is especially true of the later stages of the disease when the CD4 cell count is low and other types of infections are also more common.

Herpes simplex can be spread to others, but many people already have had it, and others who get it develop only trivial problems. When sores are active, it is reasonable to exercise restraint in contact such as kissing and to avoid sharing items that might have saliva on them.

The usual treatment is with acyclovir (Zovirax). Acyclovir is available as an ointment to place on top of sores, as a pill to take by mouth, or as an intravenous preparation. Administration by mouth or by vein is usually preferred, though the choice between options depends largely on the severity of the sores. Because herpes simplex infections tend to recur when treatment is discontinued, long-term treatment with acyclovir by mouth is sometimes advocated once the sores have healed.

Aphthous ulcers. Aphthous ulcers are open sores that may look like herpes simplex sores, occurring in the mouth, usually on the inside surface of the cheeks, on the gums, and on the tongue. Aphthous ulcers are usually very painful, especially when touched or when food or liquids pass over them. The pain can severely limit a person's desire to eat. Like thrush and herpes, the ulcers may extend to the esophagus and impair the ability to swallow. The ulcers can occur in people with or without HIV infection, but they are more common and severe in those with HIV infection.

Aphthous ulcers are often mistaken for herpes simplex infection, which they resemble. But laboratory tests of aphthous ulcers do not show any specific microbe, and the treatment for herpes simplex infection is unsuccessful in treating aphthous ulcers. The cause of these ulcers is not known. Aphthous ulcers are not transmitted to others. Aphthous ulcers may recur over a period of many years.

The usual treatment is to rinse the mouth with viscous lidocaine (2 percent concentration) or the combination of viscous lidocaine and benadryl taken by mouth. Both of these drugs are available without prescription. Severe ulcers may require prescription drugs such as corticosteroids given either as a pill or as a gel that can be applied to the surface of the ulcer. Aphthous ulcers in the esophagus are usually treated with corticosteroids and usually respond well.

Bluish or Purplish Bumps in the Mouth

Raised or thickened tissue that is bluish or purplish is a symptom of Kaposi's sarcoma (KS) in the mouth. Most people with KS in the mouth also have KS on the skin, though this is not invariably so. KS can appear anywhere in the mouth but most frequently appears on the roof, or hard palate. The tumors can cover a relatively small area or they can be spread over the entire palate. Common complications of KS in the mouth include pain, bleeding, or intrusion of the tumors onto the teeth causing tooth loss. In many cases, KS in the mouth causes few problems; it either remains stable for prolonged periods or simply grows very slowly.

The diagnosis is made by examining, under the microscope, tissue taken by biopsy. Most of the time, however, the appearance of the KS is so distinctive that no biopsy is necessary. This is especially true when KS in the mouth occurs along with KS on the skin.

In the absence of pain, bleeding, or intrusion of KS onto the teeth, there is little reason to treat the tumors. When treatment is appropriate, the KS tumors can be surgically removed if small, or treated with radiation, lasers, or chemotherapy using cancer drugs. Which treatment is used will depend on the location of KS tumors, on the severity of the symptoms, and on the bias of the physician. The person with KS obviously needs to agree to the treatment the physician recommends; agreement should be based on an explanation of the benefits, the costs, the convenience, and the side effects of various treatments.

Bleeding Gums

Bleeding gums are usually a symptom of gingivitis. *Gingiva* is the medical term for the gums, and *itis* means inflammation. Some people have severe bleeding of the gums, severe pain, and severe gingival disease with rapid tooth loss over a period as short as two or three months. This rapid loss of the structure that supports the teeth is called *periodontitis*. Periodontitis and gingivitis both are more frequent and severe in people with HIV infection.

The cause of gingivitis and periodontitis is not clearly established. Most dentists think the cause is the same bacteria normally present in the mouth which have, for some reason, gone out of control. Like other conditions, gingivitis is also common in people without HIV infection, but it is more frequent and more severe in those with the infection.

Care must be taken to distinguish gum bleeding caused by gingivitis from bleeding caused by the low numbers of blood platelets that are a part of ITP, which is an entirely different complication of HIV infection. The distinction between the two is easily made by a blood test that counts the number of platelets, or by a consultation with a dentist who will identify diseases of the teeth and gums.

For gingivitis and periodontitis, the treatment is usually mouthwashes containing germicides. One such mouthwash is chlorhexidine in a concentration of 0.12 percent, known as Peridex. Another is povidone-iodine, or Betadine. Both can be purchased in most pharmacies; Peridex requires a prescription, Betadine does not. Chlorhexidine has a high alcohol content that can cause pain in people with advanced gum disease. In this case, it is probably more appropriate to apply povidone-iodine, which is less painful, for several days and then switch to chlorhexidine mouthwashes when they can be better tolerated. For people who have extensive periodontitis, the dental procedure usually recommended is removal of plaque by planing and scaling, a procedure done by dentists. In many cases, antibiotic treatment with metronidazole (Flagyl) is also recommended.

These treatments should be accompanied by rigorously doing what your dentist has always told you to do: use dental floss, brush regularly with a soft toothbrush, and see a dentist regularly.

Problems of the Digestive System

The digestive system includes the mouth; the tube through which food passes after being swallowed, called the esophagus; the stomach; the small intestine, where food is broken down and absorbed; the large intestine or colon, where unabsorbed material is stored for elimination; and the anus. The whole system, taken together, is responsible for digestion of food and elimination of waste. This section will discuss all parts of the digestive system except the mouth: the mouth, which is a common site of problems, has been given its own section.

HIV infection can affect any part of the digestive system, and does so commonly in the later stages. The symptoms are often a clue to which part of digestive system is being affected. Painful or difficult swallowing is usually a symptom of problems with the esophagus. Pain in the abdomen, nausea, and vomiting are usually symptoms of problems with the stomach. Diarrhea, pain, and malnutrition from the failure to absorb nutrients are all symptoms of problems with the small intestine. And pain, diarrhea, or constipation are symptoms of problems with the colon.

Many of the problems in the digestive system also interfere with nutrition. Anything that interferes with nutrition is especially important to someone with HIV infection, because HIV infection itself causes weight loss and nutritional deficiencies. Severe malnutrition also seems to further weaken the immune system. Anyone with HIV infection and such problems with the digestive system should be under the care of a physician.

Loss of Appetite

Loss of appetite has several possible causes. One cause can be HIV itself, which somehow causes an altered sense of taste: food just doesn't seem to taste good. Other causes are depression, drugs, opportunistic infections, or infections of the mouth.

Treatment depends on the exact cause. When the cause is HIV and an altered sense of taste, the best treatment is to learn your preferences and eat accordingly. A person with an altered sense of taste often has a particular problem with protein-rich foods, particularly with red meat. The solution in that case is to find other sources of protein: poultry, fish, eggs, and cheese are all excellent sources of protein. So are dried beans and rice. A person with an altered sense of taste also seems to have the best appetite in the morning: try to eat large, nutritious breakfasts. If you have a preference for foods at different temperatures, indulge your preference. Try eating foods that smell good: the senses of smell and taste are closely connected. Try adding herbs, bacon, garlic, olives, cheese—anything that livens up the flavor of the food and doesn't disagree with you.

Some opportunistic infections of the mouth (thrush, herpes, aphthous ulcers, and Kaposi's sarcoma), discussed in the preceding section, cause pain with eating. When eating hurts, people often lose their appetites. In this case, avoid foods that cause pain. Stay away from salt and seasoned salts; from hot spices like pepper, chili pepper, and paprika; and from acidic foods like vinegar, citrus fruits and juices, tomatoes, pineapple, and pickles. Try food at moderate or cool temperatures. Try foods that are soft and won't irritate the mouth: mild cheeses, cottage cheese, yogurt, cooked eggs, cream soups, ice cream, puddings, popsicles, ground meats, baked fish, bread, noodles and pastas, and cooked or canned fruits (see also, below, the foods that are least troublesome if you have pain on swallowing).

Another cause of appetite loss is the emotional reaction to having HIV infection. At times, people become anxious or depressed and lose interest in eating. Both anxiety and depression can occur at any stage of this infection, but they are especially common at the time the person first learns of a positive blood test, and at the time of the first opportunistic infection. One way to fight this might be to make eating a special event: put on some music, prepare the food so it looks attractive, think of a meal as a break from your worries, relax, take your time with the meal. Eat your favorite foods. Keep snacks around: ice cream, cheese, canned fruit, crackers, peanut butter. Small meals are less filling; try several small meals a day. Eating is often a social event, and many people enjoy food best in someone else's company.

Still another cause of loss of appetite is fatigue: people are simply too tired to eat. Fatigue can also interfere with their ability to prepare a meal if they live alone. If you eat less because you are tired, be careful to eat meals especially high in calories and proteins, so that even if you eat less, you get the same level of nutrition. Try milkshakes, dried fruits, peanut butter, ice cream, cheese, sour cream, hot chocolate, custard, cream soups, scrambled eggs or an omelet with cream cheese, noodles with cheese and cream. Preparing main courses that are high in protein and calories and then freezing them also saves energy: spaghetti sauce, chili, pot roasts, beef or chicken or lamb stews, and soups all taste good made in large amounts, frozen, and reheated; they freeze well. High-protein main courses are also sold prepared and frozen in grocery stores. In either case, frozen food can be reheated on the stove or in a microwave oven. Keep ready-to-eat and nutritious snacks on hand. Many communities also have organizations that will prepare or deliver meals.

Drugs can also be the cause of an altered appetite. Virtually any of the drugs listed below as causes of nausea and vomiting can reduce the appetite, and the list is certainly incomplete.

In general, the treatment for appetite loss depends on the situation: if you have a sore mouth, get treatment for the sores; if drugs are responsible, consider alternatives to those drugs; tailor meals to your own tastes; and accommodate meals to fatigue. When appetite loss is temporary, try to get in as many calories as possible without regard to the nutritional value: you simply are not going to become malnourished in a few days. Try fortifying foods with oil, butter, mayonnaise, a little dried milk, grated cheese, cream. Try making shakes out of combinations of different foods: milk, ice cream, instant breakfast, buttermilk, bananas or strawberries or peaches or apricots or pears, fruit juice, yogurt, honey, cocoa, chocolate syrup, peach or pear or apricot nectars, ginger ale, brown sugar.

Most important is drinking enough fluids: healthy people can survive over one hundred days without food, but no one can survive more than a few days without fluid. Drink fluids that are high in calories and protein—milk, shakes—instead of diet drinks, coffee, or tea. Routinely stir some dried milk into your milk.

If people with HIV infection eat poorly for weeks or months, a physician should be consulted. In some cases, the physician may prescribe an appetite stimulant such as Megace. In extreme cases, the physician may use a feeding tube—a tube placed through the mouth and into the stomach, or through the abdomen and directly into the stomach—so nutrition is maintained despite the inability to eat. An alternative, discussed in a later section on wasting, is to feed people intravenously.

Painful Swallowing

Some people find eating unpleasant and good nutrition difficult because they have pain when they swallow. Sometimes the pain is in the back of the mouth; usually it is in the chest and is a result of esophagitis, an inflammation of the esophagus. The most common cause is infection with *Candida albicans,* the fungus responsible for thrush. Other causes are infections with viruses; some have no known cause but appear similar to aphthous ulcers of the mouth (see above).

The treatment of esophagitis depends on the cause. The probability of *Candida albicans* is so great that physicians often treat for *Candida* without testing for it. If the person with esophagitis does not respond to treatment or if the cause is obscure, an endoscopy—a special procedure in which a specialist (gastroenterologist) puts a tube into the esophagus and takes a sample of tissue—is often advised. If the cause is a viral infection, esophagitis can be treated with antiviral drugs. If the cause is aphthous ulcers, the ulcers in the esophagus, like those in the mouth, often respond to corticosteroids.

Anyone with painful swallowing should see a physician. Despite painful swallowing, it is important to maintain nutrition. Eat foods that are soft or liquid: milkshakes, milk, oatmeal, puddings made with milk or cream, custard, jello, ice cream, cottage cheese, cooked and pureed bland vegetables, popsicles, ground meats, baked fish, melons, bananas, scrambled eggs, omelets, French toast, cream soups, noodles, mashed potatoes. Try drinking through a straw. Such a diet, though easy on your throat, can cause loose stools; liquid supplements, like Enrich, Sustacal with fiber, or Metamucil, are sources of soluble fiber that can help prevent loose stools.

Nausea and Vomiting

Nausea and vomiting have a number of causes, the most common being the drugs taken for complications of HIV infection. Drugs whose side effects include nausea and vomiting are: trimethoprim-sulfamethoxazole (Bactrim, Septra), pyrimethamine (Daraprim), ketoconazole (Nizoral), amphotericin B, pentamidine (Pentam), acyclovir (Zovirax), ganciclovir (DHPG), dapsone, and trimethoprim.

Usually the nausea and vomiting are dose-related, meaning that reducing the dose of the drug will reduce the nausea and vomiting. Or the drug can be taken at times that will not interfere with meals. Or, for many conditions, alternative drugs can be prescribed. Consultation with a physician will usually reveal which drug is likely to be the cause, which is expendable, which can be safely reduced in dose, and which can be safely substituted.

Some of the opportunistic infections—particularly infections that affect the head or the digestive system—can also cause nausea and vomiting. People who have nausea and vomiting, who are taking no medication, and who have additional symptoms such as fever or diarrhea should see their physicians.

In general, the person who has nausea or vomiting should eat small, frequent meals, and eat slowly. Avoid greasy, high-fat, and spicy foods. When symptoms are not severe, follow a soft and bland diet that is low in fat: rice, noodles, pasta, mashed potatoes, clear soups, jello, clear fruit juice, ginger ale, crackers, pretzels, tea, dry toast, oatmeal, boiled eggs. For breakfast, eat crackers, dry cereal, or dry toast. Cold meals that have little odor are often easier to eat than hot meals. When symptoms are severe, it is important to replace the liquids and electrolytes lost: try saltines, pretzels, clear fruit juices, ginger ale or colas, caffeine-free Gatorade, clear soups. All liquids should be clear—that is, they should not be thick liquids like vegetable juices, citrus juices, some fruit juices, or milk. Drink them between meals rather than during meals.

Many drugs reduce nausea and vomiting. Some can be given by suppository in the event that nothing is retained when taken by mouth. Such drugs should be timed to meals; take them as directed, but try taking the drug after eating meals. Some useful drugs do not require a prescription; these include Dramamine and Pepto-Bismol. Other drugs require a prescription: antihistamines (such as Phenergan, Haldol, or Vistaril) or phenothiazines (such as Compazine), which are drugs that also reduce anxiety. Most of these drugs cause drowsiness.

Diarrhea

Diarrhea is a relatively common complication of HIV infection. It can be acute, meaning that it begins suddenly and lasts for a short time, or it can be chronic, meaning that it persists for several weeks or months. Diarrhea has a number of causes. Many people have diarrhea simply as a result of anxiety. Some people have recurrent bouts of stomach pain and diarrhea, called *irritable bowel syndrome,* that go on for years without any identifiable cause. Some people have diarrhea because of HIV itself. Some people have diarrhea because they do not have the enzyme called *lactase* that is necessary to digest a milk sugar called *lactose.* Some people with HIV infection who were once able to tolerate lactose become unable to tolerate it. In lactose intolerance, the diarrhea occurs after people eat food containing lactose, including milk, ice cream, cheese, instant coffee, chocolate, cream, cocoa, and cream fillings. Yogurt, however, is tolerated by some people who are otherwise lactose intolerant, and is worth trying because it is a good source of protein and calcium. Other symptoms of lactose intolerance are cramping and gas.

Another cause of diarrhea is the drugs commonly used by people with HIV infection. In fact, probably almost any drug used to treat an infectious disease can cause diarrhea. Some antibiotics only cause what is called nuisance diarrhea: a few loose stools most days. Other drugs can cause severe diarrhea accompanied by fever and cramps. The antibiotics that most commonly cause severe diarrhea are ddI, clindamycin, ampicillin, amoxicillin, and a group of drugs called cephalosporins. Drugs that less commonly cause diarrhea are trimethoprim-sulfamethoxazole, erythromycin, penicillin, and ciprofloxacin. Any person who has severe diarrhea while taking such drugs should discontinue the drug immediately and notify the physician. Less serious forms of diarrhea are often dose-related, that is, diarrhea can be reduced simply by reducing the amount of the antibiotic. Or the person can be prescribed another drug.

Diarrhea in people with HIV infection is also caused by infections of the digestive system, primarily infections of the small bowel and the colon. Infections are especially likely if the diarrhea is accompanied by a fever. Acute diarrhea can be caused by a number of microbes that are either easily treated with antibiotics, or that go away without treatment, or that progress to chronic diarrhea. Acute diarrhea is often due to food poisoning, viral infection, or anxiety, which are occasional problems for everyone, with or without HIV infection. Perhaps the most common cause of chronic diarrhea in people with AIDS is *Cryptosporidium*, a parasite that is easily detected by stool exam. Diarrhea caused by *Cryptosporidium* is usually prolonged and intermittent. At times, it can be severe, causing watery diarrhea ten to twenty times a day; other times it is better. Other common infectious causes of chronic diarrhea are a tiny parasite called *Microsporidium,* cytomegalovirus, and *Mycobacterium avium.* These latter microbes cause a diarrhea that persists for months, and that, unlike most of the opportunistic infections in HIV infection, cannot be successfully treated with antibiotics. A substantial portion of the people with HIV infection have a chronic diarrhea for which their physicians can establish no clear cause.

Call your physician if the diarrhea is severe, or if it is accompanied by severe pains in the abdomen or by fever, or if it persists. Chronic diarrhea is less common, often occurs late in the course of the infection when the CD4 cell count is low, and is often accompanied by severe weight loss and malnutrition.

The first test to diagnose severe or chronic diarrhea in a person with HIV infection is an analysis of the stool for infectious microbes. If no microbes are found, and if the symptoms are severe, it is often recommended that the digestive system be examined directly with an instrument called an endoscope. An endoscope is a long tube that can be passed through the mouth to look at the small intestine, or passed through the rectum to look at the colon. The physician who performs the test is a gastroenterologist, a specialist in digestive diseases. Endoscopy permits not only a direct view of the wall of the intestine, but also removal of a small piece of tissue (a biopsy) of any area that appears abnormal. The tissue can then be examined under the microscope to identify the nature of the problem. A number of x-ray procedures also allow a look at the intestine. The person should be forewarned that these types of specialized tests tend to be unpleasant and expensive. Endoscopy of either the colon or the small intestine, plus the professional fee of the gastroenterologist, plus the pathologist's interpretation of the results will cost between $1,000 and $2,000.

The treatment of diarrhea depends largely on the severity and cause. When drugs are responsible, a physician will reduce or discontinue the drug. Regardless of the cause, it is important, first, to drink enough fluids and, second, to eat enough food. The usual recommendation is to eat small, frequent meals and to drink fluids between meals. Avoid insoluble fiber: seeds, brans, nuts, whole wheat bread, the skins of fruits and vegetables. Avoid anything that causes gas: carbonated drinks, beans, cabbage, spicy foods, gum. Avoid fats, milk, cheese, ice cream. Since caffeine is a bowel stimulant, avoid coffee, tea, colas and some sodas, hot chocolate, and chocolate.

Soluble fiber, like pectin, counters diarrhea: oatmeal, jello, apples, bananas, mangoes, melons, fruit nectars, and cooked and skinned fruits and vegetables are sources of soluble fiber. Try white bread, white rice, noodles, and pastas. Drink plenty of liquids: water, clear fruit juices, clear soups, broth, ginger ale and caffeine-free colas (stir out the bubbles). Dietitians call such a diet a BRATT diet: bananas, rice, applesauce, tea (caffeine-free), and toast. The BRATT diet, though helpful in controlling acute diarrhea, lacks many nutrients and should not be continued for more than a week. In addition, avoid drinking fluids during meals; fluids should be taken between meals. As with nausea and vomiting, it is important to replace lost electrolytes: try saltines, pretzels, clear fruit juices, Gatorade, ginger ale or caffeine-free colas, potatoes, bananas, clear soups.

When diarrhea is unrelated to food, there may be an advantage to adding foods containing soluble fiber—as listed above—in an effort to add bulk to the diet.

With severe diarrhea, when malnutrition becomes a worry, supplement the diet with special high-nutrient fluids such as Ensure, Sustacal with fiber, Enrich, or Magnacal. High-nutrient fluids, which can be obtained in grocery stores and pharmacies, provide a rich source of calories and protein. (Note: some people cannot digest high-nutrient fluids, and their symptoms worsen until they stop drinking the fluids.) For people who have a severe disease of the small intestine that interferes with their ability to absorb food, such as severe cryptosporidiosis, their physicians may prescribe an (expensive) food supplement of predigested nutrients such as Vivonex T.E.N. All of these dietary decisions are best made with the advice of a physician and a dietitian.

Drugs may also be used to reduce diarrhea. Some drugs that reduce diarrhea are available without prescription: Donnagel, Kaopectate, Lactinex, Pepto-Bismol, loperamide (Imodium), and the like. None of these seems to work well most of the time, but they may be worth trying. If the diarrhea is caused by a microbe, your physician will prescribe drugs to eradicate the microbe, if it can be treated; the specific treatment will depend on the microbe found. As noted, however, many microbes do not respond to antibiotics, and sometimes no microbe is found at all. In these cases, diarrhea is treated with prescription drugs—including diphenoxylate (Lomotil), tincture of opium, and paregoric—that quiet the motion of the muscles of the intestines. Other drugs used to treat diarrhea—like ibuprofen, indomethacin, or somatostatin—seem to work, but no one knows why.

When a person with HIV infection has diarrhea, the caregiver should use common sense to avoid unnecessary exposure to stool. The stool of a person with HIV infection seems to contain no virus, and stool is not thought to be a source of transmission of HIV. The only infectious diseases that might be transmitted to others through stool are *Cryptosporidium* and salmonella; both are uncommon, and when they do infect people with intact immune systems, the diarrhea is only temporary.

Gynecological Problems

The gynecological problems that women with HIV infection get are the same that all women get. But certain problems are more common or more severe in women with HIV infection: vaginal yeast infections, pelvic inflammatory disease, and cervical cancer.

Cervical Cancer

Cervical cancer, which has no symptoms in the early stages, is a major concern in women with HIV infection. It is now also considered an AIDS-defining diagnosis. Cervical cancer is associated with infection by a virus called the human papillomavirus, or HPV. HPV also causes warts in the genital region. But the HPV that causes genital warts—easily seen as fleshy growths—and the HPV that is associated with cervical cancer are different strains of HPV. Cervical cancer is detected by Pap smears. Pap smears turn out to have abnormal results far more frequently in women with HIV infection that in those without. As a result, it is now recommended that women with HIV infection have Pap smears every six to twelve months. Those with abnormal Pap smears should have a cervical biopsy; some physicians recommend a cervical biopsy for women with HIV infection even without an abnormal Pap smear.

Vaginal Discharge, Severe Genital Itching

A discharge that often resembles cottage cheese and severe genital itching are symptoms of vaginal yeast infections. Vaginal yeast infections are common in all women but are especially common in women with HIV infection. A yeast infection is an opportunistic infection caused by the same fungus, *Candida albicans,* that causes thrush. Yeast infections occur at a relatively early stage of HIV infection, often when the CD4 cell count is over 500. The usual treatment is a cream applied locally to the vagina, like Gyne-Lotrimin. These creams are available at drugstores without prescription. Women with more advanced stages of HIV infection are likely to find that local creams do not work very well, or that the yeast infection may recur rapidly when treatments are discontinued. Management of this problem will often require consulting a gynecologist who might prescribe such drugs as ketoconazole, fluconazole, or itraconazole.

Vaginal Discharge, Pelvic Pain, Painful Sexual Intercourse

Vaginal discharge, pelvic pain, and painful sexual intercourse are symptoms of pelvic inflammatory disease, or PID. PID is an infection of the upper part of the genital tract: the uterus, fallopian tubes, and ovaries. The usual causes are sexually transmitted microbes like gonococcus and Chlamydia. In its later stages, PID can lead to infertility, high rates of ectopic pregnancies, and chronic abdominal pain. PID may occur in women who do not have HIV infection as well as in those who do, but women with HIV infection appear to have PID more frequently and more severely. The diagnosis and treatment require evaluation by a physician, including a pelvic examination and prescription drugs. The standard drugs, antibiotics, are highly effective in the short run but may not prevent the infertility and pain of the later stages of PID. Because of this, many physicians recommend that women with HIV infection and PID be hospitalized for treatment of PID.

Eye Problems

People with HIV infection do not usually have problems with their eyes, and when they do, the problems are often the usual ones that accompany the aging process. But there are some eye problems that indicate serious complications, and a physician must be notified. The most common and serious is cytomegalovirus retinitis.

Blurred Vision

Blurred vision, along with several other symptoms and a low CD4 cell count, may indicate an infection of the eye called *cytomegalovirus retinitis.*

Cytomegalovirus (CMV) retinitis. In addition to blurred vision, other symptoms of CMV retinitis can include a blind spot, pain in the eye, and "floaters." Floaters are spots that float across the line of vision as a result of inflamed cells in the middle of the eye. In many instances the person with CMV retinitis notices no symptoms at all.

CMV retinitis is caused by a virus called *cytomegalovirus,* or CMV, that, like the viruses that cause chickenpox or herpes, infects most people and then remains dormant in the body. Because CMV lives in blood cells, it can circulate to all parts of the body. In this case, CMV has infected the retina, the layer of cells in the back of the eye that, like the film of a camera, is responsible for recording images. The specific symptoms a person has will depend on which area of the retina is affected. CMV retinitis occurs in 10 to 20 percent of people with HIV infection. It does not occur until the CD4 count is severely lowered; it virtually never occurs when the CD4 cell count is over 150 and usually occurs when it is less than 50.

The diagnosis can be made by a physician using an *ophthalmoscope,* an instrument that permits the physician to see the retina. What part of the retina is infected determines how much vision is lost. On the central part of the retina, where images are focused, a small area of infection can cause complete loss of vision. On the periphery of the retina, a large infection can cause no apparent vision loss.

CMV retinitis can occur in one eye or in both eyes. If the infection in one eye is left untreated, it will often affect the other eye as well. If both eyes are infected and left untreated, the usual result is blindness. Loss of sight caused by cytomegalovirus cannot be corrected with glasses. With early treatment, vision can usually be saved before blindness occurs. Treatment is with the antiviral drugs ganciclovir and foscarnet, which slow or stop the progression of the infection. Both drugs are given intravenously, and treatment must continue indefinitely, because the infection recurs when the treatment is stopped. With either drug, there is often relapse. One drug sometimes causes side effects, necessitating use of the other drug.

Head and Nerve Problems

The nervous system has two parts: the central nervous system and the peripheral nervous system. The central nervous system is made up of the brain, where thinking takes place, and the spinal cord, which is a bundle of nerves that carries directions from and to the brain. The peripheral nervous system is composed of the nerves that bring sensory messages to the brain and deliver commands to the muscles. Both the central nervous system and the peripheral nervous system can be affected by HIV infection.

The central nervous system—primarily the brain—is somewhat more likely to be affected than the peripheral nervous system, either by HIV itself or by an opportunistic infection or tumor. The most common symptoms of central nervous system involvement are (1) mental slowing, with memory loss and impaired concentration; (2) seizures; (3) weakness or paralysis; (4) poor coordination; and (5) headache that is often severe or different from the usual headache. All of these symptoms suggest infection in the brain or meninges (the membrane surrounding the brain) and require medical treatment. In many instances, the person with these symptoms will then be referred to a neurologist, a specialist in diseases of the nervous system.

The most frequent and serious diseases of the central nervous system are opportunistic infections or tumors associated with a weakened immune system, and an infection caused by HIV itself, called HIV-associated dementia. The most common of the opportunistic infections are toxoplasma encephalitis and cryptococcal meningitis; less common are lymphomas of the brain, Kaposi's sarcoma, cytomegalovirus, progressive multifocal leukoencephalopathy, *Mycobacterium avium,* tuberculosis, and the herpes viruses.

All these diseases cause similar symptoms. Diagnosis, therefore, requires special tests. The tests usually done begin with a neurologic examination that includes a physical examination of the nervous system to determine coordination, strength, sensations, reflexes, and mental functioning. An important laboratory test is a lumbar puncture, also called a spinal tap. The lumbar puncture is done to obtain the cerebrospinal fluid that surrounds the spinal cord and brain; the fluid is then examined for any inflammatory cells or microbes that will provide clues to the diagnosis.

Other major laboratory tests are computerized tomography (CAT scan) and magnetic resonance image (MRI) of the brain. Both tests are methods of viewing the brain in three dimensions to look for specific changes. These changes indicate the location of the problem and its probable cause. Diagnosis of central nervous system problems, then, is based on the symptoms, the results of a neurologic examination, the results of examination of the cerebrospinal fluid, and any changes in the images of the brain.

Many diseases of the central nervous system can be treated successfully, especially early in the course of the disease. Many of the symptoms suggesting central nervous system infections, however, occur even when there is no problem in the central nervous system at all. Weakness, seizures, and mental changes, for instance, can be caused by medications, changes in the balance of electrolytes in the blood, and fever due to some other infection. Particularly difficult to sort out are headaches: 90 percent of all people, with or without HIV infection, have periodic headaches.

The final part of this section on head and nerve problems will discuss the problems HIV infection causes with the peripheral nervous system.

Headaches

Headaches are extremely common. In most cases, headaches bother the person who has them far more than they bother the physician who treats them. This is because headaches rarely indicate severe or progressive disease. Most headaches occur when the muscles that cover the top of the skull contract. These headaches, called tension headaches, occur off and on in everyone. They go away either by themselves or with simple drugs such as aspirin, acetaminophen, ibuprofen, or any of a multitude of drugs that contain combinations of these drugs.

A less common but more painful type of headache, called a migraine or a cluster headache, results when the arteries of the scalp contract. These headaches may be severe, may involve only one side of the head, and may occur along with nausea, vomiting, and changes in vision. Such headaches tend to recur and often require prescription drugs that relax the contractions of the arteries.

Another common cause of headaches is a generalized illness such as influenza or infections in the sinuses or ears. Sinus headaches are especially common in people with HIV infection, who frequently have sinusitis.

Finally, headaches may result from certain drugs, including AZT, trimethoprim-sulfamethoxazole, rifampin, ketoconazole, amphotericin B, and acyclovir.

All of these headaches go away by themselves, leave no impairment behind, and do not indicate any serious underlying disease.

Certain headaches, however, require a doctor's attention. Like other focal neurologic symptoms and like fever and stiff neck (see below), headaches can be a symptom of an infection of the brain or the meninges. Headaches associated with infections of the brain or meninges have the following characteristics:

1. They are unusually severe or last unusually long.

2. Either the character of the pain or the location of pain makes the headache different from headaches the person usually has.

3. They occur along with problems with vision.

4. They occur along with weakness of an arm or leg, with dizziness, or with impaired coordination.

5. They occur along with stiff neck, nausea and vomiting, or extreme lethargy or sleepiness.

6. They are severe and occur along with an unexplained fever.

The major infections that cause such headaches in people with HIV infection are toxoplasma encephalitis and cryptococcal meningitis. Both these infections, as well as a multitude of other infections of the brain and meninges, are relatively easy to diagnose. They are also treatable. A less common cause of headaches in people with HIV infection is lymphoma.

Toxoplasma encephalitis. The symptoms of toxoplasma encephalitis are what physicians call focal neurologic symptoms: paralysis or weakness on one side of the body, loss of speech, loss of coordination, and certain kinds of seizures. Such symptoms occur generally when there is a problem in a specific part of the brain.

Toxoplasma encephalitis is caused by a parasite called *Toxoplasma gondii* that is usually acquired by eating undercooked meat or by contact with cat excrement; the parasite is not transmitted from one person to another. About 20 to 30 percent of American adults are infected with *Toxoplasma gondii,* and most of them are, and will remain, unaware of it. The parasite causes severe disease primarily in people with severe immunosuppression. It seems to be most common in people with AIDS when the CD4 count is less than 100.

Toxoplasma encephalitis can be diagnosed with a blood test that detects antibodies to *Toxoplasma gondii,* but the best test is one of the methods—CAT scans or MRI scans—for imaging the brain. Either of these will show a characteristic pattern of inflammation in the brain. Some people whose symptoms are unusual and who fail to respond to standard treatment might require a brain biopsy.

The standard treatment for toxoplasma encephalitis is an antibiotic, pyrimethamine, given in combination with other antibiotics, either sulfonamides or clindamycin. These drugs are given initially by vein and then by mouth in relatively high doses. Most people improve within two weeks; brain scans two to four weeks after treatment begins generally show reduction in the size of the area of inflammation.

Toxoplasma encephalitis is one of the many infections in people with AIDS that responds well to treatment but recurs when antibiotics are discontinued. For this reason, in the majority of cases, antibiotics are continued indefinitely.

Lymphoma. Another common cause of focal neurologic problems in people with HIV infection is lymphoma. Lymphoma is a tumor of lymph cells that occurs in 1 to 3 percent of people with HIV infection. Almost any part of the body can be affected by lymphoma, but the brain is one of the parts most commonly affected.

Lymphoma is often suspected if treatment for suspected toxoplasma encephalitis is ineffective. Lymphoma can be diagnosed by taking a small sample of brain tissue, a test called a brain biopsy. Treatment is with radiation and the chemotherapy drugs used to treat cancers. (See also below, under "Problems Affecting the Whole Body.")

Cryptococcal meningitis. Meningitis means inflammation (itis) of the meninges, the fibrous membrane that surrounds the brain and spinal cord. The symptoms of meningitis are usually fever and stiff neck; other symptoms can include seizures and double vision.

Cryptococcal meningitis is caused by a fungus called *Cryptococcus* that is found throughout the world and is transmitted when the fungus is inhaled. The infection itself cannot be transmitted from one person to another. *Cryptococcus* usually causes either a trivial disease or no disease at all until the immune system is weakened: it is the most common cause of meningitis in people with HIV infection. Cryptococcal meningitis is both serious and treatable, so it is important to see a physician as soon as symptoms appear.

The test for cryptococcal meningitis is a spinal tap. A spinal tap is done so that a sample of the cerebrospinal fluid can be examined for evidence of inflammation and for *Cryptococcus*. Treatment usually consists of the antibiotics amphotericin B (given by vein) or fluconazole (given by vein or by mouth) or a combination of both. Treatment is usually successful, but the infection tends to recur when treatment is discontinued. For this reason, treatment is usually continued for extended periods.

Slowed Mental Processes

Slowed mental processes, including forgetfulness, loss of recent memory (that is, the person can remember childhood experiences, but not the morning's events), and difficulty concentrating, can be symptoms of HIV-associated dementia (HAD), which used to be called AIDS dementia complex. HAD is a mental deterioration that accompanies HIV infection and has no other apparent causes. Other symptoms are irritability, social withdrawal, and apathy. Occasional symptoms are weakness in the legs or arms, tremor, poor coordination, and loss of balance. The onset of these symptoms can be either gradual or abrupt. HAD is found in 20 to 30 percent of people in the late stages of HIV infection.

The cause of HAD is unknown. Evidence suggests the cause might be HIV in the brain: the cerebrospinal fluid that bathes the brain often shows evidence of HIV early in the course of the infection before the person shows any symptoms. The symptoms of HAD can also be caused by an opportunistic infection or tumor, and by depression.

People with HIV infection and these symptoms should see a physician, who will often consult a neurologist. Tests to diagnose HAD include tests of intellectual functioning; neurologic tests for coordination, strength, and reflexes; and MRI or CAT scans of the brain.

Treatment of HAD is usually a drug like AZT that inhibits HIV. In addition, stimulants like dextroamphetamine or methylphenidate (Ritalin) can sometimes counter apathy and lethargy.

Because of the importance of HAD for both the person with HIV infection and the caregiver, the next chapter deals with HAD alone.

Numbness, Tingling, or Pain in the Feet

The symptoms listed so far in this section on head and nerve problems have dealt with problems in the central nervous system. People with HIV infection also have symptoms of problems in the peripheral nervous system, the network of nerves that bring sensory messages to the brain and deliver commands to the muscles. The most common symptoms are numbness, tingling, or pain in the feet and legs, and less commonly, in the arms or the fingers. The symptoms in the feet may worsen, to the point that wearing shoes becomes intolerable and walking becomes impossible.

These symptoms are caused by what is called *painful sensory neuropathy,* that is, painful sensations due to damaged nerves (neuropathy). Painful sensory neuropathy can occur relatively early in the course of HIV infection, but is more common later, after opportunistic infections have begun appearing. In general, the causes of painful sensory neuropathy are poorly understood. The known causes include diabetes, alcoholism, and medications. The medications include some of the drugs used to treat HIV infection, especially ddI and ddC. These drugs must be stopped promptly when these symptoms occur, since continued use will cause progression of the symptoms to the point of irreversibility. Report the symptoms of painful sensory neuropathy to your physician to determine the cause and to begin treatment.

Treatment is mainly to relieve pain. Wear no shoes at all, or loose, soft slippers. If blankets and sheets cause pain, build a sort of bridge at the foot of the bed that lifts up the blankets and sheets. Nonprescription drugs that may help include aspirin, acetaminophen, and ibuprofen. In some cases, a physician will prescribe narcotics or drugs called *tricyclic antidepressants,* such as nortriptyline (Pamelor). Side effects of the drugs include drowsiness, so these drugs are best taken at night. Some creams, like HEET or those like Zostrix that contain capsaicin, also relieve the symptoms. HEET requires no prescription; creams with capsaicin require a prescription.

Muscle Weakness

Weakness in the large muscles, especially the muscles of the thighs and shoulders, can be a symptom of myositis. Myositis is an inflammation (itis) of the muscles (myo). Similar symptoms are caused by opportunistic infections of the central nervous system, by profound fatigue, and by some drugs (including AZT).

The diagnosis of myositis is usually based on a neurologic examination and a blood test for an enzyme produced by the muscle. Sometimes a muscle biopsy is recommended.

Treatment depends on the cause. If the cause is AZT or another drug, the drugs should be discontinued. If the cause cannot clearly be identified as a drug, the drug can be discontinued on a trial basis to see if the myositis improves. If the cause is HIV itself, treatment with ibuprofen or corticosteroids is usually successful.

Problems Affecting the Whole Body

Symptoms that affect the whole body, or constitution, are called *constitutional symptoms*. Constitutional symptoms include fever, night sweats, weight loss, fatigue, lethargy, and malaise. All these symptoms are relatively common both in the general population and in people with HIV infection. People with HIV infection tend to have constitutional symptoms when the CD4 count is low, unless the people are also depressed or have some unrelated medical problem like influenza. Some of these symptoms—fatigue, lethargy, malaise—are subjective and difficult to measure. Others—fever, severe weight loss (wasting)—are more objective.

Two of these constitutional symptoms—fever and wasting—deserve additional discussion.

Fever

Physicians always want to know when a person with HIV infection has a fever: fever is an objective indication of a problem that is not just a day-to-day variation in health status. Fever, especially prolonged fever in people with low CD4 counts, is usually the result of infections.

In people with HIV infection, the infections that are most likely are tuberculosis, sinusitis, *Mycobacterium avium* infection, cytomegalovirus infection, fungal infection, pneumocystis pneumonia, and lymphoma. Drugs may also cause fever. Nearly all drugs may do this but those that do it most commonly are sulfa drugs like trimethoprim-sulfamethoxazole (Bactrim or Septra). The best way to tell is to stop suspected drugs and see if the fever disappears, which usually occurs within 24 to 48 hours.

Most people with fever are aware of it. They cannot tolerate the usual range of heat and cold that most people consider normal room temperature; they have chills and sweats. In people with HIV infection, fevers often begin gradually, occurring off and on for extended periods of weeks or months. The fever is often accompanied by sweating at night, called night sweats, that may be severe enough to require the person to change pajamas and sheets.

It is important to measure the fever. The body temperature that is normal differs for different people and at different times of the day. The average temperature is 97 degrees F at 3:00 A.M. and 99.3 degrees F at 5:00 P.M. In general, temperatures are about two degrees higher (on the Fahrenheit scale) in the late afternoon than they are in the morning. A fever usually exaggerates this daily variation, and the highest temperature usually comes after 6:00 P.M. For this reason, people with HIV infection who think they have a fever should take their temperatures several times during the day, when they feel feverish, and in the late afternoon. Although there is no general agreement on the precise definition of fever, most physicians consider 99.6 degrees F or 100 degrees F to be a fever. (Temperature is measured on two scales: the Fahrenheit, or F scale, commonly used in the United States, and the centigrade, or C scale, used in the rest of the world and in some hospitals in the United States. A temperature of 98.6 degrees F corresponds to 37 degrees C.)

Fever is basically treated by treating whatever is causing it. Treating fever itself is a little controversial. Fever actually has advantages: the immune system works better at higher temperatures, and fever is an important indicator of the course of the disease and of the effectiveness of treatment. But fever is also unpleasant for the person who has it and increases the metabolic rate, burning more calories and making good nutrition more difficult. Otherwise, there is little evidence that fever is harmful.

When the decision is made to reduce fever, the usual drugs are aspirin, acetaminophen, or ibuprofen. The fever decreases or disappears when people take one of these drugs, but returns when the effect of the drug wears off. For people with persistent fever, these fluctuations in temperature can be more unpleasant than a steady, if high, temperature.

For this reason, people with persistent fevers are often advised to take these drugs regularly, every four to six hours, without waiting for the fever to recur.

Wasting

Wasting is the somewhat unfortunate term given to unintentional weight loss. Wasting that results in the unintentional loss of 10 percent of the body weight, with no explanation other than HIV infection, has been accepted by the Centers for Disease Control as an AIDS-defining diagnosis.

People with HIV infection lose weight for different reasons: difficulty eating, lack of appetite, apathy and depression, prolonged diarrhea, nausea and vomiting, HIV itself, opportunistic infections that affect various organs of the body, and fever. Fever can contribute to wasting because fever increases the rate at which the body metabolizes food by 7 percent for each degree F: a person with a temperature of 103 degrees F through the day will have a metabolic rate that is increased by 30 percent. Wasting is commonly accompanied by protein-caloric malnutrition (see above, "Problems of the Digestive System").

Treatment of wasting depends on the cause. If the cause is difficulty eating, the sores and ulcers in the mouth or esophagus that cause the difficulty should be treated with drugs, and the person should eat foods that are soft, easy to swallow, and bland. If the cause is lack of appetite, appetite stimulants like Megace might help, and the person should eat foods he or she likes. If the cause is apathy, the caregiver needs to encourage the person with HIV infection to eat, and a stimulant like Ritalin might help. If the cause is prolonged diarrhea, the infection causing diarrhea should be treated with drugs; the diarrhea itself can also be treated with drugs like Lomotil, loperamide, or paregoric. If the cause is nausea and vomiting, the person should eat small meals frequently, avoid aromatic foods, and eat food that is easily digested; nausea and vomiting can also be treated with drugs. If fever is a factor in wasting, treatment will try to reduce fever with aspirin, acetaminophen, or ibuprofen and will try to eliminate the cause of the fever.

For more about all these treatments for wasting, see above, "Problems of the Digestive System." In general, cater to individual tastes, eat small and frequent meals, and eat foods that contain a lot of calories and protein. For the short term, anyway, don't worry too much about a balanced diet and eat snack foods that carry large numbers of calories: peanuts, peanut butter, nuts, raisins, sunflower seeds, M&Ms, Oreo cookies, pizza, milkshakes, potato chips, Fritos, macaroni and cheese,

Big Macs, most candy bars, fudge sundaes, marshmallows, and many others. Try asking a licensed dietitian.

When people cannot eat enough to compensate for losses, supplements will help. Supplements like Ensure, Sustacal, Enrich, and Magnacal (approximately $1.50 per can) are rich in calories, complex carbohydrates, and fat. The various supplements are similar in nutritional value. They are available in grocery stores and pharmacies. If the supplements are taken in addition to meals, the person will need a few cans a day. If the supplements are the only nutrition the person is getting, the person will need about ten cans a day. Most people don't try to get all of their nutritional needs with these supplements, but they use them to supplement a diet of foods that are more pleasurable and diverse.

When people have problems that prevent the small intestine from absorbing food, different supplements which are predigested and ready to absorb will help. Supplements like Vivonex T.E.N. cost about $6 to $8 per can. If these supplements are taken in addition to meals, people will use three to six cans a day; if the supplement is the only source of nutrition, the person will need six to nine cans a day.

All nutritional supplements are available without prescription. But if a prescription is written nevertheless, Medicaid and some insurance plans will cover the supplement's cost.

On the rare occasions when the intestines quit digesting and absorbing food, nutrients might need to be provided by vein—a procedure called parenteral (meaning by vein) hyperalimentation. Most physicians prefer to use parenteral hyperalimentation for only a week or two to get past a temporary problem, though occasionally they use it for longer periods.

Causes of Constitutional Symptoms

The causes of constitutional symptoms are diverse. Sometimes the cause is anxiety and depression (see Chapter 4). Sometimes the cause is the common aches and pains—colds, influenza, gastroenteritis, nervous stomach, headaches—that affect everyone.

Sometimes the cause is one of the opportunistic infections. When constitutional symptoms are accompanied by cough and shortness of breath, the cause may be pneumocystis pneumonia. When constitutional symptoms are accompanied by headache or other symptoms of central nervous system infection (see above, "Head and Nerve Problems"), the cause is probably toxoplasma encephalitis or cryptococcal meningitis. When constitutional symptoms last for weeks or months, the cause is probably tuberculosis, *Mycobacterium avium,* cytomegalovirus, lymphoma, fungal infections, drugs, or HIV itself.

Tuberculosis. Tuberculosis (TB) is an infection of the lungs by a bacterium called *Mycobacterium tuberculosis.* Though the symptoms are usually those of lung infections—cough, bloody sputum, shortness of breath—occasionally the person with TB has only constitutional symptoms—fever, night sweats, and weight loss. In people with HIV infection, TB occurs more frequently and with greater severity; it can also spread to parts of the body other than the lungs.

TB can be active or inactive. If TB is active, the bacterium is multiplying and invading tissue; the person with active TB has symptoms. If TB is inactive, the bacterium is dormant and the person has no symptoms. Most of the people who have active TB have previously had inactive TB for several years.

Anyone who has TB, active or inactive, is likely to have a positive skin test. People with HIV infection, for whom TB is more frequent and more serious, should routinely get skin tests. Because the skin test relies on an immune response, it is most reliable early in the course of HIV infection and less reliable later when the immune system has weakened. If the skin test is positive and the person has inactive TB, a drug called isoniazid or INH will prevent TB from becoming active. If the skin test is positive and the person has active TB, isoniazid combined with other drugs will control the disease.

TB, when active, can be transmitted to others. Anyone living with someone who has active TB should take the skin test. (See also above, under "Lung Problems.")

Mycobacterium avium (MA). MA is a bacterium related to *Mycobacterium tuberculosis,* but is not transmitted from one person to another. People who do not have HIV infection also get infections with MA, but only in the lungs. In people with HIV infection, MA usually occurs late in the course of the infection when the CD4 count is low, and may spread widely throughout the body. In the liver, MA can cause hepatitis; in the lung, pneumonia; in the intestines, diarrhea. Accompanying all of these infections are constitutional symptoms.

How MA is transmitted is unclear. It is not passed from one person to another. It is found in nature, often in water supplies that we all drink, and contact with MA is probably universal.

Treatment is difficult because MA resists many antibiotics. This resistance previously made it necessary either to ignore MA infections or to treat them with five or six drugs whose side effects were so severe that the treatment was worse than the disease. Fortunately, the treatment of MA has changed greatly in the past few years because new and more effective drugs are available: rifabutin, clarithromycin, and azithromycin. As a result, many physicians now advise using these drugs to prevent MA infections in people with HIV infection with CD4 counts lower than 150 or 100.

Cytomegalovirus (CMV). CMV infections, like the related herpes simplex infections and chickenpox, occur early in life. Each virus remains dormant until a weakened immune system allows it to flourish. Like MA, CMV infections are spread throughout the body, almost always when the CD4 count is less than 200, usually less than 100. In the liver, CMV causes hepatitis; in the intestines, diarrhea; in the esophagus, difficulty swallowing; in the lung, pneumonia; on the skin, herpes-like sores; in the eye, retinitis. In many people, however, CMV infection only causes constitutional symptoms, including fever, fatigue, and wasting.

One of the most serious of these infections is CMV retinitis, which, if left untreated, can cause blindness (see above, under "Eye Problems"). CMV is transmitted the way HIV is, through sexual contact or contact with blood. Most people do not know when they were infected, and the initial infection usually does not cause symptoms. For these reasons, CMV is not considered a health threat to others.

CMV infection is difficult to treat because it resists most antibiotics. The drugs used—ganciclovir and foscarnet—must be given intravenously. CMV retinitis responds well to treatment; CMV at other places in the body responds less predictably. (See also Chapter 3.)

Lymphoma. Lymphomas are tumors of the lymph glands that can occur in anyone but are more common and more severe in people with HIV infection. In some people, the only symptoms of lymphoma are the constitutional symptoms. In other people, the symptoms of lymphoma are very large lymph glands in the neck, under the arms, or in the groin; these symptoms are more commonly caused by persistent generalized lymphadenopathy (PGL) (see Chapter 3). In some people, the symptoms of lymphoma differ according to where in the body lymphoma occurs: lymphoma in the intestines causes pain and diarrhea; in the brain, focal neurologic problems (see above, "Head and Nerve Problems"); in the lung, pneumonia.

In people with HIV infection, lymphomas often progress rapidly, more rapidly than they do in other people. Treatment is with radiation and with chemotherapy using the same drugs used for other types of tumors. The treatment is given by specialists, either radiation therapists or oncologists. The success of the treatment is variable; some people do extremely well. Curing lymphoma is increasingly likely, so talk to your physician about the side effects and potential benefits of each treatment.

Fungal infections. Constitutional symptoms can also be caused by fungal infections, including *Cryptococcus neoformans, Histoplasma capsulatum,* and *Coccidioides immitis.*

Cryptococcus neoformans usually causes pneumonia, then spreads to other areas of the body. It spreads most commonly to the meninges, where it causes meningitis (see above, under "Head and Nerve Problems"). It can also cause only constitutional symptoms.

Histoplasma capsulatum is found primarily in the central and eastern parts of the United States, especially in the Mississippi, Ohio, and St. Lawrence River valleys. Most people with histoplasmosis have been in the areas where it is common, but they may have been in those areas years earlier. In most people, it causes infections of the lungs. In people with HIV infection, it causes infections spread throughout the body.

Coccidioides immitis is found in the southwestern United States (California, Arizona, or Texas), where it causes a lung infection called valley fever. As with histoplasmosis, HIV-infected people with coccidioidomycosis have usually visited or lived in the areas where the fungus grows. In people with HIV infection, *Coccidioides,* like *Histoplasma,* tends to spread throughout the body.

All three fungal infections are diagnosed by detecting the fungus. They are usually treated with amphotericin B, given intravenously.

Drugs. Constitutional symptoms can also be caused by drugs. People with HIV infection take many drugs either to treat or to prevent infections, and to treat anxiety, depression, fever, aches, and problems with sleep and appetite. Many of these drugs have side effects, ranging in seriousness from drowsiness (from antihistamines) to kidney damage and anemia (from amphotericin B). The only side effects of many drugs are constitutional symptoms, particularly fever and rash.

For reasons that are unclear, side effects are more common in people with HIV infection. For instance, trimethoprim-sulfamethoxazole (Bactrim or Septra) causes side effects in 10 percent of the people without HIV infection and 50 percent of those with HIV infection.

Finding out which drugs are causing side effects and stopping the side effects requires the advice of a physician. The physician will either advise what is called a drug holiday—discontinuation of all drugs—or will stop drugs one at a time. (See Chapter 9, under "Side Effects of the Drugs.")

HIV infection. Some people have constitutional symptoms that cannot be attributed to an opportunistic infection or an opportunistic tumor, or to the side effects of drugs. In such cases, HIV itself might be responsible.

Constitutional symptoms with no causes other than HIV usually occur late in the course of the infection. The treatment is drugs directed at HIV—like AZT—or drugs that simply relieve the constitutional symptoms—aspirin, acetaminophen, ibuprofen, or similar drugs. These drugs are often given on a trial basis, in varying combinations and increasing doses.

Table 3. Conditions Commonly Associated with HIV Infection

Condition	Symptoms	Comments
Asymptomatic infection	None (*asymptomatic* means *without symptoms*)	May have abnormal laboratory tests often indicating suppressed immunity (low CD4 count), abnormal blood count
Persistent generalized lymphadenopathy	Nodules like marbles under the skin, in the neck, armpits, and groin	Swollen lymph nodes do not represent progressive disease but are sites of virus growth; about 10 to 15% of people will complain of tender swellings in the neck
Early symptomatic HIV infection		These include conditions previously called AIDS-related complex, or ARC
Thrush	White patches in the mouth	80 to 90% of people with AIDS have had or will have thrush; more common when taking antibiotics
Oral hairy leukoplakia	White patches usually along sides of tongue	15 to 25% of people with AIDS have had or will have OHL. There are usually no symptoms.
Herpes zoster	Painful blisters, usually on specific part of the body on one side	Caused by same virus that causes chickenpox
Idiopathic thrombocytopenia	Bleeding, especially from gums, rectum, urine, into the skin, & with minor cuts	May occur relatively early in HIV infection
Constitutional symptoms	Chronic diarrhea, weight loss, night sweats, fever, fatigue	All are common complaints with a variety of illnesses unrelated to HIV; but the difference with HIV infection is that they last a long time, usually over one month

Table 3. (*Continued*)

Condition	Symptoms	Comments
Late symptomatic HIV infection, or AIDS		This includes AIDS-defining conditions
Pneumocystis pneumonia	Dry cough, shortness of breath, fever	Most common first serious AIDS-defining diagnosis; 80% of people with AIDS eventually develop pneumocystis pneumonia unless preventive medicine is taken
Kaposi's sarcoma	Purplish or black nodules on skin	Frequency is decreasing
Candidal esophagitis	Difficult or painful swallowing	20 to 30% of people with AIDS get candidal esophagitis; most common with thrush; same symptoms may be caused by other organisms
Cryptococcal meningitis	Severe headache & fever; may have double vision or stiff neck	8 to 10% of people with AIDS eventually get cryptococcal meningitis
Cryptosporidial diarrhea	Diarrhea for over one month	3 to 8% of people with AIDS eventually get cryptosporidial diarrhea
Cytomegalovirus infection spread throughout the body	Symptoms depend on location of the infection. Intestine: pain & diarrhea Lung: pneumonia Liver: hepatitis Eye: abnormal vision Blood: fever & malaise	80 to 90% of people with AIDS eventually develop this complication

(continued on next page)

Table 3. *(Continued)*

Condition	Symptoms	Comments
Mycobacterium avium infection throughout body	Symptoms depend on location of the infection. Intestine: pain & diarrhea Liver: hepatitis Lungs: pneumonia Blood: fever	30 to 50% of people with AIDS eventually develop this complication
Toxoplasma encephalitis	Headache, seizure, fever	5 to 15% of people with AIDS eventually get toxoplasma encephalitis, in the absence of preventive treatment
Herpes simplex	Blisters on skin lasting over 1 month, especially around anus, genitals, or mouth	10 to 25% of people with AIDS develop serious Herpes simplex infections
Tuberculosis	Cough, blood in sputum, shortness of breath, fever, weight loss	Tuberculosis rates are high in urban areas and among racial minorities and IV drug users
Wasting syndrome	Over 10% weight loss with diarrhea or fever lasting over 1 month	Becoming increasingly common as the initial AIDS-defining diagnosis
HIV-associated dementia	Memory loss, apathy, inability to concentrate, inability to control arms or legs	See discussion, Chapter 7; 20 to 30% of people with AIDS develop HAD
Lymphoma of brain	Seizure, impaired function of arm, leg, speech, etc.	Lymphoma of other parts of the anatomy may also indicate AIDS

HIV-Associated Dementia: HIV and the Central Nervous System

- Mental changes
- Attitude change
- Problems with self-care
- Motor problems
- To the caregiver

People with HIV infection often worry about dementia. In fact, people are sometimes so worried that every time they forget something or have trouble concentrating, they wonder if they are in the early stages of dementia. Many of these people can be reassured: losing memory and concentration is common and normal when people are also anxious, depressed, or overextended. Nearly everyone has, at one time or another, locked the keys in the car, forgotten an appointment, or been unable to pay attention to a TV show as a result of being stressed or worried. Usually, such lapses are temporary and a sign only of preoccupation.

HIV-associated dementia, usually shortened to HAD, used to be called AIDS dementia complex. HAD occurs in 30 to 50 percent of the people with HIV infection, usually in the late stages. The cause of HAD is not understood. Physicians who specialize in HAD suspect it is caused by HIV invading the brain directly. It is rare before the late stages of HIV infection. After the immune system is profoundly weakened, dementia becomes relatively common.

Dementia causes noticeable changes in a person's mental abilities, attitude, and muscle control. The changes usually follow a certain pattern. At first, people with HIV infection or their caregivers notice mental slowing: they say they are less "sharp," or they are "not as quick," or their thinking is "cloudier." They take longer to organize their thoughts, to respond to questions. They have some days of being slower, other days of being clear and sharp. Later, mental slowing progresses and can be accompanied by apathy and withdrawal. Most people with HAD eventually have problems controlling their muscles. They walk unsteadily, and they trip or fall easily; their legs are often weak. Their coordination is reduced, and they have problems with eating and writing. Eventually, people with HAD may progress rapidly to the point where they are totally withdrawn.

Some people with dementia experience a mild mental slowing that never becomes more serious; for these people, dementia has only a small impact on their lives. For others, dementia progresses rapidly and mental impairment is severe.

Someone with the symptoms of HAD should be examined and tested to exclude the possibility that the symptoms are caused by depression or by an infection of the central nervous system. Diagnosis of dementia will often be made by specialists: neurologists or AIDS physicians. The tests for dementia include a series of tests of mental abilities, a neurological examination, a spinal tap, and a brain scan. The purpose of the tests is to find out what the person can and cannot do mentally, to determine the severity of the dementia, and to exclude other causes—like cryptococcal meningitis, toxoplasmosis, or lymphoma of the brain—that could be causing the same symptoms.

So far, there is little in the way of specific therapy for HAD. AZT, unlike many antibiotics, does get into the brain. Furthermore, some studies have shown that AZT and other drugs will slow or prevent the onset of HAD. And AZT clearly helps some people who take it by slowing the course of the dementia. Antibiotics similar to AZT, which also inhibit the reproduction of HIV, might be similarly helpful in treating dementia, but they are still being studied.

A note of caution: For reasons medical scientists do not yet understand, most drugs that act on the central nervous system, including drugs for sleep, antidepressant drugs, and antianxiety drugs, have a greater than usual effect on people with dementia. These include alcohol and all benzodiazepines: Valium, Librium, Xanax, and Ativan. Physicians must be made aware of the diagnosis of HAD so they can prescribe and monitor drugs carefully.

People with a confirmed diagnosis of HAD need appropriate medical care for this and other aspects of HIV infection, need support in their living arrangements, and need to do some longterm planning. Making some decisions becomes necessary. Some of these decisions include assigning a durable power of attorney, writing wills, and writing living wills and a medical order not to resuscitate (see Chapter 10). They must also consider when to stop driving a car, especially if they feel their motor abilities or reaction times are impaired, or when they notice people blowing horns, or when they start getting tickets, or when they forget where they are, or because they worry about hurting others. They consider stopping work, especially if they think they are doing sloppy work or can't work as well or can't remember what they need to. Quitting work or stopping driving does not automatically mean that they are dependent and useless, or that life can't be enjoyable.

The rest of this section discusses in more detail the symptoms of HAD and the strategies people have worked out for living with those symptoms.

Mental Changes

Loss of Memory

The major change in mental abilities is an increase in forgetfulness, a loss of memory. People often have problems remembering only the recent past, not the distant past, and the problem is usually more annoying than profound. People nonetheless find it distressing. They can remember childhood experiences but not what they had for breakfast. They have trouble telling their doctors their recent histories. They forget why they entered a room, or where they parked the car, or what they wanted at the grocery store, or what they did that day. They forget appointments and become confused about time or place.

People deal with memory problems by finding ways around them. Dean Lombard, who kept forgetting to take his medication and to eat crackers before he took it, bought an inexpensive pillbox equipped with a beeper that beeped when he should eat, and then again when he was to take the medicine. Other people put their medications into pillboxes that are organized by days of the week. Lisa Pratt repeated anything she wanted her husband to remember several times over a period of days, and that seemed to help him retain it.

Some people keep lists, in notebooks or in pocket calendars, to remind themselves of calls they want to make or dates to keep or things to ask the doctor. Dean bought a memo book that fit in his shirt pocket. "I always carry it," he said. "I know enough to write something down immediately if I want to remember it: pick up the parts at Sears, pick up my mother. The minute I know, I write it down." In general, people try to limit the number of things they carry in their heads: "I don't deal with twenty things at once," said Dean.

Difficulty Concentrating

Another change in people's mental abilities is difficulty in concentrating. People's attention spans become short, and they have to work harder to follow the situation in a TV show or the plot in a book. They reread paragraphs and pages over and over. Conversation jumps from topic to topic with no transitions, or just stops in the middle. People seem not to be paying full attention to the conversation or seem to lose the train of thought in mid-sentence. They say their minds wander no matter what they're doing.

Difficulty with concentration also means that people become confused easily. They can't think of the time or the date. They can't seem to work out the steps of doing something. Mental tasks that were once routine—like balancing a checkbook or giving directions—take longer to do or become impossible to do. Someone may want to apply for disability insurance but not be able to think through how to do it. Someone can be worried about making plans for young children but be unable to make the plans.

Difficulty with concentration can be helped in several ways. One is by taking in only a limited amount of information at a time. When Lisa's husband wanted to read, he read only short pieces—newspaper articles, short stories, even the *TV Guide*. "If there's a book he wanted to read," she said, "I read it to him, one chapter at a time. After each chapter, we'd sit and talk about it. That would seem to get it into his mind." Dean noticed that if a doctor asked him several questions at once, he could not answer or his answer would be wrong. Lisa's husband had a similar problem: if she talked too fast, he couldn't understand. Instead, she'd talk slowly, sometimes write it down for him to read, and break up what she was saying into small parts. "He'd need me to have just one thought per sentence, not three or four thoughts per sentence," she said. "If I wanted to say to him that our friend called and wants to come over and borrow the lawnmower, I'd have to break it up. First I'd say, 'Barbara called.' Then I'd say, 'She's going to come over,' and we'd talk about that for a minute. Then I'd say, 'Her lawnmower's broken,' and we'd talk about that too. Then I'd say, 'She wants to borrow our lawnmower.' By that time, he could respond reasonably, something like, 'When will she bring it back?' If I didn't talk to him that way, he'd be lost."

Lisa's solution was a good one: talk slowly, in sentences with no more than one thought in them; discuss the thought a little to let it sink in, then go on to the next thought. In fact, Lisa even used the same method to have arguments with her husband. "One time I wanted to buy a new sofa," she said, "and he didn't. He couldn't argue with me very well, so one by one, I said all his reasons for not wanting one—I thought of it as starting his thought processes for him. Then I said all my reasons for wanting one. All this took two or three days. Then he finally said he didn't want a sofa, and I felt he really meant it and I had to go along with him."

Another effective way of helping someone with concentration problems is repetition and reminders. Repetition helps people understand something that seems complex and confusing. Lisa's husband used to watch John Wayne movies repeatedly; Lisa said she thought repetition was his way of understanding the movie. Dean was talking to his insurance agent one night and couldn't follow what the man was saying. Dean said to him over and over, "I can't picture in my mind what you're saying. Please tell me again." The agent repeated until Dean understood.

People having trouble concentrating also have trouble with generalizations: they need their information to be specific. "I'll see you this afternoon and we'll go out" is too general, leaves too many possibilities open. "I'll come to your house at 2:30; I'll drive you to the museum" is much clearer.

Attitude Change

The biggest change in people's attitudes is an increase in apathy. People with dementia gradually become less responsive, harder to talk to, emotionally flat. They lose interest in their jobs, their family and friends, their homes, even themselves. Perhaps some of the problems of memory loss and difficulty concentrating are caused by apathy. Lisa said her husband, Glen, lost his "sparkle" and became less affectionate, gave short answers to questions, and couldn't get interested in a conversation. She described a typical conversation: "I'd say, 'What are you thinking about?' He'd say, 'Nothing.' I'd say, 'What did you do today?' He'd say, 'Rested, watched TV, read the newspaper, that's about it.' I'd say, 'Anything interesting on the TV or in the paper?' He'd say, 'I can't say so.' I'd say, 'Are you hungry?' 'No.' 'Are you thirsty?' 'Hard to say.'"

Lisa's daughter agreed: "Dad was always happy to see me, but he'd lose interest. He was real dull, not enthusiastic about anything. He just seemed to go through the motions. When I'd call him on the phone, we'd talk a minute and he'd just hang up. We used to talk for a while. If I didn't call him, we wouldn't talk for a week." Caregivers routinely report that people with dementia seem content just to sit and stare.

When people are in the later stages of dementia, their apathy becomes even more distressing for the caregiver. People with dementia gradually become disconnected from the world, stop laughing or empathizing or showing affection, and finally become so disconnected that they will not speak.

Even though apathetic people seem depressed and unhappy, they say they are not. They are satisfied with their quietness. They are not sad, not frightened, not lonely, only disconnected.

In the early stages of HAD, people who are apathetic can often be drawn out. Mental health professionals say they do not know whether being drawn out decreases apathy or just makes the situation less distressing for the caregiver. In any case, they say, it can't hurt. Lisa found that trying to draw her husband out often helped: "I'd try to talk to Glen about recent events, or someone I saw that day, or what happened around the neighborhood. That often got him talking. When he became less affectionate with the grandchildren, I'd remind him of the good times we'd had with them, and then bring them over, one at a time, and that seemed to work. When he got less affectionate with me, I began sitting on the arm of his chair and snuggling against him, and he seemed to like that. Or I'd talk about our memories, like when we were dating or got married, and that got him talking too. But sometimes I just let him be disengaged. I think he needed some of it." Dean says he doesn't socialize well any more and that other people do more of the talking, though he enjoys listening to the talk. "But I can't handle strange social situations," he says, "no company picnics, no big parties."

Because people with dementia are both apathetic and have difficulty concentrating, they need help making decisions. They can't pay attention for long, they become confused, and they don't care much about the outcomes; as a result, they make decisions slowly or not at all. Lisa's husband needed several days to make a decision. "If a friend called and asked us to eat dinner that night," she said, "he couldn't answer because he couldn't make a decision that fast. In those cases, I made the decisions. When the decision was important or when we had two or three days to make it, then he could make up his mind."

When the decision is important—like deciding when to apply for disability insurance or how to provide for children—the person with dementia has difficulty both making the decision and acting on it. Caregivers need to present the options one by one, slowly, discussing each one, the way Lisa did with the decision to lend the lawnmower. They should repeat the options until the person with dementia understands, even if that takes days or weeks: "Should the child live with your mother? Your sister? Should the child be adopted?" Once the person has made the decision, caregivers need to write down the list of things to do, the steps to take, one simple step at a time. If the person seems to have trouble carrying out the decision, the caregiver should remind him: "We talked about this and I know you want it done. Shall I call the lawyer for you? Shall we do it together tomorrow? Shall I come over at ten?" Decisions may need to be repeated, gently and sympathetically, for days.

Problems with Self-Care

Along with apathy come problems with self-care. Eating, drinking, dressing, and staying clean all come to mean less and less. "Some days I'd come home from work," said Lisa, "and he'd be sitting in a hot house in the middle of summer with the windows closed, no fan on, and he hadn't eaten all day, or just ate junk food. Once I made hard-boiled eggs and he made himself an egg-salad sandwich. But usually if I made extra for supper so he could heat it up the next day, he forgot it, or would think cupcakes were easier."

Eating and drinking are the most immediate problems with self-care, because people with AIDS need to eat good meals. People with dementia lose the internal drive to eat and drink. Lisa complained that she made food for her husband, then asked him if he'd eaten. Her husband would say he had, that it was easy and all he had to do was put the food Lisa left him into the microwave. But in fact, Lisa's husband did not eat—somehow, he couldn't think of the steps involved in taking the food out of the refrigerator, putting it into the microwave, taking it back out, and eating it. Or else he didn't notice he was hungry or didn't care. Caregivers have to try reminders—to make phone calls or set up routine supper dates. They also need to make eating and drinking as convenient as possible—a dorm-sized refrigerator or a cooler full of juices and snacks by the bed keeps food and drink within easy reach.

Staying clean can also be a problem. "Sometimes my husband was not as clean as he should have been, and would go days without a bath," Lisa said. "He'd say, 'I don't need a bath,' and would resist my reminding." Lisa found that the only thing that got him into the bathtub was bribery. "Compliments didn't work," she said. "Sweet talk did sometimes. But bribery was the best. He'd need to see some concrete benefit—I'd usually bribe him with bread pudding. I'd say, 'I've got some bread pudding in the kitchen. Why don't you get a bath, and put on your robe, and we'll eat that bread pudding?'" Other people are not as resistant to bathing as Lisa's husband and will respond to "You haven't had your usual bath. Need any help?"

Making certain the person changes clothes regularly can be accomplished easily: clothes that have been worn can simply be put in the laundry and fresh clothes set out. "Every morning I'd lay his clothes out," said Lisa, "and every night I'd throw them in the hamper. Otherwise, he wore the same clothes."

Sometimes, in the later stages of dementia, apathy gets the better of the person in the midst of bathing or dressing. Lisa would put her husband in the shower and he would not bother to come out. Or she'd help him with one sleeve of a shirt, and he would not put his arm in the other sleeve. Sometimes people seem to lose their sense of modesty and don't dress appropriately. At these stages, the caregiver needs to be around fairly constantly, and to remind or help the person to finish up the process that was started.

Motor Problems

Another effect the virus has on the brain is to cause motor problems. People begin to drop things, their handwriting deteriorates, their hands tremble. Their legs get weak, they have difficulty walking, and they lose their balance easily. Lisa's husband, whose hobby was carving wood ducks, "couldn't get the feathers right any more," Lisa said. For a while he carved things with less detail, and finally he had to stop carving.

For quite a while, these motors problems are extremely annoying but not disabling. Certainly, however, at this point, people stop driving cars. In the later stages of HAD, people can't use drinking glasses or spoons, can't dress themselves or button a shirt. People begin to live on one floor of their homes, or mostly in one room. They keep their clothes in one closet, keep food nearby.

Incontinence

A related problem in the later stages of dementia is bathroom behaviors. One effect the virus has on the brain is to reduce the sensation of needing to go to the bathroom. The necessary signals don't get through, and the brain doesn't know when the bladder is full. Caregivers describe how accidents often occur; they take the person they're helping to the bathroom, leaving the person there until he says he's finished, and help him back to bed—and then he wets the bed. Eventually, people with HAD become incontinent and lose control of their bladders and bowels. Again, this is a result of changes in the central nervous system and is not something the person has any control over. Caregivers should try not to take this personally. Urinals and bedpans and bedside commodes should be kept nearby. Some people will need diapers, which are readily available in drugstores and hospital supply stores.

This form of advanced HAD is not common, but it requires extraordinary compassion and understanding from caregivers.

To the Caregiver

To a caregiver, these symptoms—forgetfulness, lack of concentration, apathy, lack of self-care—often seem to be an emotional response to having AIDS. Caregivers often believe the symptoms would clear up if the person just paid attention, just cheered up a little, just got involved, just tidied up, just tried a little harder. But these symptoms are not an emotional response to the disease; they are the disease itself. The virus is affecting the parts of the brain responsible for attention, interest, and memory. The person with the virus cannot control its effects.

Because the person with HAD has less control, caregivers should try hard not to take away whatever sense of control the person has left. This means finding the line between helping someone out and taking away his initiative. Caregivers have had to find this line all through the course of the disease, but it may be more difficult now. People with dementia can change from day to day. Sometimes they seem unable to care for themselves, sometimes they are the people they've always been: "I never knew when the dementia was going to be there," said Lisa. Caregivers say it's like being on a rollercoaster. They have to assess from day to day what the person they're caring for needs and does not need them to do.

Though dementia makes it more difficult to balance helping with taking away control, the same principles apply as in other aspects of the infection (see Chapter 5). Probably the most important principle is to allow the person to set the limits on what he can and cannot do. "My A-number-one priority was, my husband felt in control," said Lisa. Lisa's husband resented it if she tried to fix household machines, so she stopped trying, and although he took all day and the lawnmower never worked quite the same afterwards, he did fix it. "I found that he worked around a lot of his own impairment," she said.

Later on in the course of the dementia, when apathy and motor problems are more severe, caregivers take over more and more responsibility. They find that people with dementia seem to do best in an environment of structure and routine: eight o'clock is always breakfast, nine o'clock is always bath; sweaters are always on the top shelf; Fred comes to visit on Tuesdays. They find that they feel better if they try to stimulate or divert the person with dementia, and the person with dementia seems to act better. They talk about the day's events, turn on the radio, watch TV together. Caregivers gradually come to terms with the reality of the limitations of the person they're caring for. "I learned to accept his apathy," said Lisa. "When it was important, *I* did it. If not, I let it go."

Eventually, accepting the limitations of the person with dementia means being a full-time caregiver. The people with dementia can finally no longer stay home alone—they fall downstairs or burn themselves in the kitchen or wander out of the house. Eventually, caring for a person with dementia is like caring for a small child.

Rarely, the person becomes extremely agitated or frightened or convinced that people are trying to hurt him; he may start hearing voices. In that case, call your physician, who will call a psychiatrist or neurologist to assist in selecting medications to control these symptoms.

All this is hard on the caregiver. Lisa said she felt her husband was disengaging from her: "I took it personally at first, though I knew he was just more apathetic and withdrawn. I felt like I was going through a divorce. So many of the things we used to do to feel close, he lost interest in. I was really hurt by that. It was hard to get past this."

Lisa and other caregivers gradually began taking on the role of parent, and gradually began living as though they were single. Lisa joined AAA to get the car fixed, and she took out a maintenance plan on the furnace. Now, especially, caregivers need to surround themselves with people who give them sympathy and support. Much of the course of dementia is harder for the caregiver than for the person with dementia. Caregivers need to remember that a person with dementia is not feeling lonely or rejected; he or she seems untroubled and truly content to look out the window. When caregivers need to go to work, or take a break, or continue their lives, they can forgive themselves.

Most caregivers will need to use such outside resources as community-based health organizations or AIDS-advocacy organizations that provide patient services. Many will benefit from support groups intended for caregivers. Support groups offer the opportunity to talk with others who face similar situations, and to learn of special resources or techniques that have helped others in similar circumstances. Social workers provide special expertise on programs like occupational therapy and day care services, which occupy the person with dementia and give caregivers a break.

Some of these resources are available through public funds for people with HIV infection, some are available from insurance plans, and some are available from volunteers at community-based health organizations. The individual needs and resources available to each caregiver are highly variable. What is clear is that the caregiver of the person with advanced HAD, no matter how committed and loving, needs respite, assistance, and resources.

Some will find that their desire to achieve a structured and caring environment in the home is simply unrealistic. Similar structure and care can then be achieved in nursing homes or hospices.

Chapter 8

Options for Medical Care: Medical Personnel and Procedures

- Limits on your options for medical care
- Physicians
- Comprehensive care programs
- Case management
- Hospital care
- Glossary of hospital people and practices
- Patients' rights in hospitals
- Alternatives to hospital care

A person with HIV infection is confronted with questions about medical care that are as confusing as they are important. What kind of physicians treat HIV infection? What kind of medical care is available? What kind of hospital provides the best care? This chapter outlines the options for medical care available to a person with HIV infection and provides some general guidelines for people considering those options; provides a general guide to hospitals and describes the rights people have when they are patients in a hospital; and outlines the alternatives to hospitalization.

In general, medical care is provided by different kinds of people offering different services in different settings. The providers of medical care are professionals: they are physicians, physician's assistants, and nurse practitioners. The setting in which care is provided can generally be divided into two components: *outpatient facilities* and *inpatient facilities*. Outpatient facilities are individual physicians' offices, clinics staffed by physicians who practice as a group, Health Maintenance Organizations (HMOs), and public health department clinics. Inpatient facilities, which are primarily hospitals and nursing homes, are generally used by people who need more intensive care.

In recent years, because hospital care in the United States is now enormously expensive, there has been a growing demand for alternatives to hospitals. These alternatives now include chronic care facilities (like nursing homes), home care programs, hospice care facilities and programs, and outpatient clinics. Some of the alternatives provide the services—including transfusions and other infusion services and same-day surgery—previously provided only in hospitals.

Financing for this complex network of resources varies: the principal modes of funding are Blue Cross/Blue Shield and other insurance companies, HMOs, self-pay, and the government programs for assistance with medical bills (Medicaid and Medicare). Chapter 10 will discuss how to finance medical care—since financing is obviously a major factor in deciding which option to choose.

Regardless of which option for medical care you choose, it is important to have:

—a close physician-patient relationship;

—the services of medical specialists as they are needed;

—the services of psychiatrists, psychologists, or support groups as they are needed;

—emergency medical services;

—a hospital with appropriate resources;

—such alternatives to hospital care as home therapy, chronic care facilities, and hospice care.

It is particularly important to have access to a physician or hospital or clinic that will provide the special medical resources and skills needed to treat people with HIV infection. The treatment of HIV infection is a fast-moving field: medical therapy now makes a substantial difference in the progress of the disease, and new treatments are continually being developed.

Limits on Your Options for Medical Care

Your options for medical care will depend on where you live. The kind of care specific to HIV infection is likely to be better in a big city: most big cities offer many options for treatment of HIV infection. Smaller cities and rural areas are likely to offer fewer options, and the physicians in these areas are likely to be less familiar with HIV infection. This is because most of the people who became infected in the early stages of this epidemic lived primarily in large cities like New York, San Francisco,

Los Angeles, Miami, and Washington, D.C.; disproportionately fewer people living in smaller cities and rural areas were infected. As a result, physicians who trained or who practice in small cities or rural areas often lack experience in treating HIV infection.

As a consequence, when people with HIV infection who live in small cities and rural areas want medical treatment or periodic consultation about medical treatment, they often travel to the nearest physician or clinic specializing in HIV infection (see below, under "Choosing a Physician"). Some people also travel to more distant clinics or physicians to get the anonymity they cannot get locally.

The options for medical care may be substantially fewer for people who belong to HMOs, for people receiving Medicaid, and for people who have limited financial resources and no health insurance. HMOs and city health clinics offer medical services that vary in quality, some very good and some not so good. Large urban areas have Title 1, 2, and 3 grants with federal funds from the Ryan White Act to provide medical care and support services for people with HIV infection. The range of services offered and the quality of those services are both variable. Most people served under this act are uninsured or underinsured and have limited financial resources. Some HMOs do not allow patients to see physicians other than those physicians who participate in the HMO, or do so only on a case-by-case basis. People enrolled in those HMOs therefore have no choice in what specialists they see. HMOs can also limit the hospitals people may be admitted to.

The process of selecting among medical options begins with finding out what your finances allow and what publicly funded resources are available. This disease is expensive, and HMOs, insurance plans, and Medicaid will each pay for some things and not for others. In addition, HMOs, insurance plans, and Medicaid all differ in what they will and will not pay for. Many insurance plans especially restrict the outpatient services they cover. Medicaid covers a broad range of services but reimburses physicians at so low a rate that most physicians refuse to accept patients paying through Medicaid. Many employers offer a choice between joining an HMO or being reimbursed by the insurance company, and you may be able to switch back and forth as your needs dictate. In any case, you need to know your options. You can begin by finding out what your HMO, insurance company, or government medical assistance will allow (see Chapter 10), and then discussing these issues candidly with your physician or with a social worker.

Physicians

Most people receive medical care for HIV infection from one or more kinds of physicians: primary care physicians, AIDS physicians, and specialists.

Primary Care Physicians

Primary care physicians are usually family practice physicians or internists who have broad medical knowledge, and who may or may not have a special interest in HIV infection. Many people have gone to their primary care physicians for medical care for years and have developed close relationships with them. For a person with HIV infection, however, whether this relationship continues depends on whether the primary care physician feels able or willing to care for HIV infection and how much confidence the person with HIV infection has in the adequacy of that care.

Some primary care physicians practice in groups of between three and ten. Physicians in such groups usually have different areas of expertise: some treat stomach problems, for example, and some treat lung problems. The person with HIV infection will usually see the same physician for general health care, but will see other physicians for specific problems. The advantage of group practice is that these physicians are all under the same roof, and communication between physicians with specializations is good. Group practice is especially useful when one member of the group becomes skilled in AIDS care and becomes the primary physician or a consultant for people with HIV infection.

Most primary care physicians, whether they practice alone or in groups, received their training before HIV infection was known. Furthermore, new diagnostic tests and drugs and other therapies emerge constantly, so that many physicians have found it difficult to maintain their knowledge of both this field and the rest of medicine as well. As a result, some primary care physicians simply do not accept patients with HIV infection and will refer their previous patients who have become infected with HIV to another physician. Other primary care physicians provide medical care during early stages of the infection when medical complications are few and the guidelines for treatment are relatively simple.

During later stages of infection, the primary care physician will often either refer the person with HIV infection to a specialist or consult with a physician more experienced in HIV infection. If the primary care physician is in group practice, the referral may be to another physician in the group; if the physician practices alone, the referral may be to a completely different physician, to a clinic specializing in the care of HIV infection, or to a teaching hospital (see below). In any case, the person with HIV infection will often see physicians informally called AIDS physicians.

AIDS Physicians

AIDS physicians are physicians who devote most of their time to caring for people with HIV infection. By strict definition of the word *specialist* there is no such person as an "AIDS specialist": rather, some physicians simply adopt the treatment of AIDS and HIV infection as a special interest.

A little background on what makes a specialist:

Physicians practice in a variety of specialties, including family practice, pediatrics, internal medicine, surgery, and obstetrics and gynecology. Becoming a physician requires graduating from medical school, doing postgraduate training as a resident, passing standard tests, and getting a license through the state licensing board. By law, a physician requires a license to practice medicine. The type of postgraduate training determines the specialty.

Becoming a certified specialist requires certification by a professional specialty board within the American Board of Medical Specialties. Certification requires postgraduate training for a specified number of years in an approved training program, followed by passing an examination in the specialty called a *board examination.* To be certified as a cardiologist, for example, the physician must take three years of postgraduate training in internal medicine, then pass the board examinations to be certified as a specialist in internal medicine, then take three additional years of postgraduate training in cardiology, and then pass the board examinations in cardiology to be certified in cardiology. Any physician can claim to be a cardiologist, but only those who satisfy these requirements can call themselves board-certified cardiologists.

There are no recognized accredited training programs for specializing in HIV infection and no board examinations to certify competence in treatment of HIV infection. This means there is no medical specialty in HIV infection, and there is not likely be one in the foreseeable future. Instead, physicians with different kinds of training and with different specialties have adopted AIDS as a special interest. To repeat, these are physicians informally called AIDS physicians.

The specialty that has provided most of the AIDS physicians is infectious diseases, which, like cardiology, is a subspecialty of internal medicine. Specialists in infectious diseases become AIDS physicians because HIV infection is an infectious disease, and because most of the opportunistic infections are those commonly encountered during infectious disease training. Some specialists in infectious diseases primarily treat people with HIV infection; some treat people with other infectious diseases plus people with HIV infection. Most infectious disease specialists have the appropriate expertise to treat people with HIV infection.

Other medical specialties also supply AIDS physicians. Some specialists treat AIDS because of the nature of their specialties: oncology, pulmonary medicine, dermatology. Others, like gay physicians, treat AIDS for more personal reasons.

AIDS physicians keep current with this fast-moving field by attending medical meetings dealing with HIV infection and by subscribing to several of the forty to sixty medical journals devoted to HIV infection. Their practices may be limited almost exclusively to people with HIV infection, and they are themselves often leaders in the community in social, medical, and political issues that relate to HIV infection.

Treatment of HIV infection has attracted some of the country's most competent and compassionate physicians. It has also attracted some physicians who promote what many other physicians would consider ill-advised or even risky treatments. Remember, any physician can claim to be an AIDS physician, and no reputable professional group has certification requirements to substantiate the claim.

Unfortunately, at present, the numbers of AIDS physicians are inadequate to serve the increasing numbers of people with HIV infection. As a result, many people with HIV infection receive medical care from primary care physicians who call on AIDS physicians to help with the more difficult complications of the disease. The greatest liability in this plan is that general practitioners may not be able to provide state-of-the-art care in a disease for which management guidelines seem to change every month.

Other Specialists

HIV infection directly or indirectly affects virtually every organ of the body, and no physician, regardless of training, can alone treat all the conditions associated with HIV infection. As a result, people with HIV infection, especially people with AIDS, are likely to be referred to such specialists as neurologists, psychiatrists, oncologists, gastroenterologists, ophthalmologists, dermatologists, and pulmonary specialists. Referrals to such specialists almost always come from the primary care physician or the AIDS physician. These physicians will select specialists based on the reputation of the specialist within the medical community, on their previous interactions with the specialist, and on the specialist's specific interest or expertise in AIDS.

Choosing a Physician

What is the best way for someone with HIV infection to go about selecting a physician? Begin by asking your primary care physician if he or she feels comfortable caring for a person with HIV infection. If not, ask for an appropriate referral: the medical community has an effective communication network, and your physician will either know or can easily find out who has a good reputation within the profession for the care of people with HIV infection. Physicians are the best source of advice about other physicians.

If you do not already have a primary care physician, another source of information is by word of mouth from other people with HIV infection, although some caution is called for here: watch out for people who confuse medical competence with a good bedside manner. What impresses patients and what impresses physicians are often quite different, and your highest priority is competent and comprehensive care.

Other sources are AIDS hotlines, community organizations devoted to AIDS, nurses, and the centers that run tests for antibodies to HIV. The yellow pages may have listings for physicians with a special interest in AIDS, but the relevant listings are more likely to be of physicians specializing in infectious diseases. You can then contact the infectious disease specialists directly and ask for either an appointment or a referral; they will know well the available local resources for treating HIV infection. City, county, and state medical societies often have lists of physicians with specialized interests; however, these lists may reflect those who have paid their dues and need the patients, rather than those who offer high-quality services.

In general, to choose a physician, ask another physician, check certification, be cautious about a physician who advertises medical services, find out his or her reputation among their peers, and look for a physician who has privileges to admit patients to a good hospital. Hospitals review physicians carefully before allowing them the privilege of admitting patients, and hospitals of good quality will accept only reputable physicians.

Some people with HIV infection select an AIDS physician for conditions related to HIV infection, and continue to see their primary care physicians for all other conditions. To repeat, primary care physicians are increasingly treating people with HIV infection during the earlier stages and calling in infectious disease specialists or AIDS physicians when treatment becomes more complicated or specialized. Either plan for medical care is appropriate if the care offered keeps pace with rapidly evolving developments.

Regardless of what kind of physician you see or where you live, if you have questions about your medical care, you can ask for a second opinion or get a consultation with another physician. That is, you can go to another physician or clinic that specializes in the treatment of AIDS and ask to have the program of your medical care reviewed. To have the program reviewed thoroughly, you need to bring (or send) copies of all your hospital records and your physician's office records. These records will include the results of x-rays, scans, biopsies, and any other tests, plus the diagnoses and treatments. This not only simplifies the consultation but prevents unnecessary duplication of visits or tests.

You need not worry that you will offend your own physician by asking for such a consultation. In normal medical practice, second opinions are often encouraged and, for many procedures, are sometimes required. Moreover, given the seriousness of HIV infection and the speed with which recommendations for treatment change, second opinions are often considered a very good idea.

Comprehensive Care Programs

Some hospitals, clinics, and HMOs, especially those in large urban areas, have comprehensive programs of care tailored to the specific needs of people with HIV infection. The goal of comprehensive care programs is to provide all the care needed by a person with HIV infection in one setting and under one roof.

The type and extent of services provided, and the type of specialists available, vary from one program to another. The people and programs in comprehensive care programs can include HIV counselors, medical specialists, support groups, home therapy programs, dietitians, psychologists and psychiatrists, social workers, case managers, hospice care programs, drug rehabilitation programs, and dental care. Most comprehensive care programs will have some but not all of these services.

HIV counselors are specifically trained to provide information about HIV infection, especially information about the progress of the disease, the meaning of a positive blood test, and information on preventing transmission. These counselors also give advice on where, in a local community, to go for legal advice, for financial advice, and for personal planning services.

Medical specialists associated with a comprehensive care program are the same experts a primary care physician is likely to consult about some of the complications of HIV infection that require specialized knowledge or a specialized procedure. The specialists most likely to be consulted are neurologists (brain and nerves), ophthalmologists (eyes), gastroenterologists (intestines), dermatologists (skin), oncologists (tumors), psychiatrists (mind), obstetricians (pregnancy), gynecologists (women's health), and pulmonary physicians (lungs). The specialist in a comprehensive care program may deal primarily with the specialty as it applies to HIV infection. That is, instead of a gastroenterologist who deals with all problems of the digestive system, you may find one who has a special interest in the gastroenterological problems of people with HIV infection.

Support groups offer, to a person with HIV infection, emotional support in the company of people facing similar problems (see Chapter 12). The support groups are ideally made up of no more than five to eight people affected by HIV infection who have common interests and concerns. The groups are often led by a mental health professional. The benefit of a support group is sharing experiences and problems—medical and nonmedical—that are not easily shared with others.

Home therapy programs extend comprehensive services to the person's home. These services are most useful to the person whose physical condition is stable and who may be staying in the hospital only to receive certain types of treatment, like intravenous drugs. Nurses working in home therapy programs can give intravenous drug treatments, can draw blood for necessary laboratory tests, and do general nursing care—all at home, and all much less expensively than in the hospital. In most instances, the person with HIV infection or the caregiver is taught how to administer the drugs intravenously by him- or herself, so that visits by a trained professional are few. This style of giving intravenous drugs may sound somewhat risky, but it has now become commonplace in medical practice.

A dietitian's job is to help people with HIV infection solve the eating problems which can interfere with proper nourishment. Eating problems may result from depression, altered taste, opportunistic infections in the mouth or swallowing tube (esophagus), side effects from medications, dental problems, severe diarrhea, or HIV itself. Dietitians teach people with eating problems how to deal more effectively with nutritional needs depending on the cause of the problem.

Psychologists and psychiatrists treat the array of emotional difficulties that face people with HIV infection. Some of these difficulties are serious, some short-lived; some are treatable with medications, some are best treated by talking them out. Psychological social workers, psychologists, and psychiatrists—three kinds of mental health professionals who provide somewhat different services—can determine the severity of the emotional difficulty and can decide on the best course of treatment (see Chapter 12, under "Mental Health Professionals").

Social workers and case managers help sort out many of the nonmedical problems people with HIV infection face: dealing with hospitals and insurance companies, keeping finances straight, sorting out living arrangements, and much more (see the sections in this chapter on case management and on social workers).

The services offered in comprehensive care programs are more likely to be extensive in metropolitan areas and in hospitals or clinics that serve large numbers of people with HIV infection. Some people, especially those in the early stages of the infection, have no need for such a complex network of services. Some AIDS physicians work in private offices but have established a network of referrals that is comparable to a comprehensive care program. Some people with HIV infection prefer the simplicity of a single physician; others prefer the availability of many specialized services. The people who most benefit from the advantages of a comprehensive care program are either those who need more complicated and specialized care or those whose primary care physicians are uncomfortable treating many of the complications of HIV infection.

Case Management

Case managers are usually social workers or public health nurses who help coordinate the lives of people with HIV infection. People with HIV infection are in extraordinary need of help with work, home life, medical care, medical insurance, legal issues, finances, and psychological problems. Furthermore, people with HIV infection are subject to so many sudden changes in health that planning becomes difficult. Fortunately, the complexity of their needs has been recognized, and increasing numbers of organizations, programs, and other resources now satisfy these needs. The quality and quantity of these resources vary. Case management is a way of linking the people with HIV infection to the resources in their own communities.

Working together with medical care providers, case managers commonly make two plans for each person with HIV infection: a medical care plan and a social work plan. The medical care plan includes plans for a range of continuing medical services, including home care, care in a clinic, hospital, nursing home, or hospice, and, when necessary, care in an addiction program or a mental health program. The social work plan includes financial plans, insurance benefits, benefits from publicly funded programs, resources for drugs, housing plans, and employment plans. The social work plan also links the person with HIV infection to community organizations that provide such services as support groups, home health care, companionship, meals in the home, and the like.

The primary goal of the case manager is to be an advocate for the person with HIV infection. This means obtaining for the person with HIV infection all the services that are available and appropriate. A second goal is to obtain the best services at the lowest price. In short, a case manager knows the system, and his or her job is to make the best use of it.

Case management services are sometimes funded by state health departments, by other sources of public funds, or by foundations. Insurance companies will sometimes pay for case management services. You can find out how to arrange funding for case management services by talking to the case manager or to a social worker.

Both the availability and the quality of case management services vary widely in different communities. Some are not run as well as others. Some may not be networked into both the agencies that provide social services and the agencies that provide health care services for people with HIV infection. And even those that seem to be run well and be well networked are difficult to evaluate. Case management has been used to care for the elderly, for the mentally ill, and for crippled children; evaluations of the usefulness of these programs have been quite variable. As for HIV infection, there is probably no other disease in medicine where the fundamental philosophy of case management is more sound, at least in theory. In practice, it is not clear that case management has successfully achieved any of its major goals: improved quality of life, prolonged survival, or reduced cost of care.

Case managers can increasingly be found not only in comprehensive care programs but also in hospitals, clinics, state or city health departments, and community organizations dedicated to HIV infection. To find a case manager, ask if your hospital employs a case manager, and if not, if it will refer you to one. AIDS physicians and social workers will also know the names of the good case managers.

Hospital Care

Most people with HIV infection are admitted to a hospital at some time during the course of the infection; most will be hospitalized two to four times, spending an average of thirty to sixty days, total, in the hospital. They may or may not have a choice of what hospitals they are admitted to. As discussed in a later section, the choice is largely dictated by the type of insurance they have and the hospitals to which their physicians have admitting privileges. People are often frightened about going to a hospital—to be sure, hospitals are confusing places. This section discusses hospitals, and their people and practices, in an attempt to lessen the fear and confusion.

Teaching and Community Hospitals

Hospitals differ in the services provided and the style of care. One of the biggest differences is between teaching hospitals and community hospitals. Teaching hospitals are generally larger hospitals that provide on-the-job training for medical residents and often for medical students as well. Teaching hospitals are often affiliated with medical schools, the physicians are often on the medical school faculty, and physicians may be responsible both for patient care and for research programs.

The advantage of teaching hospitals is that their resources for testing and treatment are both extensive and up to date. This is important in a field that changes as rapidly as research in the treatment of HIV infection. Teaching hospitals are also more likely to have comprehensive programs for the care of people with HIV infection. A survey of physicians by *U.S. News and World Report* in 1992 showed that all the top-ranked hospitals for the care of AIDS were teaching hospitals. In order of rank, they were: San Francisco General Hospital, Massachusetts General Hospital in Boston, the Johns Hopkins Hospital in Baltimore, the UCLA Medical Center in Los Angeles, the University of California San Francisco Medical Center, Memorial Sloan Center in New York City, and the National Institutes of Health in Washington, D.C. This list is of particular interest because it was made up by physicians; these are the hospitals the physicians themselves would choose for AIDS care.

Community hospitals tend to be smaller hospitals with fewer resources and whose staff physicians often have less experience with HIV infection. Nevertheless, many community hospitals have devoted physicians who provide excellent care in an environment less overwhelming than that of a large teaching hospital.

Experience counts, however. Surveys of hospitals caring for people with HIV show that survival is better and the length of stay is shorter in hospitals which treat many people with HIV, compared to hospitals which treat few people with HIV infection. Still, there is no doubt that many of the common complications of HIV infection can be easily managed in a community hospital.

AIDS Units

Many hospitals, both community hospitals and teaching hospitals, have established specialized units, informally called AIDS units or wards, for people hospitalized with HIV infection. AIDS units usually deal with all facets of care: they offer not only medical expertise but also social services, psychological support, advice on nutrition, addiction services, and access to AIDS-advocacy groups. In short, they offer the same services to someone in the hospital that comprehensive care programs (discussed previously in this chapter) offer to an outpatient. In many instances, the AIDS unit is part of a comprehensive care program.

The person on an AIDS unit will receive a level of expert medical care not generally available to a person with AIDS on, for example, a general medical ward. This care will often include services—like education, nutrition, social work, substance abuse counseling, and support groups—that are tailored specifically to people with HIV infection. In addition, the people providing the care on an AIDS unit have specifically chosen to work with people with HIV infection. The principal disadvantage to being on an AIDS unit is that your diagnosis is obvious to visitors. Hospitals with AIDS units usually offer the person the option of care on this unit or care elsewhere in the hospital.

Choosing a Hospital

For many people with HIV infection, choice of a hospital is limited. Participants in HMOs are required to use specific hospitals. People from small cities or from rural areas often have only one hospital near enough to choose. In medical emergencies, a public ambulance is required to take the patient to the nearest hospital, leaving the family and the patient little say in the matter, unless they hire a private ambulance.

In most instances, the physician responsible for the care of the person with HIV infection will make a recommendation depending on which hospital has the resources necessary for that person, and in which hospital the physician has admitting privileges (meaning the physician is allowed to admit and treat patients).

A large teaching hospital might best be chosen by a person who has unusual complications that require specialized services. If you have a strong wish to go to a certain hospital, you should tell your physician. In the event that your physician is not on the admitting staff of that hospital, he or she can transfer your medical care to another physician.

Glossary of Hospital People and Practices

Both teaching and community hospitals present the patient with a bewildering array of people with different titles offering different services. Hospitals also follow certain practices that may likewise be confusing. The following glossary of the people and practices a person in a hospital can expect to see might help eliminate some of this confusion.

Physician-of-Record

Your physician-of-record is the physician medically and legally responsible for your care—that is, for all medical recommendations, including decisions about diagnostic tests and about your treatment. Your physician-of-record is most often your primary care physician, but sometimes it is the physician assigned from the hospital staff. Even though you might see nurses and residents more often, the physician-of-record has ultimate responsibility for your medical care. Every person in a hospital has a physician-of-record.

Residents, Fellows, and Interns

Residents and fellows are physicians who have recently graduated from medical school but who are not yet practicing medicine on their own. Residents are still in residency, that is, they are still in training to obtain their credentials in a specialty, usually in family practice or internal medicine. Most residents receive three years of training. Fellows are physicians who have finished their residency training and are now training in a subspecialty—for example, infectious diseases. As for nomenclature, "interns" are now called "first-year residents." Residents and fellows are found in teaching hospitals that have the credentials for training specialists.

If you are in a teaching hospital, the physicians you are likely to see most often are residents in internal medicine or family practice, and fellows in infectious diseases or some other subspecialty. Their autonomy in making decisions about your medical care varies, depending on their training, the rules of the hospital, and the idiosyncrasies of the physician-of-record.

Specialists

In addition to the physician-of-record, the residents, and the fellows, the other physicians you will see in a hospital are the specialist physicians. Because AIDS affects so many different parts of the body, and because it takes so many forms in so many different people, no single physician can treat all aspects of the disease. Specialists (technically, these are subspecialists) that are most likely to be consulted in HIV infection are neurologists, ophthalmologists, gastroenterologists, obstetricians, dermatologists, psychiatrists, and pulmonary specialists. Each has a specific area of expertise that may be sought by the physician-of-record. In most instances these specialists make recommendations or provide special procedures. The person ultimately responsible for carrying out their recommendations and approving their procedures is the physician-of-record.

Physician's Assistants and Nurse Practitioners

Physician's assistants and nurse practitioners are midlevel practitioners, meaning that their responsibilities lie somewhere between those of a nurse and those of a physician. Midlevel practitioners assess medical problems, order tests, and recommend treatments. They work with varying degrees of independence, depending on state laws, the medical problems they care for, and their relationship with the other health care providers.

Midlevel practitioners often have specialized training in one area of medical care, including care of people with HIV infection. They are especially valuable in highly specialized areas of medical care because they have often acquired, through training and experience, an expertise not usually found among physicians who care for people with many different diseases. Many comprehensive care programs for people with HIV infection rely heavily on midlevel practitioners.

Physician's assistants have two years of specialized training, must pass a board exam every six years, are required to have at least one hundred hours of postgraduate education every two years, and are licensed. Physician's assistants must practice under the supervision of a physician. They may prescribe drugs in some states but not in others.

Nurse practitioners are registered nurses who have nine additional months of advanced training or have received a master's degree in nursing. Nurse practitioners do much of what physician's assistants do, but they are not required to serve under direct supervision of a licensed physician.

Nurses

Registered nurses make certain kinds of medical assessments, including assessments of patients' medical conditions, their ability to provide self-care, their psychiatric needs, and their nutrition. Registered nurses also provide psychological support, are responsible for certain types of treatments, and administer medications. Nurses can also be valuable sources of information about your care: ask them questions.

All hospitals are required to have a registered nurse on each unit of the hospital twenty-four hours a day. Each patient in the hospital is assigned a nurse for every eight-hour shift.

Nursing support techniques, licensed practical nurses (LPNs), and nursing aides are paramedical personnel who are less extensively trained than registered nurses and do many of the jobs that were previously done by nurses: these include taking pulses and temperatures, measuring blood pressure, handing out medications, bathing the patient, changing beds, handling bedpans, and dressing wounds.

Social Workers

A social worker is a college graduate with two years of postgraduate training and a Master's of Social Work. Most states require these credentials for a license to practice social work. The actual graduate training is primarily devoted to counseling. In a hospital, a social worker's primary role is to help people plan what to do when they leave the hospital. These plans, called *discharge plans*, include making decisions and arrangements for nursing home placement, home care, and outpatient care.

Good social workers also get involved with much more. They arrange for such special services as rehabilitation from intravenous drug use, treatment of alcoholism, psychiatric care, physical rehabilitation, and contact with community organizations. The job of the social worker usually ends when the person is discharged from the hospital.

Social workers can be found not only in hospitals but also in clinics, in private practice, in community organizations devoted to HIV infection, and working as case managers assigned to an individual person. All U.S. hospitals that receive federal funds must have social workers; this means essentially that all hospitals have social workers, since Medicare and Medicaid fund so much of this country's health care in hospitals.

Information about social workers or case managers may be obtained through the hospital social worker, by referral from physicians, through contact with the local health department, or through the yellow pages of the telephone directory (listed under social workers, therapists, or counseling).

Patient Representatives

Many hospitals have a public relations office with patient representatives who serve as links between the hospital and the patients. Patient representatives have varied jobs: they answer questions about bills, provide translators for persons who speak foreign languages, provide clothing for those in need. Patient representatives also serve as a complaint department. People with complaints document their concerns in writing, and the patient representative tries to deal with these concerns to the satisfaction of all parties.

Rounds

Rounds is a well-established ritual in medicine in which physicians, nurses, and often other members of the care team go "around" to see the patients every day. At the turn of the century, rounds were very formal: a professor at a teaching hospital led a parade of residents, medical students, and nurses through the wards of the hospital, reviewing each patient, writing down the findings, discussing the patient's condition, and making plans. At present, rounds are much more informal. In teaching hospitals, the rounding team usually consists of residents, medical students, and nurses, with or without the physician-of-record. In community hospitals, rounds are simpler and usually involve the physician-of-record and sometimes a nurse. Rounds are traditionally held every morning, although many private physicians find it more convenient to round in the afternoon when test results are in hand and consultants are more likely to be available. Most agencies that fund medical care require that the physician see every patient under his or her care nearly every day of hospitalization.

For the person in the hospital, rounds are an opportunity to ask brief questions about progress and plans. Long discussions with more detailed questions are probably best asked in the more private company of the resident or the physician-of-record.

Universal Precautions

Universal precautions are a set of rules to protect health care workers from certain infectious diseases. Included among those diseases are HIV infection, hepatitis, and any other infectious disease transmitted through body fluids (blood, saliva, urine). All hospitals in the United States are required to practice universal precautions.

Though the rules of universal precaution apply to all body fluids, the major concern is for blood and bloody fluids. The rules require a barrier between the health care worker and the fluid. The barrier rule means that gloves are to be worn when dressing wounds and the like. Goggles, face shields, or similar devices may be used during procedures (like childbirth) that may result in splattering of blood. Hospital gowns must be worn when clothes might be soiled. For such day-to-day care as taking temperatures and blood pressure, no gloves or other barriers need be used.

It should be emphasized that universal precautions are universal. They apply to all people participating in the care of any patient in the hospital. There are *no* precautions that are special to people with HIV infection. Exceptions are the opportunistic infections—like salmonella, tuberculosis, and shingles—that pose a threat to health care workers. But these infections require the same precautions regardless of HIV status.

The Hospital Bill

The anticipated charge for the average private or semiprivate room in a private hospital is $350 to $600 a day (in 1990 dollars), but it can be over $1,000 in such large metropolitan areas as New York City. Intensive care units are usually $1,000 to $2,000 a day. Additional charges include medications, laboratory tests, physicians' fees, and specialized procedures like bronchoscopy or operations. The hospital bill is likely to be long and full of medical jargon with lists of numerical codes for every pill, syringe, gauze pad, and procedure. Physicians' fees are billed separately from the hospital bill, except for Medicaid patients. Insurance companies determine the customary and reasonable charges for both the hospital and the physician and, on that basis, make their payments. Questions about the hospital charges should be directed to the hospital billing office or to the patient representative. Questions about a physician's charges should be directed to the physician. If finances are going to be a problem, the person should inquire about charges for various tests and their alternatives before the tests are done.

Patients' Rights in Hospitals

The medical care system is large, complicated, overwhelming, and bewildering. Everyone who is a patient in the system has a right to have questions answered. Questions about medical care are best addressed to the medical care providers—the nurse or midlevel practitioner or physician. Questions about the medical system itself are best addressed to a patient representative (see above), a patient advocate now in most hospitals and in many of the larger clinics.

People who become patients in the medical care system have specific rights they should be aware of. The following is an adaptation and amplification of the "Patient's Bill of Rights" offered at the Johns Hopkins Hospital in Baltimore, Maryland.

1. The person should expect medical care regardless of race, color, religion, national origin, source of pay, or medical condition. Specifically, no one can be denied care because of HIV infection. Early in the AIDS epidemic, some hospitals and clinics avoided providing AIDS care, on the grounds that treating people with AIDS might deter other people from using that hospital or clinic. Much of this image

problem is now in the past, but people with HIV infection should nonetheless be aware of their right to medical care in hospitals.

2. The person should expect to be treated with respect. He or she should be addressed by proper names and not be treated with undue familiarity. He or she has the right to an appropriate response to questions.

3. People should expect privacy and confidentiality in all aspects of their care. This is an especially sensitive issue for people with HIV infection. Privacy and confidentiality have some limits, however. Important diagnoses such as HIV infection or the complications of HIV infection cannot be excluded from the medical record. Moreover, these medical records are available to those who have a justified need to see them, including physicians involved in the person's care, insurance companies, Medicaid/Medicare, HMOs, and public health officials. Furthermore, all cases of AIDS are reported, by law, to the Centers for Disease Control; and many states require that blood tests that are positive for HIV also be reported to state health departments. Although this is a sensitive issue, we are not aware of a breach of confidentiality that has ever occurred as a result of such reports. And hospitals take seriously their responsibility to protect medical records from people who have no need to see them (see Chapter 10 and "Understanding Tests for HIV," pages 299–301). Insurance companies have a justified right to this information and may use it to deny subsequent policies.

4. People should know the physician who is responsible for their care. They have the right to participate in decisions involving their medical care. These decisions should be based on a clear explanation of the medical condition, the proposed procedures, the proposed treatments, and the risks involved.

5. People should expect efficient and courteous attention from all hospital personnel. They should also respect the possibility that other patients' needs might be more urgent.

6. People have the right to be interviewed and examined in surroundings that assure privacy. They also have the right to know the role of any observer and to ask observers to leave. People also have the right to restrict visitors and can do this simply by notifying the nurse or physician responsible for their care.

7. Mentally competent people have the right to reject any form of proposed treatment or diagnostic test. In particular, many people have profound feelings about resuscitation and life support measures

like breathing machines or artificial kidney machines. Uncomfortable as this subject is, decisions about life support measures should not be left until the person is too ill to participate in a rational discussion. Preferences about such issues should be discussed candidly, at the appropriate time, and should be documented in the medical record, in a living will, and by assigning a durable power of attorney for health care. This hope of empowerment for life decisions is now mandated by the Patient Self-Determination Act (see Chapter 10). In the event that there are no such provisions, and the person is not capable of making medical decisions, this role is entrusted to a hierarchy of others, starting with a court-appointed legal guardian, then spouse, child over eighteen years, parent, or sibling (brother or sister), in that order (see Chapter 10).

8. People may be asked to participate in research projects called clinical trials (see Chapter 9, under "Experimental Drugs and Clinical Trials"). Clinical trials can involve people only with their written consent and with the approval of the person's physician. Furthermore, once involved in a clinical trial, the person has the right to discontinue participation at any time.

9. People have the right to unrestricted communication with anyone. This includes physicians, lawyers, clergy, and representatives of AIDS-advocacy groups.

10. People may leave the hospital against the advice of their doctors at any time. They will usually need to sign a form entitled "Discharge Against Medical Advice." The implication of the form is that the physician will not be responsible for any harm that results from this action. In addition, the refusal of care by the person or the person's legally authorized representative may, upon appropriate notice, result in termination of the patient-physician relationship. The exception to the discharging-against-advice right is that some states have laws requiring people with certain contagious diseases who are considered potentially harmful to others to remain in the hospital. This may occur with tuberculosis, which is often difficult to control in patients with HIV infection and which is a public health risk. It is conceivable that this ruling could also be applied to people with HIV infection who are known to behave irresponsibly. We are not aware that this ruling has ever been applied in this way.

11. People may not be transferred from one facility to another unless they receive a complete explanation of the need for the transfer and the alternatives to the transfer, and unless the receiving facility accepts the transfer. People who desire transfer to another

hospital should notify their physicians, who will make the arrangements. Almost all transfers between hospitals are based on discussions between physicians, usually the physicians-of-record of the two facilities. The admitting office of the receiving hospital must also be involved to assure that the source of medical insurance complies with their requirements.

12. People who are discharged from the hospital have a right to information regarding continuing health care requirements, including recommendations for medications, nutrition, activity, return to work, and follow-up medical evaluations.

13. The person has the right to inquire about any charges by the hospital, the clinic, or a physician, and to be presented with various options for payment.

Alternatives to Hospital Care

Because hospitalization accounts for 70 percent of the health care bill and because hospitalization costs are so high, the medical profession has developed a series of alternatives to hospital care. The alternatives include expanded outpatient clinics, day care facilities, chronic care facilities, home care programs, and hospice programs. Although the motivation for these changes has been economic, the result has been humane: most people prefer almost any health care setting to a hospital.

Expanded Outpatient Facilities

Outpatient facilities—physicians' offices, clinics, or specialized facilities—now offer many of the procedures and treatments that previously required hospitalization. Examples of these procedures and treatments include blood transfusions, some intravenous treatments, specialized diagnostic examinations like CAT scans or MI scans, endoscopy, induced sputum tests to diagnose pneumocystis pneumonia, and most minor surgical procedures.

The biggest reason that outpatient facilities have expanded their services is cost: treatments done on an outpatient basis are substantially less expensive than those done in a hospital. Another reason that outpatient facilities have expanded is that insurers will not reimburse people who are only admitted to the hospital to get some types of treatments and procedures. And to make things more confusing, some insurers now reimburse only those treatments done in a hospital. The contradiction in reimbursement rules is difficult to understand but important to know about. Talk to your insurance company, your social worker, and your physician. It may be that the test you need will cost more to do in the hospital, but the final bill to you will still be less.

Home Health Care

Home health care is just what it sounds like: health care not in a hospital or chronic care facility, but in your own home. Home health care includes services such as intravenous infusions, physical therapy, and respirator treatment. The people who provide the care range from physicians and nurses to aides, physical therapists, social workers, respiratory therapists, and dietitians.

People who need home health care are those whose medical condition is stable but who need the services the hospital provides. People with HIV infection usually use home health care for intravenous administration of antibiotics, aerosolized pentamidine, nutritional treatment, and homemaker services. Services called "aids to daily living"—like feeding, bathing, toileting, or transporting—may be what the person with HIV infection needs most, but these services require "unskilled" or "custodial" care that few insurers will pay for.

The most common skilled service provided by home health care companies is the intravenous administration of antibiotics. In this case, the person with HIV infection or the caregiver (often someone who lives in the same house) is instructed in preserving and administering the antibiotic. The equipment and drugs are provided by a home health care company. Specialized services—such as a nurse to make periodic checks or someone to take blood for tests—are provided either by the medical supplier or by a licensed agency. Medical observations—including laboratory test results and nurses' reports—are sent on to the physician-of-record, who is ultimately responsible for the patient's care.

The advantage of home health care is that it permits you to remain in your own home. Though there is little scientific proof that people recover more quickly when treated at home, people being treated at home are usually happier. Home health care is also substantially less expensive, usually one-third to one-half the cost of the same treatment given in a hospital.

People usually arrange for home health care when they are discharged from the hospital. The process of arranging home health care begins with an assessment by a physician or by a physician's order to a home health care company, often with the help of a social worker or a specialist in home health care from the hospital. This assessment includes your medical status, the services you need, whether you also have a caregiver in your home, and the funds you have available.

The physician-of-record must agree that home health care is feasible. The person needing home health care should need it for a week or longer. It is not economically justifiable to train a person who will only need the equipment or the skills for less than five to seven days.

Home health care has become a big industry in this country; many cities have over thirty home health care companies. Some hospitals offer their own home health care programs. People needing the services have a large selection but no way of knowing how to make the choice. They usually depend on the hospital staff, physician, social worker, or AIDS-advocacy groups to make a recommendation. In addition, people choosing a home health care program should check for its accreditation. The organization that accredits home health care companies is the same as the organization that reviews hospitals: the Joint Commission on Accreditation of Health Organizations (JCAHO). The home health care company you choose should be accredited by the JCAHO, and most insurance companies require this accreditation as a contingency for payment.

Whether you choose home health care, and which company you choose, should depend on the stability of your medical condition, the availability of a reliable caregiver, the likelihood of medical complications, the cost of the home health care, your insurance coverage, the availability of emergency services twenty-four hours a day, and the availability of technicians, nurses, or other specialists as needed.

Financing home health care is variable and confusing. Certain home health care services are covered by Medicare, Medicaid, and the Veterans Administration. Medicare covers only services that are usually provided for hospitalized patients. Services covered include home health agencies, physical therapy, occupational therapy, and social work; the service not covered is intravenous treatment. Medicare also requires that care be under supervision of a physician, that the patient must be confined to the home, and that the patient must need skilled nursing care or physical therapy. Medicaid, though it varies from state to state, generally covers 80 percent of the cost of skilled nursing and specialized medical equipment. Blue Cross/Blue Shield, commercial insurance companies, and HMOs all have differing coverages. Moreover, the companies that provide home health care have the right to refuse to care for you, a decision often based on guaranteed payment.

Chronic Care Facilities

Chronic care facilities are nursing homes, facilities for the long-term care of people who do not require hospitalization but who cannot be cared for at home. People with HIV infection who use chronic care facilities are most likely to be those with AIDS dementia complex, those with severe nutritional problems, those who will have a prolonged convalescence from some infection, and those who are severely debilitated.

The cost of chronic care facilities usually ranges from $200 to $400 per day and up, though the costs vary by facility, location, and the kinds of services needed. Both Medicare and Medicaid will fund chronic care, but only under limited circumstances. The amount of funding provided depends on the level of nursing care you need—intermediate (the least amount of care), skilled, or chronic (the most amount of care). The level of funding is lowest for intermediate care and highest for chronic care.

Whether you are eligible for a level of care and which level of care you need is decided by the Professional Review Organization (PRO), which represents both Medicare and Medicaid, and commercial insurance companies. Once you are placed in a chronic care facility, funding continues indefinitely unless your needs change. PROs usually visit facilities and adjust levels of care intermittently.

Both you and the chronic care facility have the right of refusal. That is, you (or your guardian) can refuse transfer from a hospital to a chronic care facility if you have a suitable alternative, and the chronic care facility can refuse to accept you. Many chronic care facilities in this country have resisted accepting people with HIV infection. Their reasons are that the nursing staff is afraid of HIV transmission, that accepting people with HIV infection might deter other applicants to the chronic care facility, and that people with HIV infection often require more intensive care than the usual person in a chronic care facility. In some areas, third-party payers have increased reimbursement for people with HIV infection; in other areas, other enticements have been offered. Nevertheless, in most areas, the number of beds in chronic care facilities for people with HIV infection still falls short of the number needed.

Hospice Care

A hospice is a program of services offered to people who are dying and to their families. Hospice care provides physical, psychological, social, and spiritual care for the person for whom aggressive treatment is no longer appropriate. Hospice care was begun as an aid for people who wanted to die at home, and many hospice programs still emphasize this.

The only medical care allowed in most hospice programs is designed to make the person comfortable by controlling pain and providing hydration (liquids) and nutrition. Most hospice programs rule out treatment of new infections and complications. Most programs provide services for up to six months.

Hospice care can be provided in a facility designed for chronic care, either as part of a program serving many types of patients or as a free-standing unit. Hospice care can also be a home care program or an outpatient care program. Hospice care in a home care program, done by an interdisciplinary staff of professionals and volunteers, typically includes bathing, feeding, changing beds, and similar services, usually once a day. The hospice program's registered nurse coordinates these services. Home care hospice programs usually require that there be a caregiver in the home.

Hospice care in a facility usually costs between $200 and $400 per day. Funding for hospice care varies, depending on the services provided. Medicaid and Medicare will provide thirty days of home hospice care; other insurers vary. Most private insurers and Medicaid and Medicare will also fund care to provide the caregiver time off. They call this "respite care" and usually pay for less than 100 percent of it.

Chapter 9

Medical Treatments: The Range of Available Therapies

- Traditional medicine
- Experimental drugs and clinical trials
- Alternative medicine

In the early years of the AIDS epidemic, medical treatments could do little except relieve unpleasant symptoms. As researchers understood more about HIV—how it infects, how it multiplies—they began to find drugs that slow the infection, and even to understand how to custom-build drugs to attack HIV. The result of their understanding was and continues to be a rapid succession of new drugs to treat HIV itself.

We now know that certain drugs will delay the development of AIDS. We also know that certain vaccines and antibiotics will delay or even prevent the opportunistic infections that define AIDS. These drugs and vaccines are part of traditional medicine.

The medical care of people with HIV infection can be divided into traditional medicine and alternative medicine. Traditional medicine is traditional to us in the West—in the United States and the Western world—and is based on specific scientific standards. Alternative medicine has diverse forms: some borrow heavily from Eastern (Chinese, Japanese, or Indian) philosophy; some use methods based on the mind-body interaction; and some are based on nonapproved drugs or diets or other treatments that, measured by the standard yardstick of the science of medicine, have no established merit.

Nearly all the people with HIV infection receive traditional medical care. As many as a third of the people with HIV infection in some large urban areas receive some form of alternative treatment as well. Both traditional and alternative medicine make the same claims: the treatments kill HIV or prevent HIV from reproducing, or strengthen the immune system, or relieve symptoms. People with HIV infection hearing these conflicting claims are understandably confused.

The purpose of this chapter is to help sort out that confusion. The first section discusses the drugs of traditional medicine and their side effects, and—another source of concern for people with HIV infection—how to pay for them. The next section discusses how drugs are tested to find out whether they are useful and how best to use them. The last section is on alternatives to traditional medicine—treatments that have not been and are not likely to be tested—and whether they are likely to help or be harmful.

Traditional Medicine

Traditional medicine is a tightly controlled system of regulations, accreditation, approval, and licenses. Providers of health care—physicians, midlevel practioners, nurses—must be licensed, and their licenses depend on training, postgraduate education, and certifying examinations. The settings in which health care is provided—hospitals, chronic care facilities, and home care programs—must be accredited by the Joint Committee on Accreditation of Health Organizations (JCAHO). The drugs must be approved by the Food and Drug Administration (FDA), the federal agency responsible for judging the safety and effectiveness of new drugs. The organizations that finance health care (private insurers, Medicaid, Medicare, Blue Cross/Blue Shield) are regulated by agencies of the federal and state governments. (In a way, the financers of health care largely drive the system: they will not reimburse for care by unlicensed care providers, for stays in nonaccredited facilities, or for treatment with unapproved drugs.)

This system of controls is set up to safeguard the public. The controls are meant to stop people or programs or institutions from claiming to offer services or cures that are in fact unnecessary, useless, or unproven.

The health care providers and the health care facilities of traditional medicine are discussed in Chapter 8, and financing health care is discussed in Chapter 10.

Traditional Medicine's Drugs

Most of the drugs offered by traditional medicine have been tested by a scientific method that starts with studying the drug in a test tube and ends an average of twelve years later after studying the drug in thousands of people (see below, "Experimental Drugs and Clinical Trials"). The results of those tests are analyzed statistically, to see if some apparent benefit is actually due either to simple chance or to "outliers," those rare and exceptional cases that lie far outside the average case. Such analysis is especially important in a disease like HIV infection, because people vary so enormously in the rate at which the disease progresses and in the types of opportunistic illnesses they get. Once the test is completed, but before the drug is sold to the public, the results are reviewed by the FDA and usually sent to a medical journal for publication. The medical journal sends the results out to experts in the field, who determine if the performance and results of the trial are sound enough for publication. Physicians become aware of new treatments when the results of these trials are published in reputable medical journals or presented at medical meetings.

This process for approving drugs turns out to be extraordinarily expensive, often bureaucratic, and frequently frustrating to those who use it. Major criticisms are: the drugs cost too much, there are too many regulatory agencies, and the FDA requirements for approval are unnecessarily arduous and time-consuming. In many ways, HIV infection has called attention to these defects in the system, and as a result, the FDA now speeds up the evaluation of new drugs for HIV infection (see below, under "The Steps of a Clinical Trial").

Despite traditional medicine's ills, its accomplishments are worth celebrating. Many of the infectious diseases that once were major epidemics—as HIV is now—are no longer problems. The worst epidemic in the history of medicine, bubonic plague, claimed twenty-five million lives in the fourteenth century, and is now virtually eliminated. Other once-serious diseases now largely controlled in the Western world are cholera, polio, measles, mumps, and typhoid fever. Smallpox, once a devastating disease, has been eliminated from the earth. All this is to say that traditional medicine does work, and that the litany of breakthroughs is likely to continue.

Approved Drugs

The drugs used in traditional medicine can be classified into *approved* and *unapproved* drugs. An approved drug is a drug that is approved by the FDA and that can be sold to the public (see below, under "Experimental Drugs and Clinical Trials"). Approved drugs are further divided into nonprescription drugs, prescription drugs, and controlled drugs. Nonprescription drugs, like aspirin and cold remedies, can be bought by anyone. Prescription drugs can be bought only with a prescription or with a licensed physician's telephone call to a pharmacy. Controlled drugs, like narcotics and sleeping pills, can be physically addictive and are often subject to abuse. Controlled drugs can be bought only with a special prescription signed by a physician with a special license for prescribing controlled drugs.

Most approved drugs have two names: a generic name, which is usually also the medical name (like pentamidine), and a trade name, which is usually selected by the drug's manufacturer (like Pentam). Drugs that have been patented by a single manufacturer have only one trade name. Once that manufacturer's patent runs out, many manufacturers can make the drug, and each manufacturer now puts a different trade name on the drug. As a result, there can be several trade names for a single generic drug (trimethoprim-sulfamethoxazole is called both Bactrim and Septra).

Unapproved drugs, often called underground drugs, are drugs that are neither approved by the FDA nor in the process of being approved. They are widely taken without prescription by people with HIV infection. They are discussed further below, under "Alternative Medicine."

Types of Drugs Used for HIV Infection

People with HIV infection take three kinds of drugs: drugs against the virus, drugs and vaccines to prevent opportunistic infections, and drugs to relieve unpleasant symptoms.

Drugs directed against HIV are called *antiviral* or *antiretroviral* drugs. These drugs attack HIV itself and, in one way or another, reduce its ability to reproduce and spread. The first antiretroviral drug approved by the FDA was AZT; within three years of AZT's approval, dozens of other drugs were in the process of being tested. So many other antiretroviral drugs are being tested and the field is moving so fast that recommendations about the drugs are likely to be outdated within months. In addition, questions remain about the best time during the course of the infection to begin taking drugs, which drugs to take, and which drugs are best taken in combination with other drugs. We do know, however, that taking antiretroviral drugs is critically important during certain stages of HIV infection.

The second type of drug taken by people with HIV infection prevents opportunistic infections. A multitude of drugs prevent the most frequent and serious of the opportunistic infections, pneumocystis pneumonia; in fact, these drugs are as successful in prolonging life as AZT. Other drugs prevent other frequent opportunistic infections such as tuberculosis, thrush, pneumocystis pneumonia, and cryptococcal meningitis. Vaccines prevent influenza and pneumococcal pneumonia. As with the antiretroviral drugs, questions remain: Which drugs are best? How and when are they best taken?

The third type of drugs taken by people with HIV infection provides relief from unpleasant symptoms, including insomnia, anxiety, depression, fever, aches, problems with sleep and appetite, nausea, diarrhea, and pain. These drugs don't cure the problem causing the symptoms, but they do reduce the person's suffering. Relieving symptoms is the strategy used for most noninfectious diseases.

Side Effects of the Drugs

Many of these drugs have side effects, referred to by physicians as *adverse drug reactions, ADRs* for short. The ADRs of most drugs are well known and well defined, based on the experience of thousands of people who took the drug during its clinical trials, and on the experience of everyone who took the drug once it was on the market. Although anyone can develop ADRs, for some reason ADRs are more common in people with HIV infection. For instance, trimethoprim-sulfamethoxazole (Bactrim or Septra) causes ADRs in 10 percent of the people without HIV infection and 50 percent of those with HIV infection.

ADRs are classified as either *allergic* or *toxic*. Allergic reactions mean that the cells of the immune system have recognized the drug as foreign and have responded by causing a rash, a fever, or both—like the rashes that penicillin causes in some people. In allergic reactions, the dose of the drug is unimportant: the immune system will respond similarly regardless of the dose. Serious allergic reactions often imply that neither that drug nor any related drugs should be taken again.

Toxic reactions are caused, not by the immune system, but directly by the drug itself. An example is the drowsiness caused by Dramamine or other antihistamines or the kidney damage and anemia caused by amphotericin B. Toxic reactions are usually dose-related; lowering the dose will relieve the symptoms.

People usually develop ADRs after they have been taking the drug for one or two weeks. Some people, however, will have a serious ADR after one dose; others will have no ADRs until after they have taken the drug for months or years; some develop ADRs after repeated courses of the same drug. Therefore, ADRs are unpredictable: because a drug was taken once and tolerated does not mean that it can be taken later and cause no ADR.

Sorting out and controlling ADRs will be done by a physician. The physician will either give the person with a suspected ADR what is called a drug holiday—discontinuation of all drugs—or will stop drugs one at a time, starting with those that are most likely to cause ADRs and those that are most dispensable.

Drugs Commonly Taken by People with HIV Infection

What follows is a table of prescription drugs commonly taken by people with HIV infection, their generic and trade names, their doses, the conditions they treat, and their side effects.

Costs of the Drugs

The costs of the drugs differ, depending on the pharmacy and whether they are generic or trade-name drugs. Shop around for the pharmacy that charges least for the drugs you need. Some people prefer mail order pharmacy services for convenience, cost savings, and anonymity. Ask your physician to write prescriptions, when appropriate, for drugs under their generic rather than their trade names. Trimethoprim-sulfamethoxazole costs ten times less than the same drug under the name of Bactrim or Septra. Many drugs required by AIDS patients still have a patent; these tend to be expensive, usually $2,000–$10,000 yearly if continuous use is required.

Paying for the Drugs

The question of who pays for drugs is complicated and controversial. All insurers, public or private, differ in whether they pay for drugs, how much they pay, and which drugs they pay for. Medicaid and the Veterans Administration both provide coverage for prescription drugs; Medicare does not. Only 15 percent to 30 percent of both the commercial insurance companies' plans and Blue Cross/Blue Shield's plans cover prescription drugs.

The companies and plans that do cover drugs sometimes put limits on their coverage. They will pay only for FDA-approved drugs and sometimes only for FDA-approved drugs used for the medical conditions the FDA has approved them for. Nonprescription drugs and drugs used in alternative treatments (see below, under "Alternative Medicine") are not covered by any insurer.

Whether or not insurers will cover drugs for conditions for which the FDA has not approved the drug is still a matter of controversy. Insurers cover drugs that are in what is called "generally accepted medical practice"; they do not cover drugs that are considered experimental. The problem is that new drugs are being developed rapidly, and the FDA's approval process can take a long time; as a result, the distinction between experimental drugs and drugs used in generally accepted medical practice is vague. Some insurers make that distinction by soliciting

Table 4. Drugs Commonly Taken by People with HIV infection

Drug (other names)	Dose (adult)	Cost/wk* (dollars)	Conditions Treated	Side Effects (less frequent side effects in parentheses)
Acyclovir (Zovirax)	Mouth: 200–800 mg 2–5 times/day	25–120	Herpes simplex Shingles	(Kidney damage, headache, rash, nausea, diarrhea, liver disease)
Amphotericin B	Vein: 30–50 mg/day	115	Fungal infections: *Candida*, *Cryptococcus*, histoplasmosis	Kidney damage, anemia, nausea, vomiting, chills, fever, electrolyte disturbances, metallic taste
Ampicillin or Amoxicillin	Mouth: 250–500 mg 3–4 times/day	4	Bacterial infections: sinusitis, pneumonia	Rash, diarrhea
Ativan	Mouth: 1 mg 2 times/day	10	Anxiety	Sedation, along with memory loss, fatigue, confusion, dependency with long-term use
Azithromycin	Mouth: 250–750 mg/day	50–150	*Mycobacterium avium* Toxoplasmosis Cryptosporidiosis	Nausea, vomiting
Benedryl	Mouth: 25 mg/day	2	Insomnia Allergies	Sedation

Table 4. (*Continued*)

Drug (other names)	Dose (adult)	Cost/wk* (dollars)	Conditions Treated	Side Effects (less frequent side effects in parentheses)
Ciprofloxacin (Cipro)	Mouth: 500–750 mg 2 times/day	50–70	Tuberculosis *Mycobacterium avium* Common infections: pneumonia, infectious diarrhea	Nausea (vomiting, headache, malaise, dizziness)
Clarithromycin	Mouth: 500–1,000 mg 2 times/day	70–140	*Mycobacterium avium*	Nausea, vomiting
Clindamycin	Mouth: 300–450 mg 3 times/day Vein: 600–900 mg 3 times/day	50–70 300	Pneumocystis pneumonia Toxoplasmosis Bacterial infections	Diarrhea (rash, nausea)
Clotrimazole	Mouth: 10 mg troche 4–5 times/day	25	Thrush	Nausea, vomiting (liver damage)
Dapsone	Mouth: 100 mg/day	1	Pneumocystis pneumonia	Anemia (rash, headache, nausea, vomiting, fever, agitation)

(*continued on next page*)

207

Table 4. (*Continued*)

Drug (other names)	Dose (adult)	Cost/wk* (dollars)	Conditions Treated	Side Effects (less frequent side effects in parentheses)
ddC	Mouth: 0.75 mg 3 times/day	50	HIV infection	Peripheral neuropathy (pancreatitis, mouth ulcers)
ddI	Mouth: 125–200 mg 2 times/day	50	HIV infection	Pancreatitis: abdominal pain, nausea, vomiting, diarrhea, neuropathy with painful feet (liver damage)
Erythromycin	Mouth: 250–500 mg 4 times/day	4	Bacterial infections: pneumonia, sore throat, sinusitis	Nausea, vomiting
Erythropoietin (EPO)	Injected under skin: 6,000 units 3 times/week	220	Anemia	(Rare)
Feeding supplements	Mouth: 4 cans/day	50	Malnutrition	(Diarrhea, supplements taste bad)
Fluconazole (Diflucan)	Mouth: 50–200 mg/day	30–100	Cryptococcal meningitis Candidal infections	(Rash, nausea, vomiting, liver damage)
Foscarnet	Vein: 90–120 mg/day	500	Cytomegalovirus infections	Kidney damage (electrolyte problems with tremors, tingling, seizures, anemia, headache, irritability)

Table 4. (*Continued*)

Drug (other names)	Dose (adult)	Cost/wk* (dollars)	Conditions Treated	Side Effects (less frequent side effects in parentheses)
G-CSF	Injected under skin: 10–50 mg/day	130–170	Low white cells	(Bone pain)
Ganciclovir (DHPG)	Vein: 350–700 mg/day	170	Cytomegalovirus infections: retina, lungs, intestine	Reduced white blood cells predisposing to infections (nausea, vomiting, low platelets predisposing to bleeding, liver damage, mental changes, headache)
Halcion	Mouth: 0.25 mg/day	5	Insomnia	Sedation, along with memory loss, fatigue, confusion; dependency with long-term use
Haloperidd	Mouth: 2 mg 2 times/day	2	Delirium	Lethargy, drooling, involuntary movements, lack of coordination
Interferon	Vein: 10–20 mil units/ day	700–1,000	Kaposi's sarcoma	Flulike illness, fever, fatigue, headache, muscle aches, depression, confusion
Isoniazid (INH)	Mouth: 300 mg/day	0.15	Tuberculosis	Nausea, vomiting, liver damage (headache, rash, dizziness)
Ketoconazole (Nizoral)	Mouth: 200–400 mg/day	15–30	Candidal infections, esp. thrush	Nausea, vomiting (liver damage, reduced libido, menstrual problems, headache, dizziness, itching, rash)

(*continued on next page*)

Table 4. (Continued)

Drug (other names)	Dose (adult)	Cost/wk* (dollars)	Conditions Treated	Side Effects (less frequent side effects in parentheses)
Lomotil	Mouth: 5 mg 4 times/day	25	Diarrhea	(Rare)
Megace	Mouth: 80 mg 4 times/day	60	Poor appetite	(Rare)
Metronidazole (Flagyl)	Mouth: 750–2000 mg/day	1	Giardiasis Amebiasis Gingivitis Other infections	Nausea, vomiting, metallic taste, headache (painful feet and legs with prolonged use, reaction with alcohol withdrawal)
Nortriptyline	Mouth: 25–75 mg/day	6–16	Peripheral neuropathy Depression	Dry mouth, blurred vision, sedation, fatigue, anxiety, involuntary movements
Nystatin	Mouth: gargle 500,000 units 4 times/day	10	Thrush	(Nausea, vomiting, diarrhea)
Pentamidine (Pentam)	Aerosol: 300 mg/month Vein: 200–300 mg/day	25 500–700	Pneumocystis pneumonia	Aerosol: Cough (asthma reaction) Vein: Kidney damage, nausea, vomiting, low blood sugar, low blood pressure with fainting, rash, anemia, low white blood count predisposing to infection

210

Table 4. (*Continued*)

Drug (other names)	Dose (adult)	Cost/wk* (dollars)	Conditions Treated	Side Effects (less frequent side effects in parentheses)
Prozac	Mouth: 20 mg/day	15	Depression	Nervousness, dry mouth, insomnia, nausea, constipation
Pyrazinamide	Mouth: 1000–2000 mg/day	30	Tuberculosis	(Liver damage, joint pain, nausea, vomiting, increased uric acid: gout)
Pyrimethamine	Mouth: 25–75 mg/day	3–7	Toxoplasmosis	(Anemia, low platelets, low white blood cells predisposing to infection)
Rifampin (Rifadin)	Mouth: 600 mg/day	30	Tuberculosis	Orange discoloration of tears, urine, sweat (liver damage, rash); causes liver to eliminate some drugs faster, so doses of those drugs must increase; one of these drugs is methadone, & consequence can be withdrawal symptoms
Sulfonamides	Mouth: 2–8 mg/day	1	Toxoplasmosis *Nocardia*	Rash, fever, liver damage, low white blood count, nausea, vomiting
Trimethoprim	Mouth: 750–1400 mg/day	1	Pneumocystis pneumonia	Nausea, vomiting, rash (anemia, low white blood count)

(*continued on next page*)

Table 4. (*Continued*)

Drug (other names)	Dose (adult)	Cost/wk* (dollars)	Conditions Treated	Side Effects (less frequent side effects in parentheses)
Trimethoprim-sulfamethoxazole (Bactrim, Septra)	Mouth: 1–6 DS tablets/day Vein: 750–1400 mg trimethoprim/day	1	Pneumocystis pneumonia Other infections: sinusitis, pneumonia, infectious diarrhea	Nausea, vomiting, fever, low white blood count, liver damage
Xanax	Mouth: 0.25 mg 2 times/day		Anxiety	Sedation, lack of coordination, memory loss, fatigue, confusion, dependency with long-term use
Zidovudine (AZT, Retrovir)	Mouth: 100 mg 5 times/day	50	HIV infection	Anemia, low white blood count (headache, malaise, muscle inflammation)

*The cost figure is the approximate *wholesale* price of the indicated drug for 1993; the cost to the consumer will be higher. These prices will be generally accurate for at least 2–3 years.

advice from physicians or physicians' professional societies. Some insurers make the distinction strictly by following FDA guidelines, although the FDA has repeatedly stated that a drug can be used in generally accepted medical practice and still not be approved for that specific condition.

For more information on what insurers do and do not pay for, see Chapter 10.

Experimental Drugs and Clinical Trials

Drugs become accepted by physicians and the FDA on the basis of scientific proof of their effectiveness and safety. Scientific proof is obtained through a series of tests called a *clinical trial*. A clinical trial involves the combined efforts of the pharmaceutical company that makes the drug; the independent investigators who test the drug; and the FDA, which licenses the drug. Testing drugs through clinical trials has been standard for over four decades and has provided the foundation for most of the recommended treatments in traditional medicine.

While a drug is being tested in a clinical trial, it is considered experimental. If the drug proves effective and is not too toxic, it is then licensed and available to the public.

For people with HIV infection, participating in clinical trials has both advantages and disadvantages. Clinical trials are experiments with human lives, and special safeguards are necessary to guard both the people and the scientific procedure. These safeguards, plus the options and aspects of participation in a clinical trial, are spelled out to the participant in painstaking detail. Some trials can be seen as especially risky: they involve taking a drug with no established benefit in place of a standard drug with established merit. With other trials—for instance, the comparison of two drugs, both of which are known to work, to find out which works better—the risk is lower. The motivation to participate is an individual decision. For further discussion, see below, "Advantages of Participating in a Clinical Trial" and "Disadvantages of Participating in a Clinical Trial."

Anyone worried about the safety of a clinical trial can be reassured that the trials are conducted under the strict supervision of the FDA and a local board charged with reviewing the trial (see below, "Supervision of Clinical Trials"). Both the FDA and the local board periodically review the results of the trial. If the drug being tested proves significantly better or worse than the drugs in standard use, the trial is promptly discontinued. Moreover, a standing rule in all clinical trials is that participants may withdraw from the trial at any time.

The Steps of a Clinical Trial

All drugs used for medical therapy in the United States must first be reviewed and approved by the FDA. The FDA is responsible for assuring that all drugs, before they are sold, are sufficiently safe and effective. Accordingly, the FDA dictates that certain steps be followed from the time a drug is discovered until it is finally licensed. The process of testing drugs has several stages: a drug is tested first in the test tube and in animals, then in a few people for a short time, and then in a larger group of people for a longer time.

Preclinical trials. A new drug is first tested, not in people, but in test tubes and in animals. These first tests are called preclinical trials because they precede tests with people, which are called clinical trials. Preclinical trials determine the drug's toxicity, its pharmacologic properties, and its effects against certain microbes. Of all the drugs tested in preclinical trials, only about one drug in a thousand is ever tested in people.

If a drug shows promise in the preclinical trials, the FDA grants it the status of an Investigational New Drug (IND). IND status must be granted before the FDA allows the drug to be tested in humans.

Phase one clinical trials. Phase one clinical trials are the first round of tests in humans. Phase one trials are designed to determine the safety and dosage of a new drug. These trials usually involve a relatively small number of people, usually between twenty and eighty. The drug is given only for a short time, usually for not more than a few weeks, and sometimes only a single dose is given. Participation in a phase one trial may require staying in a research unit of the hospital, or the participant may visit an outpatient clinic which carefully monitors the trial. Participants in a phase one trial don't benefit much when the trial is for an infection like HIV because the treatment lasts for such a short time. Therefore, people who participate in phase one trials are often paid for their services, or else they participate for entirely altruistic reasons.

Phase two clinical trials. Phase two clinical trials are the second round of tests in people. Phase two trials usually involve one hundred to three hundred participants and last for months or years. The purpose of these trials is to determine the schedules for doses, to collect additional information on toxicity, and to test, at least preliminarily, the drug's effectiveness. With HIV infection, the effectiveness of a drug may be determined by the effect on CD4 cell counts, by the numbers of HIV in the blood, by the delay in progression of disease as indicated by opportunistic infections or development of AIDS, and by how the participant feels. People often participate in phase two trials for access to the drug before licensing. Or if the trial is relatively short and benefits to the participant relatively brief, people participate for payment or altruism. With some studies, the distinction between phase one and phase two is blurred, and the resulting classification is phase one/two.

Phase three clinical trials. Phase three clinical trials are the last phase before the FDA licenses the drug. Phase three trials often include two thousand to three thousand or more participants and run for months or years. In this phase, the drug is given to participants in the doses and at the intervals that the FDA is likely to consider acceptable. The purpose of these trials is to get additional information about the safety and effectiveness of the drug. People usually participate in phase three trials for access to the drug before licensing.

NDA review. The next step is to take all the information gathered during the previous steps and submit it in a New Drug Application (NDA) to the FDA. The FDA reviews the NDA and decides whether to license the drug, what the dose should be, how the drug should be administered, which side effects require specific warnings in promotional material, and what conditions the drug is useful for. This and other information is available in the *Physicians' Desk Reference,* or *PDR.* The *PDR* is published each year and is available in most bookstores for $50 to $60. There is also an edition for nonprescription drugs, like ibuprofen, cold remedies, or Dramamine, called *PDR for Nonprescription Drugs.*

It should be noted that the FDA approves drugs for the specific conditions indicated in the package insert and in the *PDR.* Despite this labeling, once a drug is in pharmacies, it may be prescribed for any medical condition. Some physicians are reluctant to prescribe beyond the labeling limits for fear of malpractice suits. The FDA acknowledges the limitations of its labeling, and most physicians believe that "standards of practice" should be the guide. Another potential problem is that some third-party payers limit reimbursement coverage to FDA indications. Such decisions are unusual because most third-party payers have no way of knowing a person's medical condition when he or she is an outpatient. When limitations are imposed, it may be possible to appeal the decision. But an appeal requires a fight with bureaucrats who often know little medicine and are paid to keep costs low.

Phase four trials. Phase four trials may be conducted after the drug is licensed in order to determine new dosing schedules, or to collect additional information about effectiveness or toxicity, or to compare the drug to other drugs. People participate in phase four trials of drugs, even though the drugs are already available in the marketplace, in order to have access to the best medical care and (sometimes) in order to receive free care.

Streamlining clinical trials. The process described above has established high standards for determining the safety and effectiveness of new drugs. Unfortunately, the process is also expensive and time consuming. The average new drug in the United States costs $230 million to develop and requires an average of twelve years to move from the laboratory to licensing. Many people with HIV infection, however, have argued that they simply cannot wait twelve years for a potentially useful drug to make it to the marketplace.

In response to this argument, the FDA has streamlined the testing process for drugs that might be useful in treating HIV infection. The process now goes faster. Drugs for HIV infection get an expedited review: this means that the FDA examines the IND and the NDA more rapidly, the phase three trials require fewer participants (around three hundred instead of the usual two thousand to three thousand), and some drugs are approved at a relatively early stage using criteria that would have been unacceptable in prior years. Drugs also are made available earlier in the testing process through a mechanism called a Treatment IND. Under the Treatment IND classification, the drug can be prescribed by physicians other than the investigators between the time the trial is completed and the time the FDA reviews the complete NDA application.

AZT was the first drug to be evaluated under some of the provisions of this streamlined process. The phase two trial began in February 1986; in September 1986, the first analysis of data showed the drug was clearly beneficial; the drug was then made available to people with AIDS through a Treatment IND, and the drug was licensed in March 1987. The entire process took thirteen months instead of the customary twelve years. The drug was approved based on studies of 282 patients instead of the usual two thousand to three thousand patients.

Although the streamlined process provided access to the drug quickly, it must also be recognized that when AZT became available, the amount of information about it was limited. As a consequence, much of the work normally done in phase three testing was actually done during the phase four, post-licensing trials. These trials indicated that the original dose of the drug was far too high, the toxic side effects consequently far too great, and the treatment was begun too late. Nevertheless, the experience with AZT showed the potential usefulness of streamlining clinical trials to get needed drugs into drugstores.

A more recent attempt to streamline the process and make new drugs more quickly available is called the *parallel program.* The new drugs may be prescribed to people with HIV infection who are not participants in clinical trials during—and therefore parallel to—the phase three trials. Early on, the parallel program with the drug ddI got mixed reviews. The good news was that twenty-six thousand people with HIV infection got access to a potentially useful drug. The bad news was that the parallel program provided almost no information about whether the drug was clinically useful. In October 1991, the FDA approved ddI based on research trials with a small number of patients whose CD4 counts increased as much with ddI as they did with AZT. At the time of approval, the FDA also demanded a proper clinical trial to show with standard clinical parameters how ddI compared to AZT. Many would argue that the parallel program for ddI was an enormous expense that notably delayed the traditional trial necessary to place the drug in proper perspective.

Participating in a Clinical Trial

Most trials are comparisons of one drug versus no drugs, one drug versus another drug, or one drug given in different doses. Participants in a clinical trial usually have to meet a specified requirement—they must have a certain CD4 count, for instance, or a certain opportunistic infection. These requirements are adhered to strictly. Though such strictness is frustrating to both the investigator and the potential participant, it is necessary for the trial to be a valid test of a drug and for the FDA to approve the drug.

Once in the trial, participants are assigned to groups called *treatment arms*. What the treatment arms are depend on what the trial is testing: one treatment arm might be high doses of a drug and another arm low doses; one arm might be one drug and the other arm another drug; one arm might be one drug and another arm no drug at all. In trials involving two or more arms, the participant is assigned to a treatment arm randomly, like flipping a coin. Random assignment is a process over which neither the participant nor the investigator has any control. This is necessary if the trial is to be scientifically credible.

The purpose of a trial is to compare one treatment arm against another. Some trials, called *placebo control trials*, compare a drug to a placebo, a pill that has no effect on the body. Placebo trials are done because people taking any pill, including a placebo, feel better not necessarily because of the physiological effect of the drug, but because of the psychological effect of taking a drug that might help. For example, 60 percent of the people treated with any drug, placebo or not, for arthritis claim that it improves their symptoms. The necessity for a placebo trial is less when the effects being evaluated are objective:

weight, blood counts, tests for the virus, or frequency of opportunistic infections. Some effects, however, are more subjective and cannot easily be measured by scientific yardsticks: the sense of well-being, the level of fatigue, the number of headaches. For these more subjective effects, a placebo control trial is more important. In most trials, the results of a trial are evaluated in terms of both subjective and objective effects.

It should be emphasized that the rule of clinical trials is that, if a drug is known to work, no treatment can be a placebo; in that case, the drug known to work becomes the standard for comparison. Furthermore, once the trial shows a clear benefit, the trial must stop. Thus, in the AZT trials, when the analysis of data in September 1986 showed nineteen deaths in the placebo arm and only one death in the arm receiving AZT, the trial was promptly stopped and everyone was given AZT. Assurance on this point is a matter of medical ethics.

The best way to make the comparison in any trial is to double-blind. Double-blinding means that neither investigator nor participant knows which drug or which dose the participant is receiving. Since both investigator and participant are likely to have biases, double-binding ensures that results will be evaluated objectively.

Although double-blinding is preferred, in some instances it is simply not realistic. For example, when the trial is to find out which way to administer the drug, by pill or by vein, proper double-blinding would have one treatment arm receive the drug by vein and a placebo by pill, and the other treatment arm receive the drug by pill and placebo by vein. But receiving a drug intravenously is inconvenient and can be risky, and it might be inappropriate for participants to receive placebo by vein simply to maintain the blind.

Not all trials are comparisons: some trials, called *pilot trials* (like pilot TV shows), simply gather enough background information to see if a larger trial would be justified. Other trials compare a new drug to an old drug tested previously—called a historical control. Many times, in an effort to gather additional information, the drug is just given with no second arm for comparison.

Advantages of Participating in a Clinical Trial

The advantages of participating in trials usually include the following:

1. New drugs: Usually, people have access to a new and unlicensed drug only by participating in a clinical trial. The exception is the parallel program, which still makes special demands on the physician and the participant to adhere to protocol requirements.

2. Good medical care: In clinical trials, the participant is monitored extensively in order to evaluate the drug's effectiveness and toxicity. The advantage to the participant is the quality of medical care that accompanies monitoring. Moreover, the research groups that conduct clinical trials are usually composed of health care providers who are devoted to controlling this disease and who are important sources of new information. Participants in clinical trials may find comfort in receiving care from health care providers who have such credentials and clear commitment, and who are working at the cutting edge of the field.

3. Free care: Most participants in clinical trials receive drugs and medical care related to the trial free of charge. The costs are usually covered by the research grant that supports the trial or by the manufacturer, who is interested either in FDA approval or in favorable publicity. However, the participant should not assume that all costs of medical care associated with HIV infection are likely to be included. Most trials provide the drug, the cost on monitoring for safety and effectiveness, and the costs for managing toxicity ascribed to the experimental drug. They do not provide the cost of care for any complications of HIV infection. Some trials are designed to provide the drug and the cost of monitoring only if the participants are not covered by insurance.

4. Altruism: The advantages listed so far provide direct benefits to the person participating. Participating in a clinical trial also serves a greater need. Medical scientists, people with HIV infection, and people at risk for HIV infection all need more information about new drugs for treating HIV infection. Even the participant who does not benefit directly will nevertheless make a contribution to the welfare of others with or without HIV infection.

Disadvantages of Participating in a Clinical Trial

Several factors might dissuade a person from participating. The most frequent concerns are:

1. Inconvenience: Many trials require extensive testing and frequent visits to the clinic. These requirements should be clearly stated in the informed consent papers (see below, "Informed Consent for the Trial"). These tests and visits can be an enormous inconvenience to the participant.

2. Risk: Clinical trials are scientific experiments. They exist because medical scientists need information about the effectiveness and

safety of a new drug, or about the safety and effectiveness of an old drug used in a new way. Some of these drugs are potentially toxic, and although trials never test drugs on humans that have not been first tested extensively in the laboratory and in animals, unanticipated side effects are always possible. The degree of risk obviously varies with different drugs and different conditions.

3. Assignment to the "wrong group": For all controlled and double-blinded trials, there is always the risk that the participant will receive the placebo, the less effective drug, the more toxic drug, or the less effective dose. Some participants attempt to break the blind and find out what drug or dose they are taking through a variety of mechanisms. The investigators understand participants' reasons for doing this, but breaking the blind destroys the scientific credibility of the trials. If enough people break the blind, the trial might as well not be done.

4. Costs: Usually drugs and costs for monitoring are provided at no expense to the participant. Some drug trials, however, expect reimbursement from the participants for the cost of medical care. You will need to establish what costs, if any, are involved before you agree to participate. In addition, if the drug is toxic, you will need to establish who pays the cost of care for any side effects.

5. Restrictions on other options for treatment: Most trials require that someone who is participating in one trial not participate at the same time in other trials. Some trials exclude people who have received other experimental drugs. Other trials prohibit the participant from using certain drugs or from receiving certain treatments. You should carefully review any such restrictions before agreeing to participate in clinical trials. A reassurance: any participant in a trial can withdraw from participation at any time.

Supervision of Clinical Trials

To be sure that the potential benefits of a trial are larger than its potential risk, the FDA requires that all trials be supervised by an independent review panel. This review panel, called the Institutional Review Board (IRB), must be composed of representatives from both the medical field and the nonmedical public. Most IRBs include representatives from law, nursing, medicine, and the clergy, as well as researchers who are expert in clinical trials. This group has the job of watching out for the participants' interests, seeing that scientific standards are upheld, and protecting medical ethics. At periodic intervals during the course of the trial, the IRB reviews the results. Any serious or unexpected toxicity must be reported immediately to both the IRB and the FDA. If the toxicity is serious and is thought to be related to the drug, all participants in the trial must be notified, and the informed consent form must be revised accordingly.

Many trials, and especially those at multiple medical centers dealing with treatments of serious conditions such as HIV infection, are also supervised by a Data Safety Monitoring Board that scrutinizes the data from the trials every six to twelve months. The Data Safety Monitoring Board, made up of experts in the field who are not involved in the trial, is also privy to unblinded results. This board is different from the IRB because it has access to data from all centers participating in the trial, not just the local center. The board's purpose is to stop the trial as soon as valid results combined from all centers emerge about the drug's effectiveness or toxicity. Six months into the phase two trials of AZT, the Data Safety Monitoring Board's review of the unblinded data convinced it to stop the trial and give all participants AZT. One year into the second big AZT trial, the data showed that the drug was beneficial when the CD4 count was below 500, and that it was less toxic at low doses; the trial was stopped and all participants with low CD4 counts were given low doses of AZT.

Informed Consent for the Trial

The most important safeguard in protecting the rights of participants in clinical trials is the informed consent process. All participants in clinical trials in the United States (and in most areas of the world) are required to sign an informed consent document. In the event that the participant is not competent to sign, this responsibility is assigned to the spouse, parent, an adult child, or a brother or sister (in that order). The informed consent document must also be signed by a witness and by the investigator.

Information in the consent form usually includes the following:

Purpose of the trial. The informed consent document must include an explanation of the scientific question the trial is to answer. It must also include an explanation of why the participant qualifies for the trial.

Procedures. Informed consent must include an explanation of the trial's design, that is, exactly how the trial will proceed. The explanation will include: the nature of the treatment arms; the method by which participants are assigned to a specific arm; the requirements for participation, including the number of clinic visits or the duration of hospitalization; the frequency and types of tests that will be done; the amount of blood that will be required; the duration of the trial; and the end point of the trial.

Risks. Informed consent must include an explanation of the drug's side effects, including their anticipated frequency and severity. It is unrealistic to list every possible side effect, or even all of the side effects that have occurred in previous trials. But certainly the most severe and the most frequent side effects should be noted.

Benefits. Informed consent must include a statement of whether the participant has any realistic likelihood of benefiting from participation. Expenses for the drugs or for monitoring, and any payment to the participant, should also be explained.

Alternatives to participation. Informed consent must include the various options people have if they choose not to participate. This generally includes the statement that a decision not to participate will not affect your care. In other words, no one at the center offering the trial will bear a grudge if you choose not to participate.

Confidentiality of records. People with HIV infection are often concerned about the confidentiality of their trial records. Some trials are done without identifiers, that is without the names, addresses, hospital numbers, or social security numbers that would connect the data to a specific person. Trials done without identifiers essentially guarantee anonymity for the participant.

Unfortunately, it is often impractical and undesirable for clinical trials that collect clinically useful data over a prolonged period to be done without identifiers. The next best option to guarantee confidentiality is to keep the records in a locked file with limited access. The FDA and the drug company that sponsors the trial can require access to these locked files, but we are not aware that this access has ever resulted in a participant's name being revealed to inappropriate persons.

In many instances, data obtained in the trial are also recorded in the participant's medical record: such data can be relevant to medical treatment. Occasionally, participants object to what they view as an unnecessary dispersal of sensitive information. The best advice is to read the consent form carefully for an explanation of how data from the trial are handled and who has access to the record. If such an explanation is not included in the consent form, ask for further information.

Further information: No consent form can provide all the information desired by all the participants. And consent forms often include technical information and medical terms that may be difficult to understand. It is expected that most participants will need to discuss any questions not answered or points not clarified with a member of the investigating team. If, either before or after signing the consent form, you have questions about toxicity, alternatives to drugs, possible participation in other studies, or compensation for injury as a result of participation, you should be answered to your satisfaction. You should not sign the consent form until you are satisfied and have no further questions. One option is to take the consent form home and list the questions you have after you have reviewed the form and discussed it with others. In addition, most consent forms include the name and phone number of an appropriate person to contact if the participant has any further questions after participation begins.

Withdrawal of consent.   Informed consent continues throughout the course of the trial, but withdrawal of consent at any time is the participant's right. Withdrawal must not have any repercussions for the participant. Withdrawal may not interfere with the availability of care.

Participation.   To find the nearest clinical trial, call the hotline at the National Institute of Allergy and Infectious Diseases: 1-800-TRIALS-A.

Alternative Medicine

Most of the medicine practiced in the United States is Western, or to us, traditional medicine. Non-Western, nontraditional medicine is usually called *alternative medicine*. Some alternative medicine—acupuncture, meditation, herbology—has its roots in the thousand-year heritage of Eastern philosophy. Some alternative medicine—psychoneuroimmunology, visualization, naturopathy, homeopathy—is more recent and is sometimes connected to traditional medicine. Most physicians who practice traditional medicine do not understand alternative medicine. What they do not understand, they cannot advocate.

Most physicians practicing traditional medicine do not understand alternative medicine for two reasons: unfamiliarity and skepticism. Physicians are unfamiliar with alternative medicine, despite the fact that the principles of some forms of alternative medicine have preceded traditional medicine by several centuries, because those principles are not taught in medical school, are rarely taught in postgraduate education, and are not published in most medical journals. Physicians are also skeptical of alternative medicine because alternative medicines have not had to pass the rigorous tests of validity imposed by the FDA when it approves drugs, or by medical journals when they approve publication. These traditional tests have to their credit most of the medical achievements of the twentieth century.

Physicians practicing traditional medicine have several concerns about alternative medicine. One is that alternative medicine might cause harm. Another is that alternative medicine might be used instead of traditional medicine. A third is that some forms of alternative medicine have an entrepreneurial element: that is, in some cases, someone is getting rich by selling treatments of doubtful benefit to people who are desperate.

Another concern is that claims are commonly made that some treatment has a specific and measurable benefit, but the benefit is not adequately documented. For example, one frequent claim is that some alternative treatment inhibits HIV in the test tube. The problem with that claim is that a drug that works in a test tube may not work in the body. There are several reasons for this: the concentration of the drug might be wrong; the drug may never get to the site of infection; or the conditions in the body are too different from those in the test tube.

Even more common are claims that some alternative treatment strengthens the immune system. Most such claims falter when scrutinized carefully. The problem is that the immune system has been studied extensively, but much of that study is relatively recent and the immune system turns out to be extremely complicated, to have many interacting parts. Many studies seem to show that almost any treatment—be it vitamins, diet, drug, or a change in behavior—has some measurable effect on some part of the immune system. HIV infection disturbs a certain specific part of this complicated immune system, and boosting a different part of the immune system may be as naive as putting oil in a car that is out of gas. In other words, claims that the functioning of the immune system has improved are true for almost any kind of treatment if you measure enough of the parts of the immune system. But no one knows how a change in one part of the immune system affects the other parts, or whether such changes in the immune system have any important effect on someone's general health.

The final concern that physicians have about alternative medicine is that people often claim that alternative treatments have been responsible for someone with HIV remaining well for prolonged periods. But, in medicine, exceptions are the rule. Studies have shown that even without medical treatment at all, 5–10 percent of the people with AIDS survive for five years. Be careful about the anecdote, the exceptional case. Remember that the history of medicine is replete with miracles that have happened in spite of treatment, not because of it. This is the reason for the strictness of the controls on a clinical trial: sufficient numbers of cases assure that differences in the results are not due to chance alone.

There are also arguments in favor of alternative medicine. First, it is presumptuous to conclude that because alternative medicine lacks scientific validity, it does not work. Alternative medicines have rarely even been tested for scientific validity. Second, people who use alternative medicine have profound faith in its benefits; such faith seems to allow people with HIV infection to gain the sense of control that is crucial not only to psychological health but possibly to physical health as well. A new field in traditional medicine, called *psychoneuroimmunology* (see Chapter 12), has preliminary evidence that physical health and immune function are partially affected by psychological health. A very well controlled trial published in the *New England Journal of Medicine*, medicine's most prestigious journal, showed that mental stress was a significant risk factor for catching the common cold. In other words, your mental health can affect your physical health, including the strength of your immune system. Psychoneuroimmunology is a new field, and no one yet knows its relevance to HIV infection. But it would be as presumptuous at this point to conclude it does not work as it would be to argue that it certainly does.

A third argument in favor of alternative medicine is that, in many cases, the drug causes no harm, the people supplying the drug are often driven by a sincere interest in the welfare of people with HIV infection, and some people with HIV infection have exhausted the approved drugs and understandably need to do something about their medical treatment.

Because of these arguments, most physicians practicing traditional medicine are willing to accept—if they cannot advocate—alternative medicine. Their acceptance has two caveats: that alternative medicine not be harmful, and that it not be used instead of traditional medicine.

Regardless of their physicians' opinions, surveys in New York City and San Francisco show that up to a third of the people with HIV infection are using some form of alternative medicine. The forms of alternative medicine that seem to be used most frequently are underground drugs, acupuncture, macrobiotic diets, megavitamin treatment, and mind work. Most people with HIV infection who use alternative medicine also use traditional medicine. Many of these people are reluctant to share this information with their physicians, and as a result, are operating without medical advice about this part of their health care.

With this in mind, the following section lists some of the most common forms of alternative medicine—treatment is a better word, since some of these alternatives are not medicines—outlines what the treatments claim to do, lists the side effects, and assesses whether the treatment is likely to be harmful.

Underground Drugs

Underground drugs are drugs made available through nontraditional or quasilegal means, such as buyers' clubs and AIDS activist groups. Underground drugs include untested drugs, licensed and unlicensed drugs, drugs produced in garages and basements outside the usual manufacturing process, and drugs that are purchased in other countries because they are cheaper than comparable drugs in the United States. Some underground drugs purchased in foreign countries are the same drugs licensed in the United States—sometimes these drugs are even produced in the United States. These drugs are bought in bulk by buyers' clubs at a lower price, and the savings are passed on to the consumer. Lists of drugs and prices are usually readily available from AIDS activist groups.

You should be cautious about underground drugs for two reasons. The first is that the source of the drug could be unreliable. An example is the street supply of ddC that preceded FDA licensing. When the FDA analyzed the street supply from various sources, it found potency ranging from 0 percent to 200 percent. In other words, some street supplies of ddC had no active drug and some had twice the amount advertised, which could be toxic. Nevertheless, many drugs from buyers' clubs are the same as those purchased in drugstores, and the cost savings can be great.

The second reason to be cautious is that people commonly and tragically have unrealistic expectations of fashionable drugs that promise miracles but have little scientific credibility and turn out to be useless. Many desperate people with AIDS went to Paris to get the Rock Hudson drug, HPA-23; hundreds went to Mexico for ribavirin; thousands were supplied with dextran sulfate from Japan; Kemron was touted as the miracle drug that Africans developed but American scientists refused to take seriously; and a few unfortunate people underwent the infamous heat treatments in Atlanta. The history of AIDS treatment, like that of cancer treatment, is replete with drugs that attracted great attention and then, with proper testing, quickly fell from favor.

Acupuncture

Acupuncture is a tradition in Chinese medicine now available from licensed acupuncturists in the United States. According to acupuncturists, HIV infection is a condition caused by the blockage of the flow of the life force, called *chi*. In addition, HIV infection might also be interpreted as a deficiency in a masculine, active quality called *yang*, as well as a deficiency in a feminine, passive quality called *yin*. Treatment is the insertion of needles at any of the 365 points along twelve body lines, which is said to permit the flow of chi. The needles are left in place for twenty to thirty minutes; treatment may continue from several days to several months.

Acupuncture is poorly understood according to the criteria of traditional medicine, although it clearly has profound biologic effects: it can, in fact, be used in place of general anesthesia for some major operations. The usefulness of acupuncture as a treatment for HIV infection has not been tested with a clinical trial, so the benefits are not established. There are essentially no risks.

Herbal Medicine

Chinese medical practitioners often use herbs to act on the twelve body lines mentioned above. Many herbs and combinations of herbs are recommended for treatment of HIV infection and are available in health food stores. The most popular herb is raw garlic; it is used for many conditions and is available as odorless capsules of garlic oil. Recent scientific studies indicate that garlic may have wide-ranging health benefits, although the usefulness of this or any other herb for people with HIV infection is not known.

Advocates of herbal medicine believe that herbs improve the immune system. Many of these herbs and combinations of herbs have side effects that include nausea and vomiting, allergic reactions, liver damage, blurred vision, dry mouth, nervousness, sedation, and hallucinations.

Dietary Modification

Dietary modification can mean almost anything. Certainly, physicians practicing traditional medicine say that good nutrition is an important part of health care for someone with HIV infection. Practitioners of alternative treatments usually define dietary modification as certain diets or food supplements that inhibit the growth of HIV or that enhance the immune system. A comprehensive guide to the relationship of nutrition and immune function for patients with AIDS is *Healing AIDS Naturally: Natural Therapies for the Immune System,* by Laurence Badgley.

Probably the most popular of the alternative diets is a macrobiotic diet. Macrobiotic diets are said to balance foods with yin (foods which form acids in the body) and foods with yang (foods which form alkalines in the body). The macrobiotic diet consists largely of vegetables and grains. It excludes red meat, commercially raised poultry, all processed foods, polished rice, dairy products, leavened breads, and sugars. Dietitians say that a macrobiotic diet lacks essential nutrients and is potentially harmful.

Other practitioners of dietary modification advocate food supplements—a list of certain substances said to inhibit the growth of HIV or enhance the immune system. None of these supplements has, by the standards of traditional medicine, established that they will help. Some of the most common supplements are the following:

Acidophilus, a bacterium available without prescription in drugstores and health food stores that is supposed to produce a healthy intestinal tract. Acidophilus is harmless.

AL721, a substance derived from egg yolk that is supposed to inhibit the growth of HIV. AL721 was tested in scientific studies; though found to be useless against HIV, it is also harmless.

Coenzyme Q10, an antioxidant that is supposed to improve the immune system. It is harmless.

Garlic, which is widely advocated in herbal medicine and is available in an odorless and tasteless form called kyolic. It is harmless.

Lecithin, which is related to AL721 and is harmless.

Lentinan, an extract from mushrooms, called mushroom power or Lentil, is said to act against HIV. It is harmless.

Vitamin C, which is often advocated in large doses for HIV infection and a whole host of other medical conditions. Advocates often recommend taking 1,000 milligrams or more a day. Vitamin C has also been studied scientifically, to see if it combats colds and cancer; it does not. The recommended daily allowance (RDA) of Vitamin C, 60 milligrams a day, is certainly good for you. Most people get more than the RDA in a standard diet. The large doses advocated in alternative medicine can cause stomach pain and diarrhea. They can also corrode the teeth—practitioners advocate taking large doses by straw.

Vitamin A, also advocated in large doses, which are said to promote the growth of CD4 cells. The RDA for Vitamin A, 3,000 International Units per day, is good you; doses of 100,000 International Units per day for three months or more can cause dry and itchy skin, sore mouth, loss of hair, vomiting, headaches, drowsiness, and liver damage.

Zinc, a metal that occurs in traces in the body. In the later stages of HIV infection, concentrations of zinc in the body seem to decrease.

Taking zinc as a supplement, however, can cause nausea and vomiting and is possibly harmful.

Selenium, another trace metal that also seems to occur in lower concentrations in people in the later stages of HIV infection. Excess selenium causes damage to cells; taking selenium as a supplement is possibly harmful.

Chiropractic Treatment

The principles of chiropractic treatment state that HIV infection is caused by a poor alignment of the backbone, which impairs nearby nerves. Treatment consists of positioning the body to correct the defect. Chiropractic treatment is probably helpful if your back hurts, probably harmless otherwise.

Homeopathic Medicine

Practitioners of homeopathic medicine believe that a substance that causes a symptom in a large dose can, when given in a small dose, stimulate the body to correct the symptom. The underlying principle is that similars correct similars. In the case of HIV infection, which weakens the immune system, practitioners of homeopathic medicine advocate using small doses of cyclosporine, a drug used in traditional medicine to weaken the immune systems of people whose bodies are rejecting transplanted organs. Homeopathic medicine uses extremely small doses of these various substances; it is harmless.

Body Work

One form of body work is endurance exercise programs and weight lifting. Another form of body work is yoga, a Hindu philosophical system of balancing mind and body through breathing and posturing exercises. A third form of body work is t'ai chi, a Chinese exercise program that achieves a balance between mind and body through slow movements. There is no evidence that body work is harmful if done within reason. It may be beneficial, and it certainly makes the people who practice it feel better.

Mind Work

One kind of mind work tries to foster favorable self-images or self-love. Books explaining this kind of mind work include *Love Yourself, Heal Yourself*, by Louise Hay; *Anatomy of an Illness as Perceived by the*

Patient: Reflections on Healing and Regeneration, by Norman Cousins; *Love, Medicine, and Miracles*, by Bernie Siegel; and *Quantum Healing: Exploring the Frontiers of Mind/Body Medicine*, by Deepak Chopra.

Another kind of mind work is visualization or guided imagery. During visualization, people imagine their immune systems attacking and killing HIV and their bodies becoming stronger and healthier.

Like body work, mind work can't hurt. And because it makes people feel more in control and happier with themselves, it can be beneficial.

Chapter 10

Practical Matters: Making Legal, Financial, and Medical Decisions

- Legal rights and obligations
- Financing medical care
- Using the social service system
- Putting your affairs in order

Many people find dealing with the practical aspects of having HIV infection almost as troublesome as the infection itself. People worry about money; about confidentiality; about dealing with the legal, medical, and social service systems; about writing wills; about removing burdens from those they love; about the possibility of becoming incompetent. Such questions about practical matters are generally best answered by two categories of professionals.

One category is composed of social workers. Social workers are found in most community agencies that deal with HIV infection: mental health centers, state and local social service agencies, AIDS-advocacy organizations, some churches, and virtually all hospitals. Hospital social workers also understand the medical system and can help you navigate it. Their job is usually to help you make plans for the short term, especially plans for leaving the hospital and returning home (see Chapter 8).

The other category is composed of lawyers. To find a lawyer, check with people you know who have lawyers they trust, with your state's bar association, or with local AIDS-advocacy agencies. Related professionals (these are often lawyers, too) handle complaints about discrimination. They can be found in your state's human relations or civil rights commission. Check in the telephone book's yellow or blue pages under the name of your state, or under social service organizations.

Legal Rights and Obligations

Federal Laws That Apply to HIV Infection

Section 504 of the Rehabilitation Act of 1973 protects all citizens of the United States against discrimination on grounds of race, sex, creed, color, or handicap. *Handicap* includes AIDS, and people with AIDS are consequently protected from discrimination. This antidiscrimination law applies to all service providers and organizations—employers, providers of health care, and providers of social services—that receive federal funds either directly or through state and local agencies. The Americans with Disabilities Act of 1990 extends federal protection against discrimination to all people with HIV infection, whether or not they have symptoms of infection. This newer law applies to all service providers and organizations, regardless of whether they receive federal funds or not.

Your rights to employment under federal law include protection against discrimination in recruitment, hiring, job assignment, sick leave, or other benefits. Your rights to health care include protection against discrimination in services offered by hospitals, nursing homes, or other health care providers. Your rights to social services include protection against discrimination in receiving welfare, Medicaid, Medicare, and other social service programs. Additional information about civil rights under federal law may be obtained by calling the Equal Opportunity Specialist in the Office for Civil Rights, United States Department of Health and Human Services, at 1-800-368-1019. When you reach that number, a computer will identify your area code and will automatically transfer your call to your regional office. For people who are deaf, hard of hearing, or speech-impaired, the TTY/TDD phone number is 1-800-537-7697.

People who feel that their rights under the federal antidiscrimination laws have been violated should file a complaint within 180 days with the Office for Civil Rights, United States Department of Health and Human Services, P.O. Box 13716, Mail Stop 07, Philadelphia, Pa. 19101, or call 1-215-596-6109. Complaints should be in writing and should include

your name or the name of the person filing the complaint on your behalf;

the service provider or organization against whom you are filing the complaint;

a statement that the complaint is based on HIV infection as the basis for a handicap;

a description of the complaint;

the time of the incident and whether the incident is ongoing;

a description of any attempt to resolve the complaint;

a telephone number where you can be contacted for follow-up information.

The representative of the Office of Civil Rights will begin an investigation. If discrimination is found, the Office of Civil Rights will ask the service provider or organization to correct the complaint voluntarily. If this request is unsuccessful, the service provider or organization may have its federal funding terminated, or other legal action will be pursued. If the complaint is not covered by law, the representative of the Office of Civil Rights will attempt to refer the complaint to the appropriate agency.

On December 1, 1991, the federal government passed a law called the Patient Self-Determination Act. This law requires hospitals to educate every patient admitted into the hospital about certain documents called Advance Directives. Advance Directives include living wills and durable powers of attorney. Living wills and durable powers of attorney are documents written by you when you are mentally competent to provide for your medical care should you become mentally incompetent. (See "Putting Your Affairs in Order," below.) The exact Advance Directives that are available to you depend on which state you live in; the federal law requires only that you be notified of those Advance Directives your state happens to recognize. Check with your hospital or your lawyer about which Advance Directives your state has and which are best for you.

State Laws That Apply to HIV Infection

Most states also have laws that protect the citizens of that state against discrimination on grounds of handicap. Whether HIV infection is included in a state's definition of handicap depends on the state: the laws that apply to people with HIV infection, needless to say, vary from state to state. The state laws against discrimination on grounds of handicap are sometimes different from the federal laws. Some people with HIV infection find it useful to pursue claims of discrimination under either federal or state laws, or both.

(Note: Some laws use the word *handicap*; others use the word *disability*. The two words mean the same thing.)

In general, state laws against discrimination govern such issues as your right to public accommodations, your right to housing and employment, your right to confidentiality, and your medical rights.

Your right to public accommodations. Public accommodations are more important than they sound. A public accommodation is any place open to and serving the public. Exactly which places are defined as public accommodations vary from state to state: some states include doctors' offices, for instance, and some do not. Depending on the state, then, public accommodations can include schools, doctors' offices, hospitals, hospices, barber and beauty shops, nursing homes, funeral homes, public transportation, restaurants, and hotels. Any place defined as a public accommodation cannot discriminate according to race, sex, creed, color, or (depending on the state) handicap. In most states, AIDS is defined as a handicap. In some states, having HIV infection but not AIDS may also be defined as a handicap.

Although all laws governing the right to public accommodations are similar, they will differ in detail according to the state. In some states, for instance, beauty shops are not allowed to treat someone with a contagious disease, and since HIV infection is contagious, those states could conceivably bar a person with that virus from a beauty shop. This is, however, an obviously unrealistic use of the word *contagious*, since the type of exposure that occurs in beauty shops carries no risk of transmitting HIV.

To find out the laws in your state, ask a lawyer. Lawyers can also draw up wills and help sort out problems with the Social Security system and with insurance companies.

Another source of information about discrimination is an agency called, in some states, the state human relations commission. In other states, it is called the state civil rights commission. If you think you have been denied public accommodations because of your HIV status, file a complaint with the state human relations or civil rights commission, and they will investigate. You will not need a lawyer to file a complaint. You will, however, need to be a pest, because agencies move slowly. You also need to remember that filing such a complaint will involve giving up the confidentiality of your HIV status.

Your rights to housing and employment. Your rights to housing and employment are the same as your right to public accommodations. In general, you have a right to whatever housing you can afford and whatever job you can carry out.

In most states, refusing someone housing or employment because they have AIDS is illegal. Most states have laws forbidding discrimination on grounds of disability; and, in most states, AIDS is defined as a disability. Whether HIV infection is also defined as a disability depends on the state: ask a lawyer. Therefore, as long as you can pay your rent or mortgage, you may not be refused housing because of the disabling effects of AIDS. As long as you can carry out your job, you may not be refused employment or fired because of the disabling effects of AIDS.

You also have a right to expect your employer to make reasonable accommodations to your disability. If your job involves heavy lifting, for instance, and you tire easily, you can ask your employer to reassign you to a less strenuous job. The general principle is that you have a right to expect your employer to modify your job in ways that do not compromise your usefulness to the job. Again, as with public accommodations, if you think you have been forced out of a job or housing because of your HIV status, file a complaint with the state human relations or civil rights commission. If the complaint involves employment discrimination, and if you win, you are entitled to back pay, attorney's fees, and damages.

Your right to confidentiality; your obligation to disclose. As a general rule, your medical record, including your HIV status, is confidential. In most states, your physician must protect your confidentiality; physicians can disclose information about patients only under certain conditions. In fact, no one with access to your HIV status—laboratory staff, hospital staff, nurses, secretaries—is allowed to reveal your name. Your name can be revealed only if you sign an authorization. The one exception, as stated below, is that some states require physicians to report all cases of certain diseases, by name, to state health departments. Otherwise, revealing your name without signed authorization is grounds for suit. If your name has been revealed, you can bring a civil law suit against the person who revealed it. If the person was a physician, the state board that licenses physicians and the physician's professional society can review the incident.

As with any law, your right to the confidentiality of your medical records has conditions. When you apply for insurance, you usually authorize the company to request release of your medical records. Your HIV status must be included in those records: medical records are, by definition, complete medical records.

If you check into a hospital, you implicitly authorize access to your medical records to all your health care providers at that hospital, including other physicians, nurses, dentists, social workers, and physician's assistants. If your physician refers you to a specialist and you accept the referral, you implicitly grant the specialist access to your medical records.

If you apply for a job, depending on the state, your prospective employer might be able to request your medical records, but your records will be released only if you authorize it. Prospective employers may not require you to authorize release.

Physicians must report every case of AIDS they treat to the state public health department. Some states require physicians to report all blood tests positive for HIV infection. Most states require that this reporting be done either by name or by such other identifiers as social security number. The state public health departments are prohibited from revealing your name. In the unlikely event that your name is revealed, most states give you some sort of legal recourse—to a lawsuit, for instance. States are required to report cases of AIDS to the federal government, but to report the cases as statistics, not by name.

HIV infection also confers certain obligations on you. You have a moral and legal obligation to notify anyone you have put at risk. In general, this includes sex partners and people with whom you have shared needles. Health care workers might be obliged to inform the institutions in which they work. If you refuse to notify those you have put at risk, or continue to place others at risk without due warning, they can sue you.

If you refuse to inform anyone you put at risk for infection, your physician may be under obligation to inform him or her. The American Medical Association has advised physicians of that obligation. In many states, the physician's obligation to inform is law; other states have legislation pending that will make this a law. Thus, whether your physician is required to reveal your name and diagnosis without your authorization depends on the circumstances and varies from state to state.

Once the obligation to inform those placed at risk is discharged, however, you have no further legal or moral obligation to tell anyone else about your HIV status. You have no obligation to tell your employer, your landlord, your psychologist or psychiatrist, your family, your friends, your co-workers, or your neighbors. Lawyers often advise their clients who have HIV infection to tell as few people as possible. Except for those whom you are obliged to tell, tell only the people you love and who will help you and respect your privacy. No one else needs to know.

Your medical rights. One of your principal medical rights is to informed consent. That is, you have a right to an explanation of any treatment or procedure before it is performed on you, an explanation of the risks of that treatment or procedure, and an explanation of the alternatives to that treatment or procedure. "Treatment or procedure" means any drugs, any tests or surgeries—anything that involves something foreign entering your body. "Risks" means material risks, that is, anything that can reasonably be expected to happen. Your doctor is not necessarily obligated to inform you of an improbable risk, a one-in-a-million chance.

Informed consent also means that you can refuse any treatment or procedure. Anyone who attempts the treatment or procedure without your consent—assuming you are mentally competent to give consent—can be sued on grounds of battery. You also have the right to refuse medication. Your right to refuse food and water is still a matter of legal argument. Your right to refuse treatments, procedures, or medication can be overruled only if you are incompetent. *Incompetent* means that you are unable to comprehend what you have been told and are unable to make decisions. In principle, the courts, guided by the advice of the physician, decide when someone is incompetent. In practice, the court system takes a long time, and competence is decided by two concurring physicians, one of whom is your physician-of-record.

You can request treatments, procedures, or medication, but you cannot demand them.

You have a right to see your medical records. Your medical records are, however, the property of the hospital. As such, the hospital can dictate under what circumstances and in whose presence you can see your medical records. You have a right to a copy of your medical records. You may not remove the original records from the hospital without the hospital's consent. In many states, you have the right to make additions or corrections to your medical records.

Hospitals, as public accommodations, cannot refuse to treat you on the grounds that you have HIV infection. Some hospitals, however, limit the kinds of treatment they offer and can refuse to treat anyone who requires services they do not offer. Any Health Maintenance Organization (HMO) to which you belong has a legal contract with you that outlines the rights and obligations of both parties.

In a hospital, you can request to be assigned another physician. The hospital is obliged to grant your request.

Some states have laws that prohibit a physician from refusing patients on the basis of race, sex, creed, color, or disability. In most states, HIV infection is defined as a disability. However, many physicians do not consider themselves competent to care for people with HIV infection and will refuse care—rightly—on this basis. Others are simply too busy to accept new patients. The first time you see a private physician, he or she can refuse to treat you. If you have previously been accepted as a patient by that physician for other medical conditions and the two of you have an ongoing relationship, she or he can still refuse to treat you, but cannot abandon you. Not abandoning you means that your physician must help you find another physician who can provide the care needed.

Similar rules apply to dental care. Many dentists are uncomfortable caring for people with HIV infection. The ethics of dental practice dictate that the dentist is obliged to provide continuing care to established patients, or at least refer them to another dentist who can provide more specialized care.

A Note on Lawsuits

The right to file lawsuits is a right no one can take away from you. But lawsuits often take years to settle. Some people decide not to file a suit because they do not want to take the time. Others decide not to file because their HIV status would then become public record. Many people go ahead and fight and win suits.

Financing Medical Care

People with HIV infection report that among their biggest worries are the problems of financing medical care. Unfortunately, many of their worries are justified. Although the average medical bill for the care of HIV infection if no greater than the average bill for most other serious medical conditions, people with HIV infection should be prepared for expensive medical care.

The average cost of medical care for HIV infection over a lifetime, in 1992 dollars, is estimated at about $100,000. Most of the costs are incurred after the first AIDS-defining diagnosis. The greatest part of this cost is for hospitalization—from $55,000 to $70,000—though expanded use of alternatives to hospital care has lowered that cost. Drug costs and supportive services account for about $30,000–$45,000.

The mechanisms for financing medical care in the United States are phenomenally complicated and full of jargon. People finance their medical care either by themselves (called self-pay), or through private insurance, or through publicly funded state and federal programs. Private insurance and public programs are together called third-party payers. Most people finance their care through a combination of self-pay and third-party payers.

Private third-party payers include commercial insurance companies, Health Maintenance Organizations (HMOs), and the nonprofit conglomerate that is Blue Cross/Blue Shield. The main public third-party payers include Medicare, Medicaid, and the Veterans Administration.

Medicare accounts for 17 percent of the financing for all health care in the United States; Medicaid for 10 percent; other government agencies for 14 percent; private insurance for 31 percent; self-pay for 25 percent; and private sponsors for 3 percent. An estimated 35 million Americans are uninsured.

Several aspects of financing medical care are unique to HIV infection:

1. People with HIV infection make up a disproportionately large number of those who receive Medicaid. By 1990, many large cities had reported that 40 percent of all persons with AIDS were receiving Medicaid; this percentage is increasing.

2. Most third-party payers will not reimburse the full range of services commonly required for people with HIV infection; services that are reimbursed insufficiently or not reimbursed at all include home care, long-term care facilities, and prescription drugs.

3. Private third-party payers have many ways—some of them devious—of avoiding reimbursement of the costs of medical care for HIV infection. They do this despite the fact that the average lifetime cost of the care of a person with HIV infection is no different than the cost of care of people with most other serious conditions.

4. Many physicians are reluctant to care for people with HIV infection because the medical care is unusually complex and because reimbursement for professional services is unusually poor due to the disproportionate number who are uninsured or recipients of Medicaid.

5. Public funds, both from the states and from the federal government, are increasingly available to people with HIV infection. However, eligibility for many of the special programs often requires a diagnosis of AIDS.

For more on paying for drugs, see Chapter 9.

The following sections go into what may strike you as tiresome detail about financing medical care. But the more you know about what is standard or required or forbidden, the better you will be able to control your options for financing care.

Private, Third-Party Payers for Financing Health Care

All private, third-party payers—Health Maintenance Organizations (HMOs), Blue Cross/Blue Shield, and commercial insurance companies—offer two kinds of plans for financing medical care: group plans and individual plans. Group plans are offered by the third-party payer to an employer, and then by the employer to the employees. Individual plans are offered by the third-party directly to the individual.

Group plans. Blue Cross/Blue Shield, HMOs, and a large number of commercial insurance companies all sell group plans to employers.

Commercial insurance companies are often national businesses that offer similar group plans to all employers throughout the country. Blue Cross/Blue Shield is a group of 77 not-for-profit, regional insurers who offer different group plans in each of their different regions. HMOs, whose rules for group plans are different from those of commercial companies and Blue Cross/Blue Shield, are discussed below.

Group plans held by companies with large numbers of employees usually do not require you to have a medical examination or to submit your medical records. Anyone with HIV infection currently working for a large company with a group plan will be covered by that plan. Smaller companies, however, are more likely to have group plans that require the employers to answer health questions about their employees.

If you are hired for a new job in a large company, the group insurance will often have a rule about preexisting conditions. To rule out people who take out insurance only when they become sick (called having a preexisting condition—see below, under "Individual Plans"), insurance companies sometimes enforce a waiting period—usually a matter of months—between the time of application and the time coverage begins. If you are hired for a new job and you have been diagnosed with HIV infection, the insurance company will usually wait for the period set by the preexisting conditions rule before covering you. This rule applies to all preexisting conditions.

Blue Cross/Blue Shield, which has a group plan offered by many employers, does not usually transfer from one employer to another. Each employer negotiates its own individual contract with the local Blue Cross/Blue Shield company. If you transfer from one employer to another, preexisting condition rules will now apply under the second employer's policy.

The insurer (whether a commercial insurance company or Blue Cross/Blue Shield) always sets limits on what the group plan covers. One of the limits is that group plans generally cover only some fraction of your medical expenses. They often cover around 80 percent of hospital expenses and about 60 percent of physicians' expenses. In addition, most of the Blue Cross/Blue Shield group plans also cover home health care, the majority also cover hospice care, and about 30 percent also cover prescription drugs.

That part of the medical bill left over after the insurer has paid its fraction is called your *co-pay*. Co-pay is done two ways, by co-insurance and by deductibles. Co-insurance is usually stated as a percentage of an annual bill; you are usually responsible for 20 percent of eligible medical expenses each year. After that, the company pays all eligible medical expenses. Deductibles are usually stated as an amount of money that you must pay before the insurance company can be billed: you must pay, for instance, the first $25 of any bill.

A second limit on what groups plans cover is that they will pay only for what they consider to be the customary charge for a service. For example, an office visit may be billed at $50, the customary charge (based on area charges by physicians for comparable services) may be $40, the coverage may be 80 percent of the customary charge, or $32, so your co-pay for this bill will be $18.

A third limit is not so much a limit as an incentive: some plans from Blue Cross/Blue Shield provide you financial incentives to choose specific "participating physicians" or Preferred Provider Organizations (PPOs). In other words, certain physicians or groups of physicians agree to lower their fees, thereby also reducing the cost to you. In general, however, the group plans offered by both commercial insurance companies and Blue Cross/Blue Shield allow you considerable freedom of choice: you can choose your own physician and hospital.

A fourth limit: most group plans limit—or cap—total lifetime payments at $1 million or $2 million.

Most insurers periodically renew their policies with employers. Most policies are conditionally renewable, meaning that insurers can refuse an employer's request to renew the policy only if the insurer refuses to renew all similar policies in that state. This means that an employer cannot be refused a renewed policy because some employees have HIV infection. They may, however, increase the rates charged for coverage of the same services.

In spite of the limits, being enrolled in a group plan through your place of employment is obviously desirable. Because group plans spread coverage over many people, many of whom make few insurance claims, insurers can afford to cover you without requiring that you give evidence of insurability (see below, under "Uninsurability").

HMOs also offer group plans. HMOs provide comprehensive services for a fixed, prepaid fee. In other words, when you join a group plan offered by an HMO, you pay a flat, fixed fee for all your health care bills, regardless of how much health care you actually get. The good news about HMOs is that they finance nearly all medical care. In particular, Kaiser, the largest HMO in the United States, provides a comprehensive program of services for people with HIV infection.

The bad news about HMOs is that, unlike commercial insurance companies and Blue Cross/Blue Shield, HMOs allow little choice in physicians or hospitals. Because competition among HMOs for employer contracts is fierce, costs must be kept low. Consequently, the HMO must carefully regulate hospital admissions, expensive drugs, and expensive procedures and must preapprove any consultation or procedure done outside the resources of the HMO. If your physician refers you to a specialist outside your HMO, for instance, the HMO may rigorously review the referral and often deny payment. As a result, many participants lack confidence in the quality of the health care providers and are disappointed in the range of services the HMO provides. Do not be persuaded by HMOs' advertisements that emphasize the services offered; in practice, many HMOs choose saving money over offering services.

You can find out the details of group plans by reading the policy or by talking to the claims and benefits office of the insurer that offers the policy. For details about group plans offered by HMOs, often the best source of information is the other people who use the HMO, especially those whose health care needs are complicated.

Continuing group plans if you can't work. A person who has been covered previously under a group plan, but who can no longer work, may have the option of continuing in the group plan for eighteen months under the Consolidated Omnibus Reconciliation Act of 1985 (COBRA). Under COBRA, the former employee would pay a premium that is 102 percent of the premium previously paid by the employer—the extra 2 percent is for administrative fees. Some states will pay these premiums for you, to delay Medicaid coverage (see below). Requirements for coverage under COBRA are as follows: COBRA applies only to businesses with twenty or more employees; the former employee must pay the premiums; the former employee must be ineligible for Medicare (see below); the employer must continue the group plan for continuing employees; and the former employee cannot join another plan.

People who are eligible for Social Security disability benefits (see below, under "Help with Income") when employment ends may obtain eleven months of additional coverage (for a total of twenty-nine months) with the same insurer, although the premium may now be 150 percent for the additional eleven months. And some states have programs that extend COBRA for people with AIDS.

People who are not eligible for COBRA because they worked for a company with fewer than twenty employees may still be protected under the Continuation of Comprehensive Benefits laws in thirty-five states; the duration of coverage of the employer's group policy varies with different states, and ranges from three to eighteen months.

The alternative to COBRA, if COBRA is not available or if it runs out, is a conversion policy: the former employee converts the group policy to a type of individual policy. Conversion policies cover less than group plans and cost more. Thirty-five states require employers to offer conversion policies to former employees when COBRA benefits run out. Premium rates tend to be high, since most people who buy conversion policies are in poor health. Nevertheless, the person with a serious disease might have few other options, and conversion policies are available regardless of health status or preexisting conditions. The remaining option is an individual plan, which costs even more than a conversion policy.

Individual plans. Individual plans are offered by third-party payers directly to individuals. About fifteen million Americans have individual plans; approximately ten million of them have individual plans with commercial companies, four million with Blue Cross/Blue Shield, and one million with HMOs.

Individual plans offer four basic kinds of policies: major medical policies, hospital-surgical policies, hospital indemnity policies, and dread disease policies. The best coverage is under major medical policies: they typically pay for hospital care, physicians' fees, laboratory tests, drugs, ambulance services, and skilled nursing facilities. Hospital-surgical policies pay for hospital and surgical services only. Hospital indemnity policies pay a fixed amount only while a person is hospitalized. Since a typical amount paid is $75 a day, and since the average hospital charge per day is ten times higher, hospital indemnity policies are regarded as a rip-off. Dread disease policies will generally not provide coverage for people who already have the dread disease.

Individual plans have different requirements for eligibility, cover different services, and reimburse at different rates than group plans. Generally, an insurer will cover some percentage of your medical costs if you continue to meet certain conditions: if you pay your premiums; if you have not reached some (usually extremely high) upper limit or cap on expenses; if you ask the company to pay for only those items they contracted to pay for; and if you do not seem to pose to them an unacceptably high risk.

For commercial insurance companies and Blue Cross/Blue Shield, risks are classified as (1) standard, for which the insurer will supply standard coverage at the usual rates; (2) substandard, for which the insurer will supply coverage at increased rates or will exclude coverage for some medical condition; and (3) denied, for which the insurer will supply no coverage (see "Uninsurability," below). For HMOs, risks are either acceptable or unacceptable: that is, HMOs will either accept you at the usual rate or they will deny your application. For insurers, virtually all people with AIDS, cancer, coronary artery disease, and diabetes pose unacceptably high risks.

To assess the risk you pose, all private, third-party payers (that is, all private insurers) use similar mechanisms. You must fill out an application, which includes a health questionnaire. Nearly all health questionnaires include questions about HIV infection: for example, Have you ever had AIDS or tested positive for HIV infection? Other questions may ask whether you have or ever had symptoms of HIV infection. Still other questions may be about drug abuse, age, and occupation: these questions are triggers for the insurer to scrutinize the application further. Questions about sexual orientation are also triggers, despite the fact that such questions violate the guidelines of the National Association of Insurance Commissioners.

When you apply for an individual plan, the insurer will request your medical records. Everyone applying for individual insurance must authorize the insurer to request medical records. The insurer might also request a statement, called an Attending Physician Statement, from your physician. Your medical records must be complete, including HIV status. Withholding or falsifying any information on a medical record is grounds for the insurer to deny payment and cancel the policy. Most insurers also require the applicant to take a medical examination.

Whether an insurer can require you to take an HIV antibody test is still a matter of legal argument. Some insurers require HIV antibody tests for all applicants for individual plans; most will require the tests if the answers on your health questionnaire merit the test. California and Washington, D.C., have banned HIV antibody testing for insurance purposes but allow insurers to use CD4 counts instead.

What insurers want to rule out with all these questions and tests and checks is what they call a *preexisting condition*. A preexisting condition is defined by the National Association of Insurance Commissioners as "the existence of symptoms which would cause an ordinarily prudent person to seek diagnosis, care, or treatment," or as "a condition for which medical advice or treatment was recommended by a physician or received from a physician within a five-year period preceding the effective date of coverage." In short, a preexisting condition is a medical condition for which you have received advice or treatment (assuming you are an ordinarily prudent person) from a physician within the last five years. Some insurers will accept an applicant with certain preexisting conditions as a substandard risk; others will deny the application for the same condition.

To be certain the applicant does not have a preexisting condition that has escaped everyone's notice, insurers usually enforce a waiting period—usually a matter of months—between the time of application and the time coverage begins. If, during the waiting period, the applicant shows no evidence of a preexisting condition, the company will accept the application and will pay eligible medical benefits. If you develop AIDS well after you enrolled in an individual plan with the insurer, that company is ethically obligated not to drop you. The company could, however, legally contest that obligation.

The bottom line: An asymptomatic person with a positive HIV blood test does not fit the definition of having a preexisting condition. Insurers nevertheless will often deny the applications for individual plans from people with HIV infection. Some of these denials are being contested in court.

Note that the preexisting condition rule affects people who apply for individual plans with a new insurer. For this reason, people with HIV infection who have a long-time plan with an insurer are often advised to stay with that insurer.

You can find out the details of individual plans by reading your policy or by talking to your insurance agent.

Uninsurability. About 8 percent of the applicants for individual plans are denied. Those whose applications are denied include virtually all people with AIDS, cancer, coronary artery disease, and diabetes. This and other health-related information obtained by insurers is recorded in the Medical Information Bureau in Boston, an insurance industry clearinghouse. Most people with preexisting conditions will find their access to individual insurance coverage limited unless that coverage comes through what is called an exclusion rider or unless they pay extremely high premiums.

People unable to purchase insurance because of preexisting conditions may have access to high-risk pool insurance at inflated prices. Pool policies are provided in twenty-three states. Requirements for eligibility include residency in the state for at least six months and a notice from an insurance company of rejection, of a high-risk rate, or of an exclusion rider. Problems with the pool policies are that only twenty-three states carry them, that waiting lists are long, and that premiums are high. Information about pool policies can be obtained from state insurance departments.

Another option is the open enrollment policies periodically available in some Blue Cross/Blue Shield plans in thirteen states. Open enrollment means that any applicant, including anyone with AIDS, is granted insurance regardless of health status. Not surprisingly, the premiums are higher, the waiting period for preexisting conditions is longer, and some preexisting conditions have limits on their coverage.

Public Programs for Financing Health Care

Help with financing health care is offered by both state and federal governments. One kind of help, called Medicaid, is available to those who are indigent; that is, people who are unable to support themselves. The other kind of help with finances is called Medicare. Medicare is an add-on to Social Security benefits. Therefore, if you are over sixty-five years old, or are disabled by Social Security standards, and if you are eligible for Social Security benefits, you should qualify for Medicare.

Medicaid. Medicaid is a combination of state and federal programs for medical care of those who are indigent. Both state and federal governments therefore dictate the requirements for eligibility and for benefits. Medicaid is the major third-party payer for people with HIV infection. Whether you qualify as indigent, what services are available, and how much money you are eligible to receive, all vary from state to state.

The definition of indigence is, in general, stringent. It ranges from an income that is 23 percent of the poverty level in South Dakota to one that is 97 percent of the poverty level in California; in thirty-four states, the definition is 50 percent of the poverty level. In other words, if the poverty level is around $7,000 per year for one person, then most states will find you eligible for Medicaid if your income is $3,500 per year or less. Some states have a definition of indigence with a higher income level for people with AIDS; that is, people with AIDS can qualify for financial help from public funds and still be relatively able to support themselves. Some states also have definitions of indigence that are substantially higher for women who are pregnant and for children.

In defining indigence, Medicaid also considers resources you have other than income. To be considered indigent, you may have liquid assets (for instance, a savings account), a car, a house, or other property only if their values are below a certain level. What that level is differs in different states.

Medicaid pays for most medical necessities but pays relatively little for each one, especially for physicians' fees. Depending on the state, it may pay for inpatient services, outpatient services, and skilled nursing home services. In some states, Medicaid also pays for home health care, private nursing, and drugs. Some states pay for as few as fourteen days of hospital care; some states have no limit. Some have special programs for people with HIV infection. Professional fees such as physicians' bills are usually reimbursed at only about 20 percent of the physicians' customary charges. As a result, unfortunately, many physicians do not accept patients who are on Medicaid. Home care, hospital care, and chronic care are also reimbursed at low rates, and some facilities will reject Medicaid patients on similar grounds.

Medicaid will pay for all drugs, but often restricts payment to drugs that the FDA has approved and sometimes pays only for conditions the drug is specifically approved for. This means that if a clinical trial shows a drug is useful, Medicaid will not pay for the drug until the FDA has approved it. If the FDA has approved the drug but has not approved it specifically for a certain condition, Medicaid may deny payment until the drug is approved for this condition.

Medicare. Medicare, unlike Medicaid, is funded entirely by the federal government. The various eligibility requirements and services do not vary from state to state but are uniform over the whole country.

Medicare is primarily for the aged, but it is also for the disabled and those with severe kidney disease. To receive Medicare, you must have contributed to Social Security, but you need not be indigent. Most of the people with HIV infection who are eligible for Medicare are over sixty-five years old or are disabled. Medicare enforces a waiting period for payment of twenty-nine months, which means that most people have enormous medical bills and often qualify for Social Security Disability Income (see below, under "Help with Income") before they are eligible for Medicare payment. During this twenty-nine months, they may also qualify for Medicaid, depending on their income and illness; if so, they will lose Medicaid when Medicare finally kicks in.

Medicare pays for hospitalization and physicians at rates that compare with the rates of private third-party payers; it asks you to co-pay for these services. Medicare does not pay for drugs. It pays little for long-term care: it will pay for 100 days a year in a skilled nursing facility (see Chapter 8). After the 100 days, you must self-pay or spend down so you are eligible for Medicaid.

Veterans Administration (VA). About thirty million Americans are veterans and are potentially eligible for care through the Veterans Administration, or VA. The VA hospital system is the largest health care system in the United States: it has 171 acute care hospitals, 133 of which are affiliated with medical schools.

Eligibility for the services of a VA hospital includes having spent time in the armed services, plus having a disability connected with that service or an income below the poverty level—for the VA, poverty level is around $18,000 for a couple. Eligibility for AIDS services includes only having spent time in the armed services and having an honorable discharge. HIV infection does *not* have to be service-connected.

The VA provides a comprehensive program of services, including hospital care, outpatient care, and medications. The VA does not require any co-pay.

The budget for the VA has not kept pace with the rising costs of medical care, so the VA has made a rigorous effort to reduce costs. The result is a corresponding reduction in services. The best quality of care is provided in the VA hospitals affiliated with medical schools, though most of this care is supervised by medical residents.

Some VA hospitals have comprehensive programs for people with HIV infection. Like most health care, the availability of resources and expertise varies in different locations.

Using the Social Service System

If you have been denied insurance, or if you have exceeded the limits of your insurance policy, you can turn to the social service system. The social service system gives financial help to the elderly, to children, to the poor, and to the disabled. You are disabled if you have a diagnosis of AIDS and if you are also unable to work. Social service money is a benefit, paid by federal and state governments, to which you are entitled as a citizen.

A problem is that many people with HIV infection are severely disabled but do not have an AIDS-defining diagnosis. Therefore, they are not eligible for many benefits that are based almost exclusively on this diagnosis.

To get into the social service system, begin by calling your city or county or state social service agencies. These agencies are listed under *social services* in the telephone book's yellow or blue pages. Or start with a social worker at your hospital, church, or AIDS-advocacy agency.

Help with Income and Medical Bills

The social service system offers several kinds of help with income. What kind of help you can get, and how much, depends on several factors. If you have worked in the past but are disabled and cannot work now, and you need financial help, you qualify for disability income. Some people get disability income as part of their job benefits. If not, the same Social Security that insures your retirement also gives you disability income, called Social Security Disability Income, or SSDI. Whether you are qualified for SSDI depends on whether you have paid into Social Security for a minimum number of annual quarters. How much you can collect depends on how long you have worked. Whether you are qualified for SSDI also depends on whether the Social Security Administration thinks you are disabled. A diagnosis of AIDS meets the criterion for disability. But the Social Security Administration will not use the new definition of AIDS. Instead, it will probably continue to use the earlier, 1987 definition. When deciding whether a person is disabled enough to receive SSDI, the Social Security Administration has traditionally emphasized how well that person functions, and many people with HIV infection and low CD4 counts function very well. For more information, call the Social Security information number, 1-800-772-1213.

If you are disabled, cannot work, and need financial help, you can also get Supplemental Security Income, called SSI. Whether you are qualified for SSI depends on your means, that is, on your income plus all your assets, everything you own. How much you can collect from SSI also depends on your means. In other words, the government says you are entitled to a certain minimum income. SSI will add up whatever you get on your own, whatever your family can give you, and whatever you get from SSDI; then they will pay you the difference between that sum and the minimum income. If you have no income and no outside means of support, SSI will pay you the entire amount of the minimum income.

If you need financial help, you may qualify for General Public Assistance, called welfare or GPA. GPA, which is offered through the states, will differ from state to state. Some states do not offer GPA at all. Other states offer it if you need financial help and if you are disabled and cannot work. Some states also offer GPA if you need financial help and are disabled only temporarily; in this case, a person with early symptomatic HIV infection who is unable to work might be able to get financial help, though only for a limited time. And some states are replacing GPA with programs that offer loans. In any case, the amount of money you can collect from GPA is small and depends on your means.

If you have children and need financial help to care for them, you may qualify for Aid to Families with Dependent Children, or AFDC. Money from AFDC can be used only for caring for your children. Notice that to qualify for AFDC, you need not be disabled. The amount of money you can collect from AFDC will be related to the size of your family and your income. You can receive income from both SSI and SSDI at the same time. You can also receive income from both GPA and AFDC at the same time. But you cannot receive income from both GPA and SSI at the same time.

If you qualify for SSI or GPA, you automatically qualify for help with medical bills. For details, see above, "Public Programs for Financing Health Care."

Navigating the Social Service System

Often people with HIV infection are unfamiliar with the large, bureaucratic social service system. They say that getting through the system is a dehumanizing and irritating experience, that the system seems to be geared more toward frustrating than toward helping people. People occasionally become annoyed enough with the system that they give up and forgo their benefits.

Getting through the system requires preparation. In a single, separate file, keep documentation of the following: proof of identity, address, and date of birth (driver's license, passport, birth certificate); Social Security card; records of income, assets, medical expenses, living expenses, and dependents, anyone living with and sharing expenses with you, record of who is responsible for you. Take this file with you when going to social services.

Keep another file of every person you talked to at social services, what date and time you talked to them, what you talked about, what you understood the outcome of the talk to be. Find out the names of the supervisors. If someone sends you away to get more information, ask them to write down what information they want; then, when you bring the information, also bring along what they wrote. Do not try to keep your diagnosis a secret: some branches of social services will speed up the system if you have HIV infection. Some benefits apply only to those with HIV infection.

Take a friend with you, especially if you're tired or ill. Some AIDS-advocacy agencies offer social workers, lawyers, counselors, or buddies who will go with you.

When to Stop Working

Often your qualification for income from social services comes down to a question of legal disability, which involves making a decision about when to stop working. Most people quit when the stress of getting to work, working, and getting home again becomes overwhelming. Some people quit work after their employers have pressed them to quit. Some people quit after they have had a specific mishap, like an assignment done badly or an accident with a machine or while driving. People usually work as long as they can.

Some people quit gradually. They work half-days for a long time, or they arrange for a leave of absence.

The importance of the decision to quit work should not be underestimated. It is one of the most difficult decisions people with AIDS have to make. Our image of ourselves as competent and useful members of society depends to some extent on our jobs. When no one pays us to do a job, we worry that we are no longer worth anything at all. Caregivers often forget the extent to which people identify themselves with their jobs. Caregivers worry about the people they're caring for and want to protect them against stress and fatigue and accidents. Because of their worries, they sometimes urge the person with AIDS to quit working before he or she is ready.

Some people welcome the chance to assess whether they really want to work. Some people decide to quit work and manage the transition well. These people see the decision not as whether to quit but as how to change. They believe that life is the process of developing one new identity after another. They want to try a new identity—to be a writer or traveler or teacher or artist or builder or musician or inventor. Many do volunteer work. Many others become AIDS activists (see Chapter 12).

Putting Your Affairs in Order

Assigning Durable Power of Attorney

Many people want to provide for the possibility that they might become unconscious or mentally incapacitated. They worry about their ability to hire help, give medical consent, sign their checks, pay their bills. Such an eventuality can be provided for by naming someone as your agent, giving him or her the power to make decisions for you. This power is called the *durable power of attorney*.

You can give durable power of attorney to anyone you trust who is over eighteen years old; that person can be a friend and need not be a spouse or relative. In general, a durable power of attorney gives that person the legal authority to sign your name if you are terminally ill or unconscious and unable to do so. That authority can cover a broad range of functions, including most financial and medical matters.

The durable power of attorney begins either when you decide it will—even before you become incompetent—or when you become incompetent. *Incompetence* is defined as it was with the right to informed consent: it is the inability to make competent decisions based on the information available to you. Two physicians decide the point of incompetence. To assign a durable power of attorney, however, you must be in capacity, that is, you must be able to make informed decisions. The durable power of attorney lasts until you die or until you revoke it. Assigning durable power of attorney generally costs somewhere around fifty dollars. AIDS activist organizations can often help you find free legal help. You can also fill out forms available from your hospital.

There are two kinds of durable power of attorney: durable power of attorney for health care and durable power of attorney for financial matters. The two are not the same. A person to whom you give durable power of attorney for your finances cannot give medical consent. Because you specify what jobs you want the person with durable power of attorney to have, you can give medical and financial powers to the same person or to different people.

Durable power of attorney for health care. The person to whom you give a durable power of attorney for health care must be at least eighteen years old and willing to serve as your agent. Health care professionals—physicians and nurses who are involved in your care—are not usually considered appropriate.

The document assigning a durable power of attorney for health care generally contains the following: a statement that you are creating a durable power of attorney for your health care; the name of the person and any alternate person to whom you are giving durable power of attorney for health care; the conditions under which this document becomes effective; a statement of what authority you are granting this person; and a list of specific wishes. The durable power of attorney generally takes effect when two physicians, including the physician-of-record, certify that you are not capable of understanding or communicating decisions about your own health; it will apply as long as this condition continues.

This document can give the person with durable power of attorney the authority to withhold or withdraw any treatments or procedures—including mechanical ventilation (respirators or breathing machines), dialysis (artificial kidneys), antibiotics, operations—that sustain life. Medical treatment that would provide comfort or relieve pain is not included in a durable power of attorney for health care. The person to whom you give durable power of attorney may access your medical records and can place you in a nursing home. The document assigning durable power of attorney can also include a section for any specific instructions you might have. For example, you could write, "In the event that I am in a coma, and have an incurable physical condition or lose my mental capacity, and have little hope of recovery, I do not want treatment that will merely prolong my life." (Also see "Living Wills," below.)

The document assigning durable power of attorney for health care must be dated and signed by you, by the person to whom you are giving durable power of attorney, and by two witnesses who are not interested parties. It is wise to have the document notarized by a notary public; some states may require this.

The original of the document assigning a durable power of attorney for health care should be kept by you or by your lawyer or by someone you trust. Copies of the document should be given to the person to whom you assign durable power of attorney, to any alternate person, and to members of your family. Your physician should know such a document exists; you may wish to consult your physician when drawing up the document.

Lawyers and hospital legal offices can provide examples of such documents that meet state laws.

Durable financial power of attorney. Much of what applies to the durable power of attorney for health care also applies to a durable financial power of attorney. One difference between the two is in the responsibilities held by the person with the durable power of attorney.

The person with durable financial power of attorney for you can pursue anything to do with business or banking, including signing checks, opening bank accounts, signing promissory notes, selling property, transferring property, signing proxies, or pursuing lawsuits. The durable financial power of attorney can be limited to any one of these jobs or can include all of them.

As with the durable power of attorney for health care, the durable financial power of attorney is in effect when you decide it should be, or if two physicians declare you incompetent—that is, incapable of understanding and communicating. It continues in effect only so long as you remain incompetent.

DNR Order

A DNR (Do Not Resuscitate) order is an order you give that you not be revived should you be near death. People with advanced HIV infection may reach a stage in the disease when either they or their physicians begin questioning whether to continue medical treatment. Medical treatment has a great deal to offer people with HIV infection, including those in advanced stages of the disease, but it would be deceptive to imply that people do not sometimes reach a point where the quality of life becomes questionable. For some people, that point might be dementia; for others, it is emaciation, or repeated or incapacitating opportunistic infections; and for some, it is simply the inability to do the things that make life meaningful.

These are the points at which people consider DNR orders. The word *resuscitate* in DNR specifically means cardiopulmonary resuscitation, or CPR. Cardio (heart) pulmonary (lungs) resuscitation (revival) means reviving a person whose heart stops beating (cardiac arrest) or whose lungs stop breathing (pulmonary arrest). All hospitals and most medical facilities have the equipment—including machines for chest compression and heart shock (defibrillation), drugs, and respirators—to respond instantly to cardiac or pulmonary arrest. The DNR order means, then, that if you have reached the point where you question the quality of life and if you suffer cardiac or pulmonary arrest, you order that you not be revived. A DNR order applies only to CPR; it does not mean that other treatment is not offered or given.

The decision to carry out DNR orders is based on your medical condition and on the quality of your life. Your medical condition is evaluated by your physician and a decision is based on the disease, the stage of disease, prior treatment, and the response to that treatment. Your quality of life can be evaluated only by you, based on your own unique values.

The decision about DNR orders should depend on several factors. One is how demanding the medical treatment to be withheld would be. For example, while intravenous fluids and commonly used antibiotics place few demands on either the hospital or the patient, dialysis, respirators, total intravenous nutrition, and major operations are considerably more demanding. Other factors affecting the decision include the likelihood of response, alternate treatment options, and the potential for relieving symptoms like pain. For example, questions that you might raise in the event of lung failure are: What is the likelihood of survival without the respirator? What is the likelihood of being able to get off the respirator once being put on it? What kind of treatments can be offered if I get over this hurdle? Will there be pain either with the respirator or without it? Is it likely that the condition causing lung failure is temporary and can be cured?

If you are medically competent (see above) and are eighteen years of age or older, you might consider making a decision about DNR orders. It is probably best to deal with this issue at a time when you and your physician can discuss the whole issue to your satisfaction and when you don't need to make fast decisions in compromised circumstances. Physicians are encouraged to discuss DNR orders with anyone who has a serious medical condition, but many are understandably reluctant to do this. If your physician does not discuss DNR orders with you, you might wish to bring up the subject.

If you are not conscious or have been declared medically incompetent by two physicians, then your representative can discuss DNR orders with your physician. Who your representative is varies from state to state. Typically, your representative will be, in rank order, your guardian, your agent as named in your durable power of attorney, your spouse, children aged eighteen or older, parent, or brother or sister.

Your representative should make decisions about DNR orders based on your anticipated desires, not on his or her own desires.

Most people have strong opinions about such decisions, and they worry that they will not be able to make rational choices at the time the choices need to be made. Two ways of dealing with such decisions in advance are to assign a durable power of attorney for health care (see above) and to make a living will (see below).

Living Wills

A living will is a legal document outlining your decisions about treatment to sustain your life should you be unconscious or incompetent. The living will is somewhat different from the durable power of attorney for health care: the person with your durable power of attorney for health care, when faced with the decision of whether to prolong your life, will usually decide to prolong life. The living will provides that person with your specific instructions for making this decision. The person with your durable power of attorney for health care can also make decisions that may not have been foreseen in your living will.

Living wills, unlike regular wills, apply only to medical treatments. The actual form and scope of a living will is established by state laws. In general, living wills specify which types of treatment you wish to have or wish not to have. Living wills also specify the physical and mental states in which you do or do not want these treatments. These treatments include transfusions, support on a respirator, operations, and resuscitation. Some states have no provision for living wills. Other states that do provide for living wills do not allow any restrictions on food and water. In most cases, a living will applies only after the person becomes incompetent and has a terminal condition. In some states, a living will applies to both terminal conditions and a kind of permanent coma called a vegetative state; in other states, a living will applies only to terminal conditions.

A living will might be written as follows:

In the event that I have an incurable disease that is certified to be a terminal condition by two physicians who have personally examined me—including one who shall be my attending physician—and these physicians have determined that my death is imminent and will occur whether or not life-sustaining procedures are used; and where application of such procedures would serve only to artificially prolong the dying process, I direct that these procedures be withheld or withdrawn, and that I be permitted to die naturally with only the administration of medication, food, and water, and any additional procedure necessary to give comfort and alleviate pain. In the absence of my ability to give directions regarding the use of such life-sustaining procedures, it is my intention that this declaration shall be honored by my family and physicians as the final expression of my right to control my medical care and treatment.

To make a living will, obtain a sample document from your lawyer, from your state attorney general's office, from a hospital legal office, or from a social worker. The content of the living will may be discussed with your physician to assure the use of proper terms and to include likely decisions. The living will must be dated and signed by you and by two witnesses. You must be at least eighteen years old and competent. The witnesses must be at least eighteen years old, must not be related to you, must not be financially responsible for your care, and may not be your health care provider or connected with the facility providing your care. You or your representative should give your physician a copy of the living will. You may revoke the will at any time, preferably by a written statement, but also by destroying the living will and notifying any persons—including the physician—who retain copies.

Stipulating What Happens to Your Property

Most people stipulate what happens to their property by making a will. No one requires that you do so. If you die without a will (called dying *intestate* your property goes automatically first to your spouse and then to your nearest living relatives. Your property will not go to friends or to unmarried partners. To assign property to friends or unmarried partners, you must make a will.

Wills apply mostly to property—money, house, car, furniture, clothes. Wills do not necessarily legislate any of your other wishes. Life insurance benefits will go to the beneficiary, even if the will states otherwise. In principle, a will may specify what your funeral arrangements are and whether you'd like to be buried or cremated, but in practice, wills are often not read until after the funeral.

Over a certain value, property left in a will is taxable. You can minimize taxes your beneficiaries will pay by setting up trusts or by giving to them a certain amount of money per year while you are still alive. Neither trusts nor gifts under a certain dollar amount are taxable.

Trusts and annual gifts also ensure that you will have property to leave. Some people, rather than use their property to finance their own medical care, decide to put it into trusts or give it to the people they love. Once they are impoverished, their medical bills will be paid by public assistance programs. Leaving your property in trust or as a gift must be done years before you need extensive medical care: Medicaid/ Medicare will check to see if money or property has been given away in recent years. To find out how and when to leave your property, see a lawyer or a financial planner.

A lawyer is the best source of information regarding what happens to your property. Lawyers also often draw up wills. State laws set the forms for wills, however, and if you know the form, you can draw up your own will.

Providing for Hospice Care

Some people want to decide where they will die. Some choose to die at home; some would rather leave their homes as a place for the living, so choose to die elsewhere. In either case, they may choose hospice care.

A hospice can be either a place or a concept, that is, either a building or a program dedicated to care of the dying. Hospice programs can be run through hospitals, nursing homes, or private organizations. Nursing agencies, like the Visiting Nurse Association, often also provide hospice care.

Both private insurance policies and medical assistance provide some level of reimbursement for hospice care, providing the requirements of the hospice are met. To find a hospice or hospice program, ask your doctor or nursing agency or hospital social worker. Your doctor can advise you on when to consider hospice services.

See also Chapter 8, under "Hospice Care."

Chapter 11

On Dying: Preparing for and Accepting Death

- Emotional responses to death
- Making decisions about the rest of life
- Other people's reactions to death
- The dying person and the caregiver
- Balancing living and dying
- Death

Dean Lombard: I've lost too many friends in too short a time. It gets stronger with each one, closer to home. I haven't been sleeping too well. I get out of bed and look at the moon. I just stand there. I don't know why I do that. I go back to bed but can't sleep. I thought I'd have a longer time. Now I think the time is shorter.

Death is hard to think about, harder to face. The thought of death is slippery, difficult to focus on, surrounded by a cloud of pain and fear. At the same time, the thought is irrepressible; it is impossible to truly ignore. No one with HIV infection ignores the thought of death altogether. "No matter how positive I am, there's a lingering dark cloud," said Alan Madison. "With a terminal illness, it's tick, tick—your time is running out. It's not like one day it's on your mind, the next day it's not. You think a lot about how it will end."

Emotional Responses to Death

Elizabeth Kubler-Ross is a psychiatrist who wrote the standard book on how all people, regardless of the causes of their death, respond emotionally to the fact that they are dying. After interviewing people who were dying, she found they have several responses in common. One is disbelief and denial that death could happen to them: as Dean Lombard said, "You feel it's not going to happen, though you know it is. You feel emotionless because it can't be real." Another is anger at having been singled out. Another is an impulse to bargain, to push back the inevitable and gain a little time: "I don't think we ever feel as though it's all complete," Steven said, "as though the world owes us nothing else." The next is depression: the loss, pain, and sorrow that come from recognition that death is inescapable. The last is acceptance, coming to terms with death: "The meaning of the diagnosis finally hit me," said Dean. "I won't be here forever. I have to make my preparations for death."

Kubler-Ross said the responses to death occurred in stages: first denial, then anger, bargaining, depression, and finally, acceptance. Later, she and subsequent researchers amended the idea, saying that perhaps the word *stages* is misleading. Not everyone has all these responses, or has them in this order. Some have several at once. For others, the responses alternate: anger, then depression, the anger again. And not only the people who are facing death, but also their caregivers, have these responses. Caregivers share the same feelings of denial, anger, depression, bargaining, and acceptance, both on behalf of the people they are taking care of and for themselves.

To anyone who has learned to live with a diagnosis of HIV infection, these responses come as no surprise. They are nearly the same emotions people experience when they learn of their diagnosis of HIV infection. These emotions are also the same as the normal responses to living with HIV infection. Perhaps this means that people with HIV infection have been facing death since the moment of their diagnosis; perhaps it means only that these are the responses people have when faced with any catastrophe.

In any case, the responses to the diagnosis serve as a rehearsal for the thought of death. People who have had these responses before are a little used to them, and know a little about how to handle them. The same strategies—strategies for refusing to fret about what will not change, for finding harmless or even helpful ways of discharging anger, for turning despair into some sort of hope for something or someone, for facing down fears, for distracting yourself with pleasure, for accepting yourself with fondness and your condition without self-hatred, guilt, or blame—still work, even against death.

People have other natural responses to the thought of death. One is fear. People are afraid of dying in pain. They fear the moment when life stops. The truth is that dying—the process that leads to the moment of death—sometimes does hurt, but doctors have medications to block the pain.

Death itself seems not to hurt. The body, either quietly or quickly, stops working. No one knows much about the moment of death, but it does seem that a built-in mechanism protects people from physical and psychological pain. As a rule, death comes peacefully.

Most of our fears about death are actually about what will happen before death. This is a universal fear; the sixteenth-century French philosopher Michel de Montaigne wrote about it in his *Essays*: "It is not against death that we prepare ourselves. . . . To tell the truth, we prepare ourselves against the preparations for death. . . . It is certain that to most people preparation for death has given more torment than the dying." Montaigne goes on to offer a sort of rough comfort: "If you don't know how to die, don't worry; Nature will tell you what to do on the spot, fully and adequately. She will do this job perfectly for you; don't bother your head about it."

Specifically, people are afraid that while they are dying they will be abandoned. They are afraid of being alone at such a difficult time. They fear they will lose control. They worry that they have been bad and deserve death. They fear physical pain and disfigurement. They worry about the people they will leave, about the relationships left unresolved and business left unfinished.

Another natural reaction to death is confusion. The thought of life ending is new territory, and people are unsure how to think about it or what to do about it. "I don't know how to just let life go on until death comes," Helen Parks said. "I'm between this pole and that pole."

It is also natural to feel a sense of loss. Through sickness, people lose the bodies they were accustomed to. They lose their abilities to do what they were good at, their competencies. They lose the healthy, active lives they shared with their friends, and to that extent, they lose a commonality with their friends. And because they are aware of dying, they lose their sense of a future, the feeling that limitless time is available to them. Accepting these losses brings anguish.

Some of the anguish in accepting losses comes from knowing that smaller losses are tokens of greater ones, of the loss of life and the entire world. Some is because losing the future also means losing the idealistic, hopeful part of you, your potential, the person you might have become. And some of the anguish is because people want so much to live. "The will to live is so great, you can't even think about it," said Dean. "You feel as though you could beat anything just by wanting to live." The anguish people feel over losing life is in proportion to the intensity with which they want to live.

People facing death also want to settle existential questions about life: What is being human all about? Do I believe in God? What will happen to the world after I die? What will happen to me after I die?

They turn to religion or spirituality or philosophy, and they think about the same questions people have been asking for centuries. Lisa's husband was not unusual in becoming religious before he died, reading the Bible and writing his thoughts in a journal.

For all the feelings and worries that dying people have in common, their progress through these feelings and worries is individual. People experience these emotions in fits and starts and at their own paces. Sometimes they want to face death, sometimes they do not. Sometimes they want to make plans and see people, sometimes they do not. Sometimes they want to take control and make decisions, sometimes they do not. Sometimes they want to talk about their feelings, sometimes they do not: Lisa's husband said, "I don't always want to talk about dying. Sometimes I want to have days when I'm just living."

Emotional Responses to Death and HIV Infection

Most of the responses to death described above are shared by all people who have time to contemplate dying, regardless of the cause of death. What makes HIV infection different is death at an early age in the midst of the deaths of many friends. Most people who die of HIV infection are in their thirties. Someone who has HIV infection probably knows many others with the disease.

Because they are young, they have worries about dying that older people do not. Young people have less time to get used to death gradually. They are not yet tired of living. They have not slowly come to see themselves as dispensable and mortal. They do not understand what to do about mortality, how to sum up and conclude their lives. "I have to face my own mortality," said Steven, "which I didn't expect to face until I was eighty." They look at their relatively short lives and ask questions they are not used to asking. "Usually people ask in their sixties, 'What have I accomplished?' Alan said. "I'm going to have to ask that earlier." They often feel resentful that they must ask these questions so early, and they feel unready to supply the answers.

They also worry about dying before their parents. They want to be able to help their parents out as their parents age. "Now I'm looking at dying before my parents," said Dean. "That changes the natural process. It hurts."

Because people with HIV infection often know others who are dying of the disease, they have concrete images of what will happen to them. They visit their friends in the hospital and think, "Is this what will happen to me? Is this what I will look like? Is this what I will feel?" "I know what the last few months are," said Alan, "and I wish I hadn't seen the suffering. Knowing what it looks like is difficult." Dean lost twenty friends in two years. "It gets stronger with each one," he said. "Closer to home." People with HIV infection say too much death surrounds them. "I have so many friends who are disappearing," Steven said. "In one year, I went to twenty-six funerals. I sit at the funerals and think how wonderful the person was, and how they looked before the end, and how long will it be before I'm there." For that reason, some, like Steven, no longer go to funerals. Alan said, "I've been to forty-seven funerals. That's my limit."

Making Decisions about the Rest of Life

People who are facing death gradually begin making decisions about the rest of their lives. They look inside themselves for reference points, for what is important to them: Which people mean the most to me? What kinds of things should I be involved in? Where should I live? They also find outside references: people, poetry, spirituality, support groups, music, books. They often talk with counselors who can help them make decisions and handle their overwhelming emotions. What they finally do is decide who to spend their time with, and how to spend it.

Some people begin by summing up their lives. Part of what Dean called his preparation for death was to look at what he had accomplished and decide what his legacy would be. Dean runs a small newspaper, and he is arranging for the smooth transfer of the business to his partners. He also thinks of the paper as his legacy: "I have to have something that says, 'Dean was here.' I'd like people to read today's newspaper in fifty years and say, 'Oh that's what it was like then.' My paper is going to go on, and people after me are going to benefit from it." Lisa's husband began talking more about an earlier divorce, how sad he was that the family hadn't been able to stay together, and for the first time in twenty years, he invited all his children to come home at the same time.

Some people decide to do the things they have always wanted to do. June Monroe's son went on a photo safari to Africa: "It wasn't too sensible," said June, "but he didn't want to die without having done it." Dean had always wanted a personal computer with which to keep track of household expenses and could never justify the cost; finally he bought one. A friend of Dean's decided he wanted to travel because he never had. He arranged his trip, arranged his sources of medical care and medicine, sold his house, and took off.

People often want to resolve relationships. They work hard to get on more comfortable terms with their parents, children, brothers and sisters, spouses, friends. Lisa's husband and his family had for a long time been unhappy with each other. When the family understood Lisa's husband was dying, Lisa said, "Everyone realized all the things they had gotten wired up about were garbage. All he had ever wanted was to be accepted for the person he was, and that's what they fought about. Finally either he let it rest, or they did, and they all seemed to accept each other. The acceptance showed as much in what they didn't talk about as what they did."

Often the person with HIV infection makes the first step toward resolution. Some people who are approached for this purpose do not react positively. Resolving a relationship with a dying person means admitting death's inevitability, and some people are intimidated by the thought of death. Sometimes they only want time to get used to the idea, and they react more positively when they are approached again a little later. In general, the person with HIV infection and the person he or she wants to talk to both want the same things. They want to reminisce and think about what good times they had. They both want to know they're loved; they want to be accepted for who they are. They want to feel comfort and warmth in each other's company. People who are dying also want reassurance that the people they love will be watched over and cared for.

Some people decide what should happen to their property. Dean said, "Finally I sat down and decided who was getting what, and wrote if down. I considered giving stuff to the people that most hated it. Then I decided not to do that." Some people decide they are uninterested in having a say about the disposal of their property, so they don't bother with it.

Some people consider suicide. Thoughts of suicide most commonly occur early in the course of the disease. People often devise concrete plans: at what point they will decide to end their lives, what method they will use, how they will keep the burden of guilt off their survivors. Mental health professionals recommend that people talk to a professional about their decision, then give it a while before doing anything. When Lisa's husband said he was considering suicide, Lisa asked him to first talk to a psychologist. She also told him she thought he owed it to her not to act without talking to her. He agreed and made those promises. Eventually, he decided against suicide. Like Lisa's husband, many people find their interest in life is stronger than their desire to die. In fact, the suicide rate among people with HIV infection is low. Perhaps the thought of suicide is a means of regaining a feeling of control over life. Perhaps suicide is a way of saying, "AIDS does not have the power of life and death over me. That power is mine."

Some people who are dying and their caregivers want to know what to anticipate clinically. They find that knowing what their bodies might do and what the treatment will be takes the mystery out of the process.

They say that the more they know, the less they invent to worry about. Other people do not want to know, and would like to distance themselves a little from the physical aspects of being sick and dying. Still others want to know a little at a time. Learn the facts only if you want, and only when you want to.

Often people decide under what conditions they would like to be allowed to die. Some refuse medication or procedures they think would prolong a life that has become distressing. A friend of Dean's who had become blind, deaf, and incontinent refused transfusions and drugs with painful side effects that might prolong his life, and accepted only pain-relieving medication. Dean's friend saw this not as giving up but as making his last days comfortable. Others refuse life support systems. Lisa spent nights at the hospital with her husband toward the end of his life. He refused the respirator, so Lisa brought him home. He lived ten days, then died as he had wished, at home. Like Lisa's husband, many people would like to die where they feel a sense of control and privacy, in their own beds. Many others feel their homes should remain a place of life and would rather die in a hospital or hospice. And some people do not want to choose beforehand but simply wait and see how they feel at the end.

Some people who are dying make funeral arrangements with the help of their caregivers. Some want to make sure their caregivers find a funeral home that won't refuse to offer services because of AIDS. Others want to give their caregivers some moral support. "I asked my partner his opinion on a cemetery plot," said Dean. "The reason is, once when I had to go away for six months, he was very upset. I helped him through that by doing everything—my planning and packing—with him. That's what I'm doing now, helping him by doing everything with him."

Other People's Reactions to Death

We are raised to think of death not as a necessity but as an enemy. When people who are still healthy are confronted with someone who is dying, they are intensely uncomfortable. They are frightened of losing the dying person, of their own deaths, and of death's finality. "Death isn't like breaking up with someone and time heals it," said Helen. "Death is death, period, and no one wants to deal."

Sometimes their discomfort, their not wanting to "deal," makes people appear insensitive. Alan was in a mall, shopping, and someone he knew came up and asked, "Why have you got all those shopping bags? Aren't you dying soon?" Alan snapped back, "How soon are *you* dying?" but he was surprised and confused and hurt by his friend's question. Dean had a friend who habitually made a joke of looking around at Dean's furnishings and saying, "Oh, that's new. Leave it to me in your will." Dean finally replied, "Okay, that's fine. Do you want the kitchen chairs too?" After that, the friend dropped the joke. Such remarks sound insensitive, as though the person is taunting you with life and health. But they are not; no one is this callous. Insensitivity is the method some people use to deal with their own pain and fear. The method is certainly inappropriate. Both Alan and Dean let their friends understand how inappropriate their remarks were and that they should be more careful in the future.

Sometimes people's discomfort with the reality of death isolates those who are dying. People facing death often find that other people are friendly and sympathetic but want to talk only about easy, comfortable subjects. When the subject of death comes up, they talk instead about what they've done recently, or about the future: "I can't wait until we get you to a ballgame." They also sugar-coat the subject: "Remember how sick you thought you were before, and a month later you were off on a trip." This is hard on the person facing death. He or she may be happy enough to talk about the weather, the news, or sports, or to gossip about mutual friends. But being prohibited from talking about the things that are of most concern makes a person isolated and sad.

On the other hand, everyone facing death knows some people who will "deal." Perhaps it is someone who also faces death or someone who has lost a person they loved, or a professional who has had training in helping people handle the emotions and problems of dying. Often it is someone who loves the dying person and is less afraid than other people of the reality of death. These people tell the person who is dying that they will not leave, they will stay as long as they can. With Alan's young nephew, that message is reversed. Alan's nephew worries about Alan's death, and Alan tries to help by telling him he won't be abandoned: "My nephew cries when he thinks about it," Alan said. "I tell him, 'I'm not going to give up easily and I'm going to try to be there for your graduation. Don't be disappointed if I can't, but I'll try.' "

The Dying Person and the Caregiver

People who are dying and the people caring for them ask difficult questions of each other, and say things they always meant to say to each other, and cry together. They find these things comforting—people feel better knowing someone else is concerned or is having the same feelings. Both the people who are dying and their caregivers find it a relief when someone sincerely asks them, "How are you?" Dying people and their caregivers want attention and companionship. They want to be taken seriously. They want to know that they need not be alone. People facing death together often grow closer.

This is not to say that their interests always converge. They have to solve some real problems. One is that they may be experiencing different "Kubler-Ross" responses at the same time. When, for instance, one person is accepting death and the other is denying it, they will probably feel alienated from each other and find communication difficult. They may solve this by accepting that the other person's feelings are as compelling as their own. They try to treat the other person's feelings as facts, at least temporary ones, that require respect. In extreme circumstances like these, people have only the feelings they can afford to have, and they feel things only when they are ready. Sometimes they have had enough of HIV infection and death, and they need to take a break for a while. Sometimes they are ready to think and feel and talk about what is happening to them.

Another problem for the caregiver is knowing when the dying person wants to talk about what is happening and when he or she needs to ignore it. The best the caregiver can do is listen for cues. Cues are when the person begins talking about his troubles or what he has read about dying or how tired she is or that she is frightened, or how to deal with the business of leaving the world. Then the caregiver can say, "How can I help? What would you like to do?"

A second problem is that the normal balance of the relationship begins to change. Dean is not yet close to death, though he and his partner are aware that he will die and they discuss it. "My partner is going through a hard time right now," said Dean. "Not only is he concerned about me, but he also just had to put his mother in a nursing home, and he doesn't get along with his father and sister. So now he's telling me, 'I need you. Don't go anywhere for a while.' "

When Lisa was in distress because her husband was dying, she found herself asking him for comfort. From the outside, this seems odd: surely the caregiver should not ask for help from the dying. But in fact, it is an entirely natural extension of the relationship between people who care for each other. People in a relationship normally take turns. Sometimes one is the comforter, the helper, the listener, sometimes the other is. The problem is that for the person close to death, this sort of give-and-take becomes too heavy a burden. When death is imminent, the balance of responsibility begins to shift to the caregiver.

Caregivers need to begin to forgo the luxury of asking for help with their own fears and worries. They need gradually to stop coming to the dying person with both minor irritations and profound troubles. They listen. They ask questions: "Are you comfortable enough? Are you upset? What do you fear?" They let the dying person cry, and are silent or cry with him. They let the dying person express her fears and fantasies, and help test fears against reality. They say, "I will try to do what you like. How can I help?" They hold and touch the dying person whenever they can and as often as the person wants.

A common ground rule is that the dying person calls the shots: when to stop working, when to get another x-ray, whether to answer the phone, which friends to see and when, whether to make decisions, when and where to talk about their feelings about what is happening to them. The caregiver can argue, but the decision rests with the person who is dying.

Balancing Living and Dying

In general, people facing death continue the process they began in response to depression and fatigue. They concentrate their energies on what is possible. They let go of some things they had wanted, mostly long-term career goals. They take control of their own attitudes: they decide how to live with their limits in life and still feel satisfied. In short, they balance living and dying.

In a way, they seem both to live and to die at once. Not only did Helen plan her trip to the beach the following summer and buy beach clothes, she also celebrated Mother's Day in December—"In case I wasn't here," she said. Steven says his life is "back to normal," and he doesn't "sit around waiting to get sick," but he doesn't "order things that will take a year to get," either. Alan says, "I'm keeping myself healthy and trying to keep the disease from getting worse"; he also says, "I won't enroll in night school, I'm afraid I couldn't finish."

These people are not contradicting themselves. They are dealing with two facts; one is that they are dying, and the other is that they are still alive. They have to live recognizing both death and life. "I need some help dying," said Dean. "But I also need help with living until I die, graciously and with dignity." In fact, people have always had to learn to do this. Everyone has to figure out how to stay alive and still be ready for death, how to approach dying and still live the rest of their lives.

Eventually people say that they have always known how. At some time in their lives, they have had to accept the inevitable with courage and grace. "If we have not known how to live," wrote Montaigne, "it is wrong to teach us how to die, and make the end inconsistent with the whole. If we have known how to live steadfastly and tranquilly, we shall know how to die in the same way." Lisa's husband said the same thing,

that he would die as he lived, by paraphrasing the Bible: "I know I came
into this world naked and I will go out naked." The person who has
lived is the same as the person who will die. If you know yourself at all,
you know how you will die.

Death

Because we have to, we accept the conditions of mortality: having means
losing, being here means leaving. Seneca, a Roman philosopher, wrote
to his old friend Lucilius, in *Moral Letters to Lucilius*: "You will die,
not because you are ill, but because you are alive." The idea, though
people have known it forever, always comes as surprise. We want life
never to end; we want those we love never to die.

But we have never been able to have everything we want. The fact
that we want what we cannot have is only a fact, not a surprise, not
cause for despair. Sooner or later, we find ways to accept it. Dean's way
is to think about his friend's future: "Each person who has fought this
disease does it with his own weapons. When the people die, they leave
their weapons behind. When I die, my friends are going to pick up my
weapons." Like Dean, people who are dying are often calm and talk
quietly about death and their lives.

For the caregiver, this hurts badly. Caregivers want to resist the pain
by trying to keep the dying person alive as long as possible. Lisa said,
"I was fighting to keep my husband alive. I just didn't want to give up.
He said to me, 'Don't you know, Lisa, it's just one sickness after another.'
I said, 'Never mind. Just keep fighting.'" After a time, caregivers become
a little better used to the death, and know they must let go. Lisa said,
"I stopped fighting about two weeks before he died. I finally let him go,
said to myself if he had to die, that would be okay. I didn't want him to
die. But I would not cling to him."

At the end, people who are dying should be able to have with them
the people they love. People who love someone who is dying should be
able to be with that person. Lisa sat with her husband while he was
dying: "I held his hands and talked to him. I think he could hear, even
though he seemed unconscious. I told him who I was and that I wouldn't
leave. I just kept talking, I said, 'I love you. I don't want you to suffer
any more. I'll take care of the kids. It'll be fine. Let go if you want.' I
did all I could. I think I helped him die."

People tell those who are dying, "I won't leave you. If I go away,
I'll come back soon." They say prayers. They read aloud, often the holy
books of their religions. Some sing: a woman June knew sang gospel
songs to her son while he died. Some, like Lisa, just talk, lovingly and

reassuringly. When they find nothing to say, they sit quietly. Most importantly, they hold, touch, caress, hold hands. For both the dying and those left behind, the physical presence of another person eases loss and loneliness. One hospital clergyman said that at death, the physical presence of another person amounts to a sacrament.

Maybe death is not so bad. We know so little about it. Why should it be worse than sleep? Socrates, a Greek philosopher who lived in the fifth century B.C., was ordered by the leaders of his state to kill himself for insubordination. Socrates acquiesced, and he died after drinking poison. Before he died, he talked about death: "Perhaps death is something indifferent, perhaps desirable. It is likely, however, that if it is a transmigration from one place to another, it is an improvement to go and live with so many great persons who have passed on and to be exempt from having any more to do with unjust and corrupt judges."

"If it is an annihilation of our being," Socrates continued, "it is still an improvement to enter upon a long and peaceful night. We feel nothing sweeter in life than a deep and tranquil rest and sleep, without dreams."

Chapter 12

On Living: Tactics for Preserving Mental Health

- Sources of support
- Taking control
- The mind-body connection

This chapter is about how to fight the disease, how to keep from giving in, how to stay in one piece. It is about how to face uncertain physical health and still preserve emotional health. Preserving emotional health in the face of HIV infection is heroic, and people do it all the time, using all sorts of tricks. They call the tricks survival strategies or mind games or mental tricks—preservation tactics, for lack of a better term. Preservation tactics allow people to function in their daily lives, to endure pain and loss, to choose how to live, and to find real satisfaction and pleasure in the process.

There are a great variety of successful preservation tactics. People use different tactics at different times, depending on their needs. Many of the tactics even seem to contradict one another: sometimes people need to confront what the disease might bring; other times they need to take a break from that. Some of the tactics might work for you; some you might need to modify. You will almost certainly make up new ones for yourself.

Some tactics come from mental health professionals, though these professionals have no firm rules for maintaining emotional wholeness. Most tactics come from the rich imaginations and enormous inner resources of the people affected by HIV infection.

These people are proud of their toughness and resourcefulness, and so they should be. Steven Charles said, "I have to deal with this whether I want to or not. A whole year has gone by since I was diagnosed with the virus. How have I come through it? I think I've come through it admirably." Neither Steven nor anyone else feels they have been admirable every minute: "It's hard to do seven days a week," he says. But on the whole, everyone who uses preservation tactics says that life is better.

Preservation tactics seem to fall into two broad categories. The first is: use your sources of support. The second is: as far as you are able, take control of your life.

Sources of Support

We accept as a standard truth that we are separate from all other people: we are alone, we are individuals, we are each one of a kind. We never truly understand what other people feel, nor do they truly understand our feelings. We are on our own, responsible for our own decisions and for solutions to our own problems. We protect ourselves first, and at almost any cost.

We accept as just as much a standard truth the opposite: that we are also interconnected. What happens to a friend seems to some extent also to happen to us. When a friend is lonely or worried or in pain, we cannot simply ignore him or her; we even feel some of her or his misery. Conversely, when we are unhappy ourselves, the presence of a friend is a comfort and relief. "For grief concealed strangles the soul," wrote Robert Burton, a seventeenth-century minister and scholar, "but when as we shall but impart it to some discreet, trusty, loving friend, it is instantly removed." Friends help us feel that someone else is interested, that we need not be alone. "Friends' confabulations are comfortable at all times," Burton wrote, "as fire in Winter, shade in Summer, as sleep on the grass to them that are weary, meal and drink to him that is hungry or athirst." Friends give us the warmth of their concern, a rest from our troubles, and a feeling that we are somehow nourished.

The point is that, for people affected by HIV infection, the support of other people is as important to their minds as medication is to their bodies. When people are sick and hurting and alienated and guilty and feeling unjustly struck, they have a greater need for other people. Even when they are alone and feeling isolated, they are comforted by the knowledge that other people care about them. Alan says, "I can fight this because I'm not fighting by myself." Over and over, people affected by HIV infection say they could not manage to preserve their emotional health without a sister or a certain friend or a support group or an aunt or a counselor. In fact, they go further and say that without these people, they would no longer know how to live.

This is not an absolute. Some people are more private than others, or would rather rely on their own resources. All people have times when they would rather be alone. Nor are other people always a treat; they can be boring or irritating or cause outright pain. Even the best of friends can get tiring. But in general, the people who do best with this or any other disease are those who have the support of their family and friends.

The principal sources of support for people with HIV infection are their caregivers: partners, parents, husbands and wives, brothers and sisters, aunts, and uncles, cousins, grandparents, friends, neighbors. Other sources of support are other relatives, volunteer buddies from advocacy agencies, co-workers, church members, and members of any other groups to which they belong. Still other sources are the professionals who tend the mental health of those affected by HIV infection: psychiatrists, psychologists, social workers, counselors, religious leaders—therapists of all kinds. Some caregivers give full-time care, some part-time care, and some check in occasionally. Anyone supporting a person with HIV infection or a caregiver is also a caregiver.

Being a caregiver is not simple. Chapter 5 discusses the tricky balances that people affected by HIV infection must maintain with each other: the balance between helplessness, dependency, and control; the balance between sympathy and intrusiveness. People affected by HIV infection must negotiate the territory between what one person needs and the other can supply. They must understand and tolerate each other's anger, depression, guilt, fears, and desires to talk or not to talk. "All the time, I put myself in my husband's position," said Lisa. "I thought, how would I like to be treated? How would I feel? I would have been afraid of being left alone, afraid of losing control over my life. I had to remember all that."

But in spite of the difficulty of maintaining all these balances and negotiations, people affected by HIV infection say that their supporters are invaluable, indispensable, fundamental to their lives. As June's son said, "My mother keeps me alive."

In general, supporters find ways to get people out of themselves, help them stay interested in life, and make them remain a part of the world. Supporters touch them, bring them things they like, and let them know they're valued. Supporters talk about themselves and by doing that, give tacit permission to the person affected by HIV infection to talk as well. Supporters listen—without criticism, without advice, without too many suggestions for improvement, and with kindness.

What follows are examples of the ways family, friends, religious leaders, AIDS-advocacy organizations, and mental health professionals have provided support. The examples can give caregivers some ideas of what support to offer and how vital that support is. The examples can also give people with the virus some notions of what support might be possible and where to get it, and perhaps a recognition of the support they already have. This is not a representative sample of all the kinds of support. People are endlessly inventive, and the ways to provide support must be nearly infinite.

Family

Families can provide a unique kind of support, some of the closest relationships people ever have. For some people, this closeness seems to make them feel as though they and their families are arms and legs of the same body. The exact kind of support families provide is not always concrete, and sometimes it is a little mysterious. Helen's face shines when she talks about her family: "Sometimes when I feel pretty much alone and discouraged, my family overpowers me. They just overpower me."

One of the most important things that members of the family do is bring with them a sense of a shared past. Families reminisce, talk about good times, retell old stories. Steven's family reminds him of the time he fell out of the tree onto the picnic table and got his mother's potato salad all over him. With such stories about the past comes a sense of being part of both the past and the future, a sense of who you are and what your roots are, a sense of continuity. Feeling a part of something larger is a deep comfort to people affected by HIV infection. Perhaps that is what Helen means when she says her family just "overpowers" her.

Families also make people feel cared about. When Steven was sick, his mother flew in from another city to cook for him. "Nothing is like home cooking," he said. "I call her up and say, 'Hop on a plane, Ma, and come cook for me.'" Dean's mother brought in meals, sat on his bed, and played cards with him. All my out-of-town relatives have come to visit," he said. "It makes me feel good, what my family does to me." June said her relatives drive a long way to see her son: "Those that can't come write letters saying the right things. My son knows he is accepted and loved in his family." Feeling cared about is not only a comfort; it can also be a reason to stay alive. Dean said that without his family, he wouldn't be here: "I would have nothing to fight for. They care about me, and because of that, it's important that I care too."

People affected by HIV infection seem to feel most free with their brothers and sisters. They often find it easier to tell their brothers and sisters about the diagnosis in the first place. They feel their brothers and sisters understand them and accept them as they are. "I've been able to talk and let loose my feelings with my sister," Dean said. June noticed that her son seemed most comfortable talking to his brother. "My son can talk to his brother especially," she said, "and his brother brings over his children." Helen's stepmother did the same thing: "My stepmother brought her little kids to visit me when I was in the hospital. I told her not to, there are germs here. But she just said, 'You're sick. We're coming.'"

In fact, many relatives, especially brothers and sisters, make a point of bringing their children to visit. Offering your children seems to be a way of offering part of yourself. And children can be so cheerful and straightforward, they are an immediate comfort. Alan said that his nephew gives him something to fight for: "I want to be here for his graduation," he says. "And seeing him with his baby sister, it's been worth every minute of the fight."

Not everyone people consider family is a blood relative. People who are distant from their families make substitute families out of their friends. They celebrate holidays and birthdays together, give each other presents, stay in touch, travel together, help each other out. Steven has an old teacher who took him into her family, introduced him to her friends, and takes him on trips and out to dinner: "She's extended family to me," he said. A friend of Alan's has a mother who, Alan said, "is like another mother to me." Family also needn't be exclusively human; many people find comfort in their pets. "My cat meets me at the door every night," said Alan. "One night, he didn't, and I missed him. I realized how much I appreciated that he usually did."

In some families, the same closeness makes them expect more of each other than they would of other people: they feel that members of their family should not be gay or use drugs, should not be depressed or even sick. Such expectations are difficult and often impossible to meet, and both sides feel disappointed and frustrated. For some people, then, the family is unable to provide much help. "My husband's family couldn't deal with his being sick," Lisa said. "For a long time, they wouldn't call, wouldn't send money, wouldn't come to visit. When they finally did come, they talked only about routine things." Notice, however, that Lisa's in-laws did come to visit, and did provide what small comfort they could by talking about routine things. Though Lisa wished they could have done more, both for her and for her husband, she recognized they had been a help. "All the same," she said, "it helped him just to hear from them."

Probably, even if your family cannot provide as much support and comfort as you would like, they nevertheless wish they could. They probably feel they should be able to make all your problems go away, and they feel guilty and helpless when they cannot. Perhaps the best thing to do is what Lisa finally did: accept what they are able to offer, and find the comfort in it.

Families are also prime sources of well-meant and unasked-for advice. Such advice can be hard to listen to, especially because the adviser rarely has experience with the kinds of problems HIV infection presents. As a result, the advice can sound annoying or distrustful or condescending or just wrong. The same principle that applies to disappointed expectations also applies to unwanted advice: ignore it, or explain you'll have to agree or disagree, and find comfort in the adviser's good intentions and concern. Dean said his rule with his family is, "No criticisms, no advice."

Friends

Another vital source of support is friends—anyone from a partner, lover, or confidant to a person to have fun with, a neighbor, a co-worker, another person affected by HIV infection, or anyone who shares interests. Sometimes, because some of these people feel less intimately connected to you than family, they actually find it easier to be good companions and sources of support. June said that with her son's sickness, she really needs her friends: "I need all the support and prayers and love I can get from anyone. My friends call and say, 'I just wanted to know how you were. And how your son is. I'm thinking of you.' My friends are such a source of strength. They're *there*."

Sometimes friends are also less intimidating to talk to than family. You choose your friends in the first place for what you have in common, and because they will not judge what you say. People commonly say of a friend, "I can say anything to her." Alan is quiet and not especially talkative, but he gets together with other people who have HIV infection and listens to them talk. "It helps to hear other people talk," Alan said. "They say your feelings for you. You relate to people who think the way you do."

Many people affected by HIV infection have found their friends more helpful than anyone else. Their friends bring them food, help them do their laundry, cook meals, clean their houses, pick up medication, bring flowers or books or videos, drive them to the doctor, get them out of the house, and are just generally on call. Dean's friends brought him a birthday party when he was in the hospital: "Balloons everywhere," he said, "and cake, cards, presents, everything. I had lost track of the date, and had forgotten it was my birthday. I felt so good I cried."

If friends honestly offer these services, do not be shy about accepting. Your friends are certainly concerned about you—and some of them love you—and helping you is a way for them to show how they feel.

Even co-workers can be a support: some people feel the people they work with are a kind of family. When Dean had his second opportunistic illness, a co-worker called his hospital social worker and asked what she and other colleagues could do. The social worker's answer was a good one to give anyone who asks such a question: "Don't leave him alone. Give him openings to talk but don't push. And stick around and don't head for the hills."

Religion

People's religions offer them two sources of support, one human, one spiritual. Priests, rabbis, ministers, nuns, pastors of all religions give the same sort of help as social workers and psychologists, but they talk particularly to people who want to talk about God. They offer advice, company, and comfort. A hospital chaplain who deals largely with people with HIV infection says, "I start by asking, 'What do you want me to pray for?' They tell me, and we talk about that. I think my presence as a representative of the church brings a sense of hope and warmth and comfort. I think I bring the rituals and the nurturing of the church."

A pastor in a large city church, when she celebrates the Eucharist at church, consecrates extra wafers and takes them along for celebration of the Eucharist at the hospital. "That's become important," she said. "The people in the hospital are getting the wafers that were consecrated when everybody has gathered together to celebrate the Eucharist. That connection becomes very important to sick people. They don't say it in exact words, but I can see it in their faces. Sometimes they cry."

Lisa's pastor used to pick up her husband at home and drive to Lisa's workplace, where the three of them would have a coffee break and a brief prayer. Lisa also found that she needed more attention from her fellow church members, but she didn't want to tell them why. So she told them instead that her husband's increasing weakness was caused by a heart condition, and that sometimes the situation really got her down. Then, she said, "they stopped being so plastic-y and I could see the real feeling in them."

The spiritual comfort of religion can be separate from the human comfort. Dean's faith brings him strength: "My greatest source of support is my church," said Dean. "It's spiritual support, having God who is greater and could intervene. I don't believe God creates these things; I don't believe any of that stuff about plagues. I do a lot of communicating with God. I say, 'Okay, I'll work it out with you.' It has a healing effect. God gives us the strength to meet each day and live it to the fullest."

Helen's faith brings her reassurance: "God loves me so much. Even when I fail in my own eyes, I don't fail in God's. God is a good parent. If someone is hungry, God sees to it that they're fed."

AIDS-Advocacy Organizations

What this book calls AIDS-advocacy organizations are organizations in the community, sometimes only local, sometimes affiliated with a national organization, that offer a huge variety of services to people with HIV infection and to their caregivers. The services these organizations offer include buddies, counselors, information on treatments, education about HIV infection, help with financial problems, home health care, help with housing problems, help with legal problems, legal services, reports on the latest medical research, support groups, political action, and transportation—to name a few.

Many of these organizations also run hotlines, which are free 800-phone numbers to call for information on HIV infection and for referrals to the organizations and services available in your local community.

To find out what's available in your community, check the phone book's yellow pages under AIDS or HIV, or the phone book's government blue pages under Health or AIDS or HIV. Or call the hotlines of national AIDS-advocacy organizations. In addition, a book put out every two years by the U.S. Conference of Mayors, called *Local AIDS Services: The National Directory*, lists, as its title implies, the local services available everywhere from Anniston, Alabama, to Laramie, Wyoming. Your physician or hospital social worker is also a good source for the resources in your own community.

For more information, and for addresses and phone numbers of national organizations and hotlines, see "Resources," which follows this chapter.

Support and Therapy Groups

Some of the best support for people affected by HIV infection comes through organized support and therapy groups. People often resist joining such groups because, they say, their families and friends and religion are sufficient, or they are embarrassed to turn to strangers, or they just don't like joining groups. Once they join a group, however, they find that talking to people who share the same experiences allows them to open up and say things they could not otherwise say. For people whose family and friends are unable to be much help, support and therapy groups are lifesavers.

Talking to people who share your situation can reduce your sense of isolation and give you a feeling of community. Listening to them talk can also give you a different perspective on your own problems. Seeing what works for other people and what does not helps you decide what might work for you. Hearing your problems described by someone else as their problems is somehow reassuring, calming—you don't feel alone with your problems; you're in good company. People say that groups give them a sense of relief from their own problems, and a sense of hope. People like the thought that they might be helping others in their group.

Support and therapy groups are found everywhere (see "Resources," following this chapter): hospitals, clinics, churches, AIDS-advocacy organizations, to name a few. Groups are composed of people with common situations. Some groups are for people who have the virus but no symptoms; some are for people with early symptomatic HIV infection, some for people with AIDS; some are for caregivers; some are for the people with AIDS and their caregivers; some are for women with AIDS; some are for black men with AIDS; some are for gay men; some are for intravenous drug users.

Though the difference between support and therapy groups is not always clear-cut, support groups tend to be for company and comfort, therapy groups for solving specific problems. The goals of support groups often include learning to reduce isolation, to share experiences, to see what works for others, to express things you might not express elsewhere, to feel accepted. Those who choose a support group are principally looking for a safe place in which to be themselves and to be less isolated. The goals of therapy groups are the same, but also include learning to confront negative patterns. Those who choose a therapy group worry about patterns in their lives with which they are unhappy: they feel they are always lonely, for instance, or that they pick the wrong sorts of partners. These are not necessarily problems specific to HIV infection, though everyone else in the group should also be dealing with HIV infection.

Both types of groups should be small, usually from five to eight people. Both groups are usually led, more or less loosely, by a qualified, experienced mental health professional. Mental health professionals say that what kind of group you get into is less important than getting into a group in the first place. Alan began going to a support group when his counselor recommended it: "The group has had a big effect on me. One of the worst things about the virus is not talking about it. When I talk to the group, my feeling of isolation is gone. The group also helps me release stress and anger. Plus you get a perspective on HIV, that it's no big thing, though I'm logical enough to know it *is* a big thing. But the perspective helps me not paralyze myself and not get into self-fulfilling prophecies. The group has been such a support."

Steven found that his group helped him feel hope and courage: "It's uplifting at the meetings. You get encouraged to keep trying to find help, to pursue all avenues. You learn that someone is out there no matter how bad it is. You learn you're entitled to help."

Support groups help people understand themselves better and find connections with other people. "Sometimes, when you finally verbalize the things that are pretty far down," Alan said, "they become a permanent part of you. I have always felt pretty isolated, and I was able to say that. One time the group leader said that we will realize the people we love, love us. I found some people who love me that I hadn't even realized did love me. That opens me up to a nonsexual loving relationship."

Mental Health Professionals

Some mental health professionals—psychiatrists, psychologists, social workers, psychiatric nurses, counselors—deal primarily with people affected by HIV infection. Psychiatrists are physicians who have specialized in psychiatry—that is, in disorders of mood and thinking; psychiatrists can prescribe medication. Psychologists have doctoral degrees, either a Ph.D. or an Ed.D., in psychology; psychologists can test and diagnose. Social workers have master's degrees plus supervised training. Psychiatric nurses have master's degrees plus supervised training. And counselors can be pastors or others who counsel people. All these professionals should be certified by the certifying boards of their respective professions. The certifying boards for counselors are variable, some good, some not so good, and as a result, counselors are not as tightly monitored as the other mental health professionals.

To overgeneralize, these professionals offer two kinds of therapy—talk therapy and medical therapy. All of them offer talk therapy. They can help you express and understand and resolve painful feelings, analyze and solve problems with other people, gain a sense of who you are as a whole person. They will work with problems that range from the specific and practical to the fundamental and philosophical. You can say anything to them. Psychiatrists alone can also offer medical therapy, drugs that restore sleep, appetite, and mood. Probably the best advice is to begin with talk therapy, but you will want to ask the professional to refer you for medical therapy if necessary. The professional who is unwilling to do this is best avoided.

If you do not know who the mental health professionals are, begin by asking the medical professionals—doctors, nurses, physician's assistants—you do know. If they cannot help, they will surely refer you to someone who can. Local AIDS-advocacy groups, the gay community, local mental health associations, and state mental health agencies all have lists of qualified, experienced mental health professionals.

Taking Control

At some level, everyone knows that, as Robert Burton wrote in *The Anatomy of Melancholy*, "[In this life, we are] subject to infirmities, miseries, interrupt, tossed & tumbled up and down, carried about with every small blast, often molested & disquieted upon each slender occasion, uncertain, brittle, & so is all that we trust unto." One of the conditions of life is that we are susceptible and vulnerable, and so is everyone else we depend on. People affected by HIV infection know that their emotions—depression, anger, fear, guilt, dependency—though painful to feel and difficult to admit, are also realistic and perhaps inevitable. They know that despite the comfort of their friends and relatives, they must resolve these painful emotions alone. Their resolutions, though varied, are at bottom the same: somehow or another, they learn to deal with the conditions of life. The twentieth-century poet Randall Jarrell wrote: " 'If you are afraid of wolves, do not go into the forest,' the Russian proverb says. We all live in the forest, and there is nothing to do but get used to the wolves."

What this means to people affected by HIV infection is that in spite of an inescapable infection and the inevitable accompanying emotions, they are in charge. They still make their own decisions and determine their own outlooks. "I'm made of good stuff," Dean said, "and the stuff I'm made of doesn't change because my situation changes." "Facing what I am up against gives me a new frame of mind," said Helen. "I expected a lot of life that I won't get. But I will do the best for myself and be an inspiration to others. I think we have more control over our lives than even we think we do."

No one says that finding a "new frame of mind" is easy. Helen said, "It's easier to say these things when you're feeling good." Easy or not, people do get used to the wolves, do gain a sense of control, do find a new frame of mind. They accomplish this with a few tricks.

Consider Changing Your Usual Tactics

Most of the tactics people use to get through their lives are appropriate to normal circumstances. HIV infection, however, is certainly not one of life's normal circumstances. So people occasionally have to consider switching their normal tactics, their usual style of living, the way they normally go about things. Alan has been a successful professional whose success was partly the result of concentrating hard, working persistently, passing tests, and solving problems until he got what he wanted. But HIV infection presents him with different kinds of problems: his job is now too demanding, and he needs more emotional support. For these problems, Alan's usual tactics—concentration, hard work, and persistence—no longer work. So he's gradually changing his tactics. He's learned to back off from his job a little, he does volunteer work with AIDS advocacy agencies, he spends more time with his friends and family.

Divide and Conquer

Cut overwhelming and insoluble problems into manageable, solvable ones. People have various ways of doing this.

Divide problems into those that have solutions and those that do not, and focus on the problems that have solutions. Helen had been thinking about dying and worrying about how her family would deal with her death. She could not annul the fact that her death would create problems for her family, so she decided to solve a smaller problem. "I am a real junk collector," she said. "I thought, if I died tomorrow, would my family want this twelve-year-old perfume? I've pitched out so much I didn't need. I had old *Family Circle* magazines since 1976. I went through them and laughed and laughed—at the prices, at the styles. I threw out two of my three corkscrews. I threw everything out. My surroundings are so much more comfortable, and now my family won't have to sort through all that junk."

Focus on short-term problems. Alan had been angry and depressed because he was just becoming established in his career when he began getting sick. After talking to his counselor and his partner, he decided not to focus on his long-term career goals—"I gave up on rich and famous," he says. Instead, he makes only short-term goals he knows he can accomplish. He has a kit for a grandfather clock he wants to build. He'd like to learn some Italian. When he accomplishes those goals, he says, he will make some more. He tries not to "get upset if the goals don't get accomplished."

What this tactic comes down to is this: avoid looking at the whole picture and trying to solve everything at once. Steven says he lives from one day to the next, and does only what is necessary to get through each day. He says he solves only small problems, one at a time, and trusts they will add up. June says that a caregiver needs to do exactly the same: "I concentrate only on making a particular day better," she said. "I just don't bother with the big picture."

Like Steven, Dean says he has learned to stop worrying about overwhelming problems. He tries to change only what he can: "I always tried so hard to change things I couldn't. Realistically I can't change my problems—the only way not to have problems is to be dead. And I can realistically change myself. I forgot I could make myself happy. I am as happy or unhappy as I decide to be. I'm surprised at how happy I am, and it's not in spite of the problems. There are happy people with problems." In short, take it a little at a time. Expect of yourself only what is reasonable. Try not to borrow trouble or worry about what might happen or cross bridges before you come to them. Be easy on yourself.

Take a Break

"With this disease," says Steven, "you need an escape hatch. Sometimes I zombie out in front of the TV. Or get a hot fudge sundae and eat it slowly." Lisa goes for long walks, reads what she describes as "trashy love stories," and drives out into the country. People go away for a weekend, plan an evening away at a play, opera, concert, sports event, movie. For a while, they let themselves drop their worries, they say, and think of nothing except the pleasure of the moment. Some, like Helen, take advantage of the mind's ability to distract itself with pleasant thoughts. She has learned to recognize these moments of pleasure as they occur and to say to herself, "At this minute I happen to be happy, so I'll enjoy this minute."

A lot of people do relaxation exercises and say that relaxation gives them the necessary distance from their problems. Relaxation exercises are part of performing artists' training, some psychotherapies, meditation routines, and yoga practices. All exercises are pretty much the same. Lie down and get comfortable. Beginning with your feet and working up to your face and scalp, muscle by muscle, first tense the muscle, then relax it. Repeat the tension and relaxation with each muscle several times before going on to the next muscle. Eventually you will notice that you breathe more slowly and regularly, that your body relaxes, and finally, that your mind relaxes. In this state of relaxation, imagine yourself in a place that is comforting to you, a place where you are free and happy, where you feel safe and calm. You can either do this relaxation on your own or buy recorded tapes that direct you through the relaxation or join a group that does the exercises together. In any case, mental health professionals often know where you can get help learning the exercises.

Caregivers especially need to take breaks. "I had no time to think of myself," said Lisa. "I couldn't get away from it, it was all-consuming. For a long time, I felt crazy. I just went five hundred miles an hour." Caregivers often feel guilty about taking breaks, but breaks are essential to good caregiving. Without breaks, caregivers start burning out. Find other supports: nurses, social workers, hospice staff, groups, buddies, home health aides, clergy, all can take some of the heat off, give you some time out. "One of the greatest things a caregiver can do," said June, "is cry for help. I see myself getting hyperactive and losing control, and I call the doctors or my pastor or my friends who know. I've learned to admit weaknesses. With all my wisdom and intelligence and backbone I'm so proud of, there are still things I can't handle."

Give Your Feelings Their Due

When you feel bad, go ahead and feel that way. Tell yourself, as Dean does, "I'm just tired of this. I don't see how I can do it any more." Cry, stare into space, refuse to talk, stay in bed, write your terrible feelings in a private journal—go off by yourself and do whatever expresses the bad feelings. "I don't believe in this crap of, 'You've got to be happy all the time,'" says Steven. "I'm not taped together as well as I thought I was, or more likely, the tape was old. Anyway, sometimes I fall apart and just feel awful."

In short, give your feelings their due. This is not giving in. It is acknowledging the reality and size of the problems you face. Somehow, such acknowledgment is easier than trying to control how you feel, or going from crisis to crisis and never feeling anything. These feelings, once acknowledged, don't last as long as you might think. They seem to wear themselves out and disappear. "After I've been feeling hopeless for a while," says Dean, "the feeling lightens up, and I feel that I've really got a long road ahead of me. I've seen too many people give up. I feel like I'd just like to keep going."

The feelings will certainly come back again—Steven says he now knows when he is likely to feel bad and sets aside time for the feelings: "I plan for falling apart," he says. But when the feelings do come back, you will have them in better perspective. That is, you will know that the feelings are both real and temporary. For good reasons, you feel bad; and after a while, for reasons just as good, you will feel better.

Learn to Deal with the Medical System

A crucial part of living well is taking control. A crucial part of taking control, for some people, is learning to deal with the medical system. The medical system is complicated (Chapter 8 outlines the system and explains who does what).

The best advice we can give both the person with HIV infection and the caregiver is to ask questions. One reason that people don't ask questions is because they feel intimidated. Medical people often don't understand they are intimidating. If you don't ask them questions, they assume you already know the answers, not that you're afraid to ask. Another reason people don't ask questions is because they worry about offending their physicians. Any good physician will not be offended by a question. Neither of these is a good reason not to find out what you want to know.

Ask how to get medical care at night and on weekends. Get pushy if you are in pain; pain is usually unnecessary. Ask what's happening with new treatments. Ask for advice on alternative treatments—treatments like acupuncture or untested drugs. Ask where you are in the course of the infection. Ask what tests you are being given, what those tests detect, what the alternatives to the tests are. Ask for a second opinion on a diagnosis or an interpretation of a test. People worry especially about asking for second opinions; but this is a reasonable and prudent request, and physicians are not offended by it.

In general, you have a right to know about treatments, medications, and procedures. Patients in hospitals have a whole set of rights; Chapter 8 outlines them.

It is a good idea to write questions down before visiting the doctor: most people forget some or most of what they want to ask. Questions about medical care are best addressed to your doctors. Questions about the medical system and resources for medical care in general are best addressed to a social worker.

Relabel the Negative; Focus on the Positive

Relabeling means redefining a troubling situation so that it seems more benign (see Chapter 5). Relabeling is related to thinking positively: any situation, no matter how bad, contains the possibility for something good. The idea is to focus on the possibilities for good and define the situation in those terms. "If I approach it with the right attitude," says Steven, "I can see the blessings."

Call something a challenge rather than a struggle, a preference rather than a need, an opportunity rather than a problem, caring rather than dependency. People who have to quit work say they are not losing their usefulness but gaining freedom and opportunity: the chance to volunteer, to read certain books, to learn to paint, to teach, learn a language, put together models, and especially, spend more time with the people they love. Helen knows that even though HIV infection is not curable, it is treatable, and seeing the disease as treatable, she says, "does a lot for me." Dean, who has lived a long time with the virus and has weathered several serious illnesses, defines himself not as a sick person but as a survivor, a winner: "I've survived a lot of illnesses, and some even the doctors thought I wouldn't," he says. "So even if I die, I'll still feel I've won."

Eat Well

Eating well helps your immune system, provides energy, and prevents muscle loss. People with HIV infection are beset with a variety of conditions that make eating difficult. Chapter 6 details which foods soothe or counter those conditions.

In general, people with HIV infection should be careful about their nutrition. Remember the four basic food groups: every day, you should have two to four servings of milk or milk products, meat or meat substitutes, fruits and vegetables, and cereals and starches. For more specific advice, ask a registered dietitian. (A registered dietitian is usually trained and licensed in nutrition and problems of nutrition; nutritionists need not be either trained or licensed.) Registered dietitians can be found at hospitals, clinics, and county health departments, and in private practice.

Dietitians often advise people with HIV infection to be careful of infections by microbes like salmonella that live in perishable food. These infections occur only rarely in people with HIV infection. If you want to be extra cautious, however, the microbes' growth can be inhibited by very hot and very cold temperatures, and by cleanliness. Keep hot food hot: cook at 165 degrees F to 212 degrees F, keep warm at 140 degrees F to 165 degrees F. Keep cold foods cold: refrigerate at 40 degrees F, freeze at 0 degrees F. Keep everything clean: wash fresh fruit and vegetables. Do not eat moldy food. Do not eat rare meat, raw fish, or raw meat, and do not drink unpasteurized milk. Thaw meat in the refrigerator, not at room temperature. Do not eat raw eggs; cook eggs thoroughly.

Encourage Yourself

Protect your physical health. Eat well, sleep enough, cut alcohol and smoking down or out. Exercise as much as possible; just going for a walk is great exercise. Relax when you can: read, watch a movie, do relaxation exercises. Take good care of your body. If you have HIV, give your body a chance to fight the infection. If you are a caregiver, you also have to take care of yourself. Lisa said, "I am very careful about exercise and food. You owe it to the people you're caring for."

Be kind to yourself emotionally. Steven gives himself pep talks:

"When I feel good," he says, "I let myself know that. I tell myself, 'Steve, you feel great today.'" Dean says that every day he rates how he feels on a scale of one to ten: "It's mostly nines and tens," he says. Helen says that her best support is herself. "Basically, it comes down to me," she says. "I want to survive this. So I have to support myself, and when I do something well, I pat myself on the back."

If an emotional problem seems too severe or does not go away, or if you are seriously considering suicide, or if you simply want someone to whom you can express all your feelings, see a mental health professional.

Confront the Possibilities a Little at a Time

Once, when Dean Lombard was in the hospital, he roomed for a while with a man who was in the advanced stages of AIDS. "I was glad to get out of that room," Dean said. "As long as I was there, I needed to confront the possibility that what happened to him would happen to me. But confronting that possibility seemed necessary, to deal with this disease as positively as I am."

Confronting the possibilities means, for Dean and others like him, understanding and admitting that the fact of HIV infection cannot be annulled. Steven said, "I have to deal with this whether I want to or not." It is now a part of life. So are the possibilities of fatigue, disability, dependency, illness, clinic appointments, and hospitalizations. And so are the emotional reactions to all this. "HIV makes me face things I didn't think I'd have to face," Helen said. Confronting the facts and possibilities and reactions is often the only way through them.

Confronting everything all at once, however, is overwhelming and unnecessary. Face what you are ready to face, and only when you are ready. When you are tired of thinking or feeling, stop and rest. Do not push yourself because you or someone else thinks you ought to be facing things. Face a little at a time.

In fact, confronting the facts means facing not only sickness but also health. If, within some amount of time, fatigue, death, or dependency are possibilities, so are strength, life, and confidence. People remind themselves that no one knows with certainty how the disease progresses in every individual.

Positive Denial

People who focus on hope rather than despair may seem to be denying the facts. But whether denial is positive or negative depends on what you are denying. Denial is negative only if people deny the facts of their infection and live inappropriately: drink too much, take drugs, practice unsafe sex, avoid seeing a doctor, or prevent a person with AIDS from talking about sickness or death.

Denial that admits both the realities of today and the unpredictability of tomorrow is positive. Alan, who bought a new car on a five-year finance plan, is denying not infection, only knowledge of the future. No one knows what will happen or when. No one knows how any one person's body will handle HIV infection. No one knows how long he or she will live or what she or he might die of. "You really have to deny some of this stuff," Alan says. "I'm sad when I lose a friend, but I'm careful not to connect that death to mine. Death happened to my friend, and I'm sad about that. But it still hasn't happened to me."

Positive denial is nearly essential in dealing with this disease. If you don't know the future, you have a certain distance between yourself and the disease: you are much more than someone affected by HIV. Your life has many aspects, many parts to it, many things you are interested in, many things and people you love; and HIV, though important, is only one aspect of your life. "I'm not denying I'm sick," Dean said. "But I've made up my mind not to act sick, not to just sit around being a sick person."

Positive denial also helps people feel feisty about the disease. They feel like they are not just victims of some virus; they are people who have some say in how their lives are run. "I'm going to fight until I can't any more," says Dean.

Find Comforts and Interests in Things Outside Yourself

"Don't lock yourself in," says Steven, "get yourself out." The world is full of pleasures, beauties, people to get to know, wrongs that need to be righted, jobs that need to be done, places to visit, adventures to be had. People find, in things outside themselves, anything from a trivial and momentary distraction to a profound interest in living. The possibilities are limitless.

Some people make their surroundings beautiful and comforting. Helen says she tries to make the place where she spends her time a space she enjoys: "I like brass and glass. I like plants—they're another life. I like a little elegance. Things should be as fine as they can be." Alan repainted his house: "I've made it warm, restful, and interesting with colors. These colors reflect a color of light that looks good on people. People look wonderful in my house. My own house is a comfort to me."

Some people find things they like to do, or things they have always wanted to do but have never done. Helen gardens: "I crave being out there. I put all these bulbs in, and now I have next year to look forward to. Plus I also have a room I want to redecorate." Steven's cousin, whom he says is like a sister to him, moved in with him. They enjoy doing the same things, Steven says: "While I'm feeling reasonably well, we'll do what we like doing—we go to museums, we play music together. We'll just enjoy the things that give us pleasure." Dean had always loved both music and teaching: "I've always been a closet teacher, and now I direct music full time. Being sick also gives me time to do what I want."

Some people teach themselves new things because learning, they say, takes them out of themselves. Dean became interested in archaeology and astronomy: "Maybe, in the light of ancient history and the immense universe," he says, "my disability insurance isn't all that important. I wonder why people worry about things that don't matter all that much."

Some people spend more time with people they love and enjoy: "Before my husband died," said Lisa. "we concentrated on putting lots of importance on kids and grandkids. You can get so busy with run-of-the-mill stuff, you don't get around to it. My husband went on a fishing trip with his son. He went to visit our granddaughter at kindergarten. He listened to his grandson's first piano piece."

Some people become activists. June runs an AIDS-advocacy agency; she says she throws herself into work. "I feel that it helps to help," she says, "to *do* something." Lisa was going to run for city council, but decided instead that she could do more putting out a newsletter, so she raised money and started one: "I think you should speak up, be visible, be yourself." Steven began doing public speaking and recommends it to others: "Get interested in legislation," he said, "in outreach; contact speakers' bureaus, call people up. I've gone from being a passive type to being a real civil disobedient type." Dean is writing a book about his experiences with AIDS, and says the book gives him a positive attitude: "It's leaving my mark. It's doing what will help other people."

Some people help others in different ways. Many become buddies or carepartners through AIDS-advocacy programs. Dean volunteered in a hospital on a floor for children with cancer. "It was hard on me to see those kids so sick," he said, "but it put things in perspective for me. I thought, 'Who am I to complain? They're so good and so happy. I've had forty good years. How can I complain?'" Helen is less ambitious but no less helpful: "I visit the woman who used to be my roommate in the hospital. She won't eat anything. I make her get out of bed, sit in a chair, go for a walk; I give her my jellybeans. I talk to her. It makes me feel good."

A Positive Attitude

People affected by AIDS agree on this, that the single most important thing they can do is to keep a positive attitude.

During one of Dean's serious illnesses, he was near death. While he was recovering, he said, "I sat and thought, 'How long can I keep this game going, denying this disease? Do I want to continue? Do I have it in me?' Then I thought, 'I fought everything else, it's up to me again. I'll beat this too.' In a way, death would have been easier. But I think about what I'd have missed—the pictures of Neptune from Voyager, my sister's baby, my son growing up."

Now Dean says he concentrates not on what he's lost, but on what he has left. "I've become more conscious of the quality of life," he says. "Now I'm concerned with living before I die, and living *every* minute. Sometimes it's like a violent smack hits me: wake up and enjoy life."

Steven has feelings that are almost identical: "I don't know where my ability to enjoy life comes from. I love life so much, I want every minute. I keep myself occupied and my mind working. I compare myself to other people—I still have advantages others don't. I've been fortunate, and it's been a good life. It has been one big education. If this is all I'm going to get, okay. It's not bad. It's pretty good."

Keeping a positive attitude can change the way people think of themselves. They think of themselves less as people with a disease and more as people who are—for the present, anyhow—alive. They say they know how to be alive and will live their lives the way they know how. They come to trust their own resources, to trust themselves. Sometimes they even become different people: "I've never liked telling anyone what's going on with me," said Alan, "but dealing with this disease has made me more open than any time in my life. I'm voicing my opinion more, am more self-confident." Along with that comes a better view of themselves: "I think I began loving myself," said Helen. "There's a difference between just taking care of yourself and loving yourself. I'm working on loving myself."

Keeping a positive attitude can also change the way people feel about the future. "I think a person should feel everything in life," Alan said, "even the negative things. But I tell myself I'm fine and I'm going to be fine as long as I can. I have this feeling, I could be here when a cure comes. I'm very strong." Helen says she's never going to settle for less than she can have. Dean says he doesn't know what will happen in the months ahead, but he doesn't want to give up: "I've worked too hard, I'm a good person, and I have a will power that won't quit. I want to make something positive out of something negative."

Dean has a motto he uses to keep himself active and interested in life: "A body at rest stays at rest," he says, "and a body in motion stays in motion." He borrowed the motto from his high-school physics class and, he says, "I say it over and over. I use it to think myself well."

People come to believe that life need not be perfect or infinite to be good, and that hope can come in little packets and delight can come from little things. "I've been able to cope and feel happy and delighted about living," said June. "A lot has to do with your attitude toward life. You like it or you don't."

The Mind-Body Connection

Your attitude toward life might in fact be related to your health. A field of research studies the intricate connections between mental state, the brain, and the immune system. The field goes by two impossible names: one is *neuroimmunomodulation*, the other is *psychoneuroimmunology*.

Specifically, stress seems to affect the immune system's ability to respond to infection. Several studies selected people under certain kinds of stresses: people whose spouses had died, people with severe depression, medical students at examination time, people under such extreme physical stresses as marathon running or dieting to the point of malnutrition. Their blood was analyzed for changes in immune response, that is, for changes in certain cells of the immune system: T cells, B cells, and white blood cells called natural killer cells.

Different studies measured immune response differently. In some studies, researchers counted the numbers of T and B cells in the blood. In others, researchers treated people's T cells with a chemical that stimulates reproduction, then counted the numbers of new T cells. In still others, researchers added natural killer cells to foreign cells, then measured the number of foreign cells not killed.

Regardless of which measure of immune response was studied, most researchers found that people under stress have immune responses that are somewhat lower than the immune systems of people not under stress. In other words, people under stress have fewer of certain immune system cells, or they have cells that reproduce less successfully, or they have cells that respond ineffectively to foreign cells.

The converse is also true: not only do people under stress have lower immune responses, but people with positive attitudes seem to have better immune responses. Some studies, done specifically on people with HIV infection, found that those who describe themselves as vigorous and self-expressive, who have ways of venting their emotions, and who exercise regularly have better immune responses. The level of T cell reproduction and the response of the natural killer cells—the same measures of immune response that had been lower with stressed people—were higher.

Other researchers have suggested theories of how stress might affect immune response. In other words, all these theories suggest how a person's mental state and the immune system might be linked. When people are under stress, their adrenal glands release hormones called *glucocorticoids* (the medications cortisone and prednisone are examples of glucocorticoids). In the immune system, glucocorticoids inhibit the release of chemicals called *interferon* and *interleukin-2*, which immune cells use to fight off fungi, bacteria, and viruses. In the bloodstream, glucocorticoids also decrease, temporarily at least, the number of certain T cells called T4 or CD4 cells, the same cells that HIV preferentially infects. And in experiments in the laboratory, another hormone the adrenal gland releases under stress, called *adrenaline* or *epinephrine*, seems to suppress reproduction of CD4 cells. In any case, because HIV specifically infects CD4 cells, anything that suppresses CD4 cells might make matters worse for someone trying to combat HIV infection.

It is hard to draw conclusions from any of these studies. The experiments with CD4 cells were done on animals or in laboratory dishes and not on living humans. The studies on humans measured different aspects of the immune system's response, they did not exclude people who were not eating and sleeping, they measured stress differently, and the stresses themselves were different and of different magnitudes.

Most importantly, many of the changes measured were small, and no one knows whether small changes in immune response are clinically important—that is, whether they actually increase the chances of getting sick. In general, take the research with a grain of salt: this field is only a few years old; it connects psychology, the brain, and the immune system; and all three systems are extraordinarily complex and not yet understood.

In spite of the studies' inconclusiveness, however, the sense in this new field is that people who are more emotionally stable may be less vulnerable to disease. When sick, they seem to do better, become less severely sick, stay alive longer.

The fact is, to people facing HIV infection, whether the research turns out to be right or wrong is irrelevant. If a positive mental state does affect the immune system, so much the better. If it does not, nothing is lost. A positive outlook makes your life more pleasant. The only trap is the possibility that people who do get sicker might blame themselves for not having worked hard enough. In view of the studies' inconclusiveness, blaming yourself is both unrealistic and unnecessary.

Resources:
Where to Go for Help

- Types of services
- Selected national resources
- Finding local services

Many organizations offer help of different types to people affected by HIV. The list of these resources, however, is a moving target. Any such list—and there are many—gets outdated fast. New organizations spring up, change the services they offer, change their addresses and phone numbers, expand, merge, or go out of business. Most lists of resources are updated every few months.

Given that, the best thing this book can do is list the types of services that can be available to people affected by HIV, list a few national resources that offer these services, and offer advice on how to find resources that are local.

Types of Services

The types of services an organization offers will depend on, among other things, the purpose of the organization and its geographical location. The range of services is immense, from problems specific to some people (e.g., Spanish-speaking educational counselors) to problems shared by everyone with HIV infection (education on preventing transmission). If the organizations do not offer the services themselves, they will recommend other organizations that do offer the services.

The following is a list of the services organizations may offer. If you need any of these services, call a national organization (see below) to find who in your local area offers the services. Or find a local resource (see below) that offers them.

Alcoholism: the national organization Alcoholics Anonymous (AA) has information on which of its local branches offer groups specific to people with HIV infection who also have problems with alcohol.

Buddy systems: buddies are volunteers, sometimes trained, who provide services that range from filling prescriptions and driving you to the grocery store to cleaning the refrigerator and holding hands.

Children with HIV infection

Counseling: can be individual or group counseling (see below, Support groups)

Drug use and HIV infection

Financial problems

Government reports

HIV testing

Home health care

Hospice care

Hotlines: toll-free phone numbers, either community, state, or national. Ask any questions about HIV infection and about services available to people with HIV infection.

Housing problems

Insurance problems

Legal services

Minorities and HIV infection, including organizations with Spanish-speaking counselors

Nursing homes

Physician referral

Political action, speakers' bureaus

Preventing transmission of HIV

Religious counseling

Safer sex

Scientific research reports

Sexually transmitted disease testing and treatment

Social workers, who help with plans for recuperating at home, with plans for finances and insurance, with recommendations to different organizations. They are hired by mental health centers, churches, social service agencies, and virtually all hospitals.

Support groups: groups can be specifically for women, gays, drug users, couples, caregivers, spouses, the worried well, and people who are HIV-positive, or who have early symptomatic HIV infection, or who have AIDS.

Transportation

Visiting nurse programs

Women and HIV infection

Selected National Resources

The following is a list of national resources, selected either because they run information hotlines or because they publish newsletters. We also include buyers' clubs. These organizations sometimes change their telephone numbers. If you call and get a message that the number is not in service, try directory assistance. For 800 numbers, the directory assistance number is 1-800-555-1212.

AIDS Clinical Trials Groups (ACTGs). These are the medical centers (discussed in Chapter 9) that are part of a national program of the National Institute of Allergy and Infectious Diseases (NIAID) to test new treatments for HIV infection. ACTGs need people to participate in these clinical trials; they are also superb sources of information and treatment. The list of ACTGs changes with time, so the best way to find the ACTG nearest you is to call the NIAID hotline at 1-800-TRIALS-A.

AIDS Treatment News, Box 411256, San Francisco, Calif. 94141, 1-415-255-0588. This is a twice-monthly newsletter on AIDS treatments.

American Foundation for AIDS Research (AmFAR), 733 Third Avenue, 12th Floor, New York, N.Y. 10017-3204, 1-212-682-7440. This organization keeps track of funding, research, and experimental treatments. AmFAR publishes the *AIDS/HIV Experimental Treatment Directory,* a directory of drugs being tested in clinical trials, updated quarterly. AmFAR also publishes *AIDS Targeted Information Newsletter,* a monthly newsletter of reports of, and comments on, the latest medical research appearing each month. It's expensive, $125 per year; 1-800-243-7909.

Buyers' Clubs: Healing Alternatives, 1748 Market Street, Suite 204, San Francisco, Calif. 94102, 1-415-626-2316; PWA Health Group,

150 W. 26th Street, Suite 201, New York, N.Y. 10001, 1-212-255-0520.

Gay Men's Health Crisis (GMHC), Department of Medical Information, 129 W. 20th Street, New York, N.Y. 10011. GMHC publishes *Treatment Issues,* a monthly newsletter on experimental drugs, which comes out ten times a year; no cost, but a donation is requested. GMHC also has a hotline for AIDS information and for peer counseling: 1-212-807-6655.

National AIDS Hotline, 1-800-342-AIDS or 1-800-342-7514. This is a 24-hour-a-day, 7-day-a-week hotline, contracted through the Centers for Disease Control. Ask them questions about types of services, about general information, and about what services are available in your local area. For Spanish-speaking callers, the number is 1-800-344-SIDA (7432) (8 A.M. to 2 A.M., Eastern Time).

National AIDS Information Clearinghouse, 1-800-458-5231. This is a sort of library for information on HIV infection; it sends publications, videos, and lists of services and community organizations for all areas.

National Commission on AIDS, 1-202-254-5125. It provides information on federal laws about funding for and research on HIV infection; located in Washington, D.C.

National Institute of Allergy and Infectious Diseases, National Institutes of Health, Building 31, Room 7A50, Bethesda, Md. 20892, 1-301-496-5717. The Institute publishes *NIAID AIDS Agenda,* a monthly newsletter about federally funded research projects.

Pharmaceuticals Manufacturers Associations, Communications Division, 1100 15th Street, N.W., Washington, D.C., 20005, 1-202-835-3400. It publishes *Update: AIDS Products in Development,* a quarterly chart of drugs, diagnostic tests, and vaccines.

PWA Coalition, 31 W. 26th Street, New York, N.Y. 10010, 1-212-532-0290. PWA stands for People With AIDS, though the organization welcomes everyone with HIV infection. It publishes the *PWA Coalition Newsline,* a monthly newsletter on alternative and experimental drugs, community-based research programs, and outreach activities; free to people with HIV infection, donation requested of all others. PWA Coalition also runs an AIDS information hotline: 1-800-828-3280.

San Francisco AIDS Foundation, P.O. Box 426182, San Francisco, Calif. 94142-6182, 1-415-864-5855. It publishes *BETA, Bulletin of Experimental Treatments for AIDS,* a newsletter about experimental treatments of HIV infection, updated periodically; no subscription price, but a donation is requested. Their AIDS information hotline is: 1-415-863-AIDS.

University of California at San Francisco, AIDS Health Project, Box 0884, San Francisco, Calif. 94143, 1-415-476-6430. It publishes *Focus,* a newsletter with practical information about AIDS research.

Finding Local Services

These organizations sometimes change their telephone numbers. If you call and get a message that the number is not in service, try directory assistance. For 800 numbers, the directory assistance number is 1-800-555-1212.

To find the services nearest to you, call or write:

Local AIDS Services: The National Directory, a book costing around $15 that lists all services for people with HIV infection everywhere in the country, from Anniston, Alabama, to Laramie, Wyoming. It is put out and updated every two years by the U.S. Conference of Mayors, 1620 Eye Street, N.W., Washington, D.C. 20006; 1-202-293-7330.

Your state, county, or city health department. Find their phone numbers in the blue government pages of the phone book under Health. Departments of health offer varying services but usually know what's available locally, including local and state hotline numbers; all state health departments have AIDS education departments.

National AIDS Hotline, 1-800-342-AIDS or 1-800-342-7514. This is a 24-hour-a-day, 7-day-a-week hotline, contracted through the Centers for Disease Control. Even though it is a national hotline, they have information on the services available in your local area, including local and state hotline numbers.

Local and state hotlines. They know local resources; to find hotline numbers, call the National AIDS Hotline or look up AIDS in the index to your phone book's yellow pages, or look up Health in the blue government pages of the phone book.

Your physician should also know about local resources; so should a social worker.

Understanding
Tests for HIV

- The tests
- Whether to get tested
- Who should get tested
- Informed consent for the tests
- Confidentiality
- Where to get tested
- What the test results mean

In 1983, the virus that came to be called the human immunodeficiency virus (HIV) was discovered in human blood samples. Two years later, researchers developed a test to detect HIV in the blood. At that time, the best use of the test was to screen people who wanted to donate blood so that blood transfusions and the blood supply would be free of HIV.

Medical researchers, however, were reluctant to use the screening test to identify people with HIV infection. First, although the test was one of the most accurate tests of its kind, occasional errors in its results created a lot of anxiety. Someone whose test result was positive might *not* have HIV, while someone whose test result was negative couldn't be certain that HIV was not present. Second, at that time, the public was not ready to accept people with HIV infection, and the newspapers were full of stories of discrimination against these people. This public response was partly due to fear and partly to our uncertainty about how the virus was transmitted. The third reason, and the most important, was that physicians had little to offer anyone who tested positive. As a result, recommendations from the medical profession and from others concerned with the epidemic about whether to get tested for HIV were ambiguous. That is, no one knew whether testing for HIV made sense or not.

Since these early times, the accuracy of the test has improved substantially, public understanding has progressed somewhat, and medical research has made a gigantic leap forward in the treatment of HIV infection. Recommendations have changed accordingly. The purpose of this chapter is to discuss the tests themselves and their accuracy, make recommendations about who should be tested, discuss the confidentiality of the tests, and help interpret the results.

The Tests

There are two general tests that detect HIV infection. Because HIV lives in blood cells, both are tests conducted on human blood, although tests using saliva and urine are expected soon. One blood test detects evidence of the virus itself; the other detects the antibody to the virus.

Tests for HIV

Three tests for HIV infection detect either the virus itself or parts of the virus in the blood. These tests are called (1) cultures for the virus, (2) P24 antigen tests, and (3) polymerase chain reaction (PCR).

Two tests (culture and PCR) are positive in about 95 percent of people with HIV infection. False positive tests results are rare. The tests are relatively expensive, usually $300 to $700 for cultures and $80 to $150 for PCR. Neither of these tests is available in most commercial medical laboratories, but most physicians who regularly treat people with HIV infection know where to get the tests done. At present, the major uses of such tests are for the rare person whose test results for the antibodies to HIV are ambiguous, and for research studies.

Tests for Antibodies to HIV

The most common method for detecting HIV infection is the test to detect antibodies to the virus. Antibodies are proteins the body makes to kill any microbe that invades human tissues. If antibodies are present, the microbe also is, or has been, present. Testing has been done to identify antibodies to many microbes for several decades; it is a common method for finding the microbes that cause a multitude of infectious diseases.

Laboratories use two standard tests for detecting antibodies to HIV: an initial screening test called the ELISA, followed by a confirming test called the Western blot. The results of the tests are positive (meaning that the antibody is present), negative (meaning the antibody is not present), or indeterminant (meaning that the test results are inconclusive).

Indeterminant, false negative, and false positive results.   The antibody test, on rare occasions, produces indeterminant or false results. Indeterminant results mean that the laboratory cannot determine definitely whether the results are positive or negative (see below, "Indeterminant Test Results"). People with indeterminant results are usually told to repeat the test in three months.

False results mean that the test results are inaccurate: they can be either falsely negative or falsely positive. A false negative result usually occurs because the test was taken too early during the course of the infection. After infection by most microbes, the body begins manufacturing antibodies within about two or three weeks. After infection with HIV, however, different people's bodies produce antibodies over widely varying amounts of time: about half the people infected will produce antibodies and have positive blood tests within six weeks; nearly all the rest will have positive tests within three months.

During this early period in the infection—after infection but before antibodies are manufactured—tests can be falsely negative, meaning that the person actually has HIV infection but the antibody test is negative.

The likelihood that a negative result is false is different for different people. A negative result is more likely to be false in people who are actively participating in high-risk behavior. A negative result is not likely to be false in people with low-risk behavior. For blood donors in general, the frequency of false negatives is vanishingly small: the standard antibody test will miss only 1 in 200,000 blood donors.

The results of the tests can also be falsely positive. The results can be falsely positive because the laboratory made an error or mixed up blood samples, or because the person has antibodies to miscellaneous proteins that incidentally resemble HIV. If the laboratory is reliable, and if both the ELISA and Western blot are done, the frequency with which the tests are falsely positive is also vanishingly small. In a study done purposefully to magnify the number of false positive results, the frequency with which tests were falsely positive was 1 in 135,000 tests.

The figures quoted above make the test for antibody to HIV one of the most accurate tests in medicine. Like other tests, it is subject to both human error and technological error. If there is reason seriously to question the results of the test, it is best simply to have it repeated. In the rare circumstance where repeat tests also leave questions, it is sometimes wise to take the test to detect the virus or parts of the virus.

Whether to Get Tested

Recommendations for testing have varied over the years. In 1985, when the antibody test was first introduced, physicians were concerned about the accuracy of the test. People with the infection were also concerned that they might lose their jobs, apartments, insurance, and even family and friends. Furthermore, in the early days of testing, physicians had little to offer in the form of effective therapy.

At that time, the most compelling reason for the test related to public health: to identify those who were infected so they could avoid spreading the virus through unsafe sex or by donating blood or organs. Although testing for public health reasons had worked well with other infectious diseases, it did not make great sense for HIV infection. The reason is that the message concerning prevention was the same for everyone. That is, people with many sexual contacts were told to practice safer sex if they had the infection—to avoid spreading the virus—and they were told to practice safer sex if they did not have the infection—to avoid getting the virus. The same type of message applied to intravenous drug users.

At present, however, reasons for getting tested are much clearer. In the first place, as noted earlier, tests are very accurate now.

In the second place, though public attitudes have not entirely changed and perhaps never will, they have progressed considerably. Some progress has been made through legislation, some through the media, and much of it through the efforts of advocacy groups. More and more, the public is coming to recognize that HIV infection now directly touches the lives of nearly everyone. In the early days of the epidemic, few people actually knew a person with HIV infection, and many thought the infection could be caught the way the common cold can be caught. As the epidemic progressed, people began to see this infection in their own friends and relatives, and the public attitude became more accepting.

In the third place, and most important, physicians can now manage the infection with treatment. (It is noteworthy that tests for syphilis at one time were similarly controversial: the discovery of penicillin more than offset the disadvantages of testing, however, so that large-scale testing for syphilis is no longer controversial.) It is now known that treatment of HIV infection and of selected opportunistic infections will substantially delay the onset of AIDS in people with HIV infection, including those who have no symptoms. At present, the medical benefits of getting tested outweigh the disadvantages.

Who Should Get Tested

The blood test for HIV infection can now be justified for virtually any person concerned about HIV infection. Most clinics that treat sexually transmitted diseases will routinely test for HIV. Some hospitals are also contemplating using the HIV antibody test as one of the routine tests for admission. The current recommendation is that in hospitals where the rate of AIDS is 1 per 1,000 admissions, any patient aged fifteen to fifty-four years old should be voluntarily tested. In a survey of hospitals, such voluntary testing revealed a large number of people who were unaware that they had HIV infection, including a sizable fraction who did not consider themselves at risk for HIV infection. Many advocate testing all pregnant women for the same reason, but also because another life has been placed at risk.

In addition, it is often recommended that the following people should get tested: those who have engaged in behaviors that run the risk of exposure to HIV; those who have medical conditions that suggest HIV infection; those who pose a risk of spreading HIV infection to others; those who want to participate in a research study or a clinical trial (see Chapter 9); and those who simply are concerned and want to take the test. The chapter next presents each of these reasons in more detail. At the end of this section is a summary of the behaviors that put people at risk for HIV infection. People with these behaviors should get the blood test for HIV infection.

Behaviors That Run the Risk of Exposure to HIV

Some of the following behaviors run a high risk of exposure to HIV, and the people who engage in the behaviors will find it in their best interests to get tested. Other behaviors run a lower risk, and the people who engage in them might want to get tested.

High-risk behaviors. The behaviors that run the highest risk of exposure to HIV are injecting drugs and having sex with gay or bisexual men. Hemophiliacs who received clotting factors before 1986 also have had a high risk of exposure to HIV. Having sex regularly with anyone who injects drugs, has gay sex with men, or has hemophilia also runs a high risk.

Among people with these behaviors, the frequency of HIV infection ranges from 10 percent to 70 percent, meaning that somewhere between 1 out of 10 and 7 out of 10 are infected. People with these levels of risk of infection should be tested.

The risks of HIV infection, and the recommendation for getting tested, differ in different parts of the country. In the Northeast, 20 percent to 70 percent of those who regularly use drugs intravenously are infected. In such areas as Denver, Tampa, and Los Angeles, only 5 percent or fewer of those who regularly use drugs intravenously are infected, a risk of 1 in 20. The risk of infection among men who have gay sex is more consistent throughout the country, ranging from 20 percent to 50 percent. For people with hemophilia, the risk of infection was constant in different parts of the country. The reason is that the clotting factors used for therapy were prepared and distributed throughout the United States from a central location. (It should be emphasized that these clotting factors are now considered safe because the blood is screened and because the factors are treated to eliminate HIV.)

In any case, those who will find it in their best interests to get tested are people who use drugs intravenously; or people who have sex with gay or bisexual men; or hemophiliacs who received clotting factor before 1986; or people who regularly have sex with any of the above or with people known to have HIV infection.

People who have high rates of infection also have different levels of risk. Among people who use injected drugs regularly, the risk is substantially higher than among those who use these drugs only occasionally. The same is true for sexual exposure: no one knows exactly what the risk is with a single sexual episode, although the number of people who have been infected after a single episode appears to be small. Those who have had sex with a lot of people have higher risks of infection than those who have had sex with fewer people. Those who have had sex more frequently with an infected partner have a higher risk of infection than those who have had sex less frequently. The risk is somewhat higher for women exposed to infected men than for men exposed to infected women. The risk of infection is also substantially higher in those who fail to practice "safer sex" or who have genital ulcers. And there may be differences according to the type of sexual practice: anal sex and sex that results in injury may be more likely to risk infection. As above, the probability of HIV infection depends on many interrelated variables. The probability by risk category may be 10 percent or 70 percent, but for the one who is infected, it is 100 percent. It is important for people to know this information so they can protect others and can obtain the best medical care.

Lower-risk behaviors.   Other behaviors, though they still risk exposure to HIV, have a substantially lower risk. These include having many sexual partners, having sex with prostitutes (prostitutes have had many sexual partners and are also likely to use drugs), and having had transfusions between 1978 and 1985.

The risk of exposure from these behaviors is relatively small, but it may be large enough to warrant testing, especially if a person is worried about the possibility of exposure.

Conditions That Are Associated with HIV Infection

Sometimes a physician requests the test because a person has certain conditions that suggest or are associated with HIV infection. Such sexually transmitted diseases as gonorrhea, chlamydia, and syphilis are associated with higher rates of HIV infection. Tuberculosis is also associated with higher rates of HIV infection. The Centers for Disease Control advocates HIV tests for anyone with a sexually transmitted disease or with tuberculosis.

Specific conditions that suggest HIV infection. Some conditions specifically suggest HIV infection, such as pneumocystis pneumonia, Kaposi's sarcoma, cryptococcccal meningitis, and toxoplasma encephalitis. These conditions are the so-called opportunistic infections that occur in a weakened immune system and, if accompanied by a positive HIV blood test, are diagnostic of AIDS. Other conditions suggest HIV infection more vaguely: unexplained weight loss, unexplained fever lasting for a month, or diarrhea lasting at least a month. Low blood counts—including low red blood cell counts (anemia), low white blood cell counts (neutropenia), and low platelets (thrombocytopenia)—also suggest HIV infection.

People with these latter conditions are also likely to have any number of other diagnoses. The physician of anyone with any of these conditions will recommend that the person be tested for HIV.

People Who Pose a Risk of HIV Infection to Others

Women who are already infected or who have a high risk of being infected, and who are contemplating pregnancy or who are already pregnant, should get tested. The reason is that the mother poses a risk to her unborn child. About one-third of all children born to an infected mother will become infected. The best way to avoid this is to prevent pregnancy through effective birth control. Once pregnant, it might be best to consider an abortion. Abortions are far more easily performed early in pregnancy, so pregnant women with HIV infection should consider this option early in pregnancy, and pregnant women with a risk of HIV infection should be tested as early as possible.

People who have been the source of blood exposure to a health care worker also pose a risk to others. That is, if a health care worker was exposed to blood, the person who was the source of the blood should get tested. Note that the major concern is exposure to blood, since no other body fluids are known to transmit the virus in job-related injuries.

The possibility that people might get HIV infection from health care workers is suggested by the case of the Florida dentist, Dr. Acer, who appeared to have infected five of his patients. As a result, the Centers for Disease Control has advocated policies regulating health care workers who perform "exposure-prone invasive procedures."

In addition, donors of blood, sperm, or organs pose a potential risk to those who receive the blood, sperm, or organs. These people will also be tested.

People Who Have Been Exposed to the Blood of Another Person

The most common way to be exposed to the blood of another person is through a "needlestick injury": a health care worker obtaining a blood sample is accidentally injured by the needle used to obtain a patient's blood. The risk of transmission of HIV, when the patient is infected, is not great: about one chance in 250. This is the risk when both patient and health care worker are injured and there is blood-to-blood contact. A few health care workers also got infected when blood splashed on their skin or mouths, but such cases are rare.

As noted, health care workers can theoretically transmit HIV infection to their patients during dental care or during surgery. The odds of health care workers transmitting HIV infection to their patients are substantially lower and may be nil. The Centers for Disease Control estimates the risk at 1 in 41,000 to 410,000 major surgical procedures if the surgeon is infected, and 1 in 100 million when all surgeons are considered.

Because the blood test is for antibodies, and antibodies will appear only after several weeks, blood must be tested for three to six months after the exposure before it is certain that infection did not take place. During this interval, those who have been exposed must avoid behaviors that transmit the virus, and in particular must practice safer sex.

Participants in Research Studies and Clinical Trials

Some people who participate in research studies of HIV infection or clinical trials of treatments for HIV will be required to take the test as part of the study or trial, unless the test has already been done elsewhere.

To Summarize: People Who Should Get Tested

Those engaging in high-risk behaviors

- Injecting illegal drugs
- Having sex with gay or bisexual men
- Having hemophilia with clotting factors administered before 1986
- Being the regular sex partner of drug users, of gay or bisexual men, of hemophiliacs, or of people who have HIV infection

Those who engage in lower-risk behaviors
- Receiving blood transfusions between 1978 and 1985
- Having multiple sex partners

Those who have conditions associated with HIV infection
- Tuberculosis
- Sexually transmitted diseases, such as gonorrhea, syphilis, chlamydia

Those who have conditions suggesting HIV infection
- Opportunistic infections that may accompany a diagnosis of AIDS, including pneumocystis pneumonia, Kaposi's sarcoma, cryptococcal meningitis, toxoplasma encephalitis
- Conditions that sometimes indicate HIV infection and are otherwise unexplained, such as weight loss, diarrhea for at least a month, or fever for at least a month
- Low blood counts for which HIV infection is one of the many potential causes

People who may pose a risk to others
- Women contemplating pregnancy, but primarily those with a higher risk of being infected, and those in cities or hospitals with a high incidence of HIV infection
- Pregnant women, especially those with a higher risk of being infected, and those in cities or hospitals with a high incidence of HIV infection
- People who have been the source of blood exposure to others
- Donors of blood, sperm, or organs

Those who have been exposed to another person's blood

Participants in research studies

Any person who desires the test

Informed Consent for the Tests

Regardless of the circumstances of testing, whether the person asked for the test or the physician did, the person being tested is usually required to give informed consent. Informed consent means that the person must understand the limitations, benefits, and risks of the test, and must agree to have the test. If the person cannot understand or agree to sign the consent form, the decision about testing should be made by a representative of that person. Informed consent is recommended by the Centers for Disease Control and most scholarly medical societies; it is required by law in forty-one states. The reason for this unusual requirement for a blood test is that the consequences of a positive test may be so harsh.

Exceptions are few: Persons donating blood, sperm, corneas, organs, or other tissue or body fluids must be tested. In these cases, the test is done to protect the recipient, and informed consent is not required. In extreme conditions when someone has been the source of exposure to a health care worker or has raped someone, and refuses to take the test, the test can be obtained without consent in some states or through a court order in others. Members of the military and the foreign service are also tested without consent.

The method of obtaining informed consent is highly variable in different places. Most places will have a standard consent form, along with a trained professional either to explain the test or to answer questions.

The information that is often included in the informed consent process includes the following: what positive, negative, and indeterminant test results mean; how accurate the test results are; how the person's confidentiality is maintained; and what resources are available for people who test positive. All this information is provided elsewhere in this chapter or in "Resources," which precedes this chapter.

In addition to being presented with this information, the person to be tested is usually offered the opportunity to ask questions, and the signed consent will often include a statement such as, "All questions regarding the test have been answered to my satisfaction."

The following is a list of questions that are often not included in informed consent forms. If they are not, the person being tested may want to ask them:

Who will pay for the test, and how much does it cost?

Will results be communicated to family members, partners, public health officials, insurance companies, and so forth?

Are test results confidential or anonymous? (See below.)

Where can an anonymous test be obtained?

How will the results be provided: in person? by telephone? by mail?

In the event of a positive test, what services are provided in terms of counseling, psychological support, and health care?

Testing carries an inherent responsibility for the medical and psychological care of people who test positive. The person tested should know in advance what resources will be provided for this type of care and support.

Confidentiality

Most people are concerned whether the results of an HIV test are confidential. Tests can be done either anonymously or confidentially. In anonymous testing, the person tested cannot be identified in any way. In confidential testing, the person tested can be identified, but the identification is considered confidential medical information.

Anonymous or Confidential Testing

Anonymous testing means there is no possibility of connecting a result, positive or negative, with an individual person by name, address, social security number, or hospital number, or by any other means. The name of the person being tested is never taken. The person is simply given a number, and the results are provided for this specific number without being linked to the person in any way that permits identification. Anonymous testing essentially guarantees that only the person tested will know the results. There are two drawbacks: First, in many areas, anonymous testing is not available. Second, important medical decisions cannot be made on the basis of anonymous tests, so tests must often be repeated in order to get necessary documentation.

Confidential testing uses a name, social security number, or other mechanism to identify a specific individual. The results of virtually all laboratory tests done in medicine are confidential, although many health care facilities have special provisions for HIV blood tests because of the sensitivity of the results. Test results called confidential are considered privileged medical information that is an important part of the medical record; such results are available to nonmedical people only by subpoena.

Confidentiality of Medical Records

Once a person consults a physician about a positive HIV blood test, the results of that test become part of the person's medical record. Simply excluding the result of HIV blood tests from a medical record is not possible: the results are too important a part of the medical record. But these results, if made public, may conceivably affect a person's job, housing, insurance status, personal relationships, and social standing. The obvious questions are, Who has access to this information? And how is it guarded? The answers to these questions differ for different institutions, different states, and sometimes even for different physicians.

In general, medical records can be reviewed by certain medical personnel. Various authorities also have the legal right to review medical records: third party payers (such as insurance companies), professional review groups, and the like. Although this sounds alarming to someone worried about breach of confidentiality, the actual number of cases in which confidentiality has been breached is nil. The reason is that the people who have access to medical records are well aware that they have ethical as well as legal responsibilities to prevent unnecessary or unwarranted disclosure.

Similar rules apply to health departments that maintain such information. All people with AIDS are reported to health authorities by law. Some states require reporting everyone with a positive blood test. To our knowledge, reporting to state or federal health authorities has never once been the source of inappropriate disclosure of the information (see also Chapter 10).

Where to Get Tested

The blood test for HIV is widely available. Virtually all hospitals, most physicians' offices, and many public clinics run by most state, county, or city health departments provide testing for HIV. These places vary in matters of price, time of results, resources available for counseling, medical care, and convenience. Some testing sites offer anonymous testing, some only confidential testing. Public clinics usually offer the test free, but they may not have hours of operation or locations that are especially convenient. Private testing centers often charge $30 to $80 for the test and often lack resources for counseling, psychological support, and follow-up care.

The test itself requires a teaspoon of blood obtained like any other blood sample. The time required in the laboratory actually to run the test is brief, usually a day or two. But the time from blood sampling until the results are available may vary substantially, often taking one or two weeks. The reasons for the delay may be that the blood needs to be sent to a distant laboratory for testing, that a preliminary ELISA test at one site needs to be verified by a Western blot test at another site, or that a laboratory does the test only on certain days.

Sites offering the test will also vary considerably in the kinds and quality of educational counseling and psychological support they offer.

The test should be done only in a setting that offers appropriate counseling before the test. The counseling should answer all questions about informed consent; this may involve a two-minute discussion in some places and a thirty-minute video in others, but the opportunity to ask questions should not be omitted. More importantly, the test should preferably be done in a setting that offers supportive care and counseling for people who have positive tests.

What the Test Results Mean

To repeat, the HIV test is designed to determine the presence of HIV infection—that is, it is designed to detect antibodies to the virus. Antibodies to the virus are present in virtually all people who are infected and absent in people who are not infected. Test results are usually either positive, meaning the antibodies are present, or negative, meaning they are absent. Occasionally test results are indeterminant, meaning that the results were neither clearly positive nor clearly negative. In this case, the test should be retaken.

Inaccurate or false test results are extremely rare. Nevertheless, as discussed above, the test is not always positive in people who are infected and not always negative in those who are not infected.

Negative Test Results

A negative result of the test generally means the virus is not present. In a few rare cases, as noted above, the negative result can be false. This can happen if the test is taken during the two- to three-month period (or occasionally longer) between the time of infection and the time when antibodies develop. Health care workers can use this early negative result if they have had an occupational exposure and want to apply for workers' compensation. A test that is negative several days after a needlestick injury and that converts to positive in six to twelve weeks is irrefutable proof of the source of infection. For the person who is concerned about false negative results, the usual recommendation is to repeat the blood test after three months.

Indeterminant Test Results

The virus is either present or not present—there is no middle ground. But like all tests in medicine, the test for antibodies to HIV does not always give decisive positive or negative results. Indeterminant test results are a gray zone, and they are an obvious source of anguish for the person tested. They could mean that the person's body is only now manufacturing antibodies to the virus. Or they could mean that the body is manufacturing antibodies to some miscellaneous protein that is unrelated to HIV.

People with indeterminant results are usually told to be tested again in three months. If the person with an indeterminant result has been exposed to the virus recently, or has participated in high-risk behavior, the results of the second test may be positive. If the person has not participated in high-risk behavior, the results of the second test are almost always indeterminant again. The reason for this is unknown. Almost invariably, however, these people do not have HIV infection.

As noted above, alternative tests may be used to detect the virus instead of antibodies to the virus. These tests, however, are not as well standardized as the antibody tests, they are far more expensive, and they are not available in most laboratories.

The usual recommendation is to repeat the test for antibodies in three months. While all this gets sorted out, the person being tested is advised to take precautions to prevent transmission, just as if the test were positive.

Positive Test Results

A positive test means that antibodies to HIV are present. If the antibodies are present, the virus is also present. The person with positive results can transmit the virus to others and needs regular medical attention.

A positive test for antibodies to HIV is not a test for AIDS; a diagnosis of AIDS requires other tests. A positive test also does not indicate the amount of time any one person might take between having a positive test and getting AIDS.

Over 99 percent of the people with positive tests know how they became infected; for a small portion of people, the source of the infection is unknown. Because false-positive tests occur occasionally (rarely), the person with a positive test who has no reason for it may request that the test be repeated. In fact, because HIV results are so important, some authorities recommend that anyone with positive results should repeat the test.

People with a positive test will understandably be upset, will need psychological counseling, will need medical care, may need ongoing psychological support, and will certainly need the support and friendship of the people they love. All this, of course, is what this book has been about.

Glossary

ACTG: ACTG stands for AIDS clinical trial groups (also called ACTU, with "units" instead of "groups"). ACTGs are a consortium of medical centers throughout the United States that conduct clinical trials of drugs for treating people with HIV infection. Specifically, the drugs are for treating HIV itself, for treating opportunistic infections or tumors, and for stimulating the immune system. ACTGs are funded federally through the National Institutes of Health. Taken together, the ACTGs are the largest trials of drugs for treating HIV infection in the world: they have the largest budgets, the largest number of investigators, and the largest number of participants.

AIDS: AIDS stands for acquired immune deficiency syndrome. AIDS is the late stage of an infection caused by the human immunodeficiency virus, or HIV. The virus infects the CD4 cell (also called a T4 cell, a T4 lymphocyte, and a T-helper cell), which is critical to immune defenses. As the numbers of these cells decrease, the immune system weakens until it becomes susceptible to what are called *opportunistic infections* and *opportunistic tumors.* These infections and tumors are called opportunistic because the microbes that cause them are opportunists, taking advantage of a weakened immune system. A person with HIV infection has AIDS if he or she has a CD4 cell count below 200 or one or more of certain specific opportunistic infections or tumors, *called AIDS-defining diagnoses,* that go along with a severely weakened immune system. The list of AIDS-defining diagnoses was drawn up by the Centers for Disease Control (CDC) in 1986 and has been modified twice, once in 1987 and again in 1993. The CDC's latest definition of AIDS includes all the old criteria and adds three new diseases and a CD4 count of less than 200. AIDS is also known as late symptomatic HIV infection.

AIDS-advocacy organizations: See *Community-based organizations,* below.

313

AIDS-defining diagnosis: A person with an AIDS-defining diagnosis has HIV infection plus a CD4 cell count below 200, or an immune system weakened enough to allow one of several opportunistic infections or tumors to occur. As a result, the person is now said to have AIDS. The opportunistic infections and tumors that make up the AIDS-defining diagnoses, according to the Centers for Disease Control, include pneumocystis pneumonia, Kaposi's sarcoma, toxoplasma, encephalitis, cryptococcal meningitis, candidal esophagitis, infection with cytomegalovirus throughout the body, and *Mycobacterium avium* infections throughout the body. These are not the only AIDS-defining diagnoses; they are simply the most common.

AIDS dementia complex: See *HIV-associated dementia,* below.

AIDS-related complex: See *ARC,* below.

Amitriptyline: Amitriptyline hydrochloride (or, e.g., Elavil) is one of a group of drugs called *tricyclic antidepressants* that are grouped together because of their chemical similarities. Other tricyclic antidepressants include amoxapine (or Asendin), desipramine hydrochloride (or Pertofrane or Norpramin), doxepin hydrochloride (or Adapin or Sinequan), imipramine hydrochloride (or Tofranil), and nortriptyline hydrochloride (or Aventyl Hydrochloride or Pamelor). Tricyclic antidepressants are used to treat depression and the peripheral neuropathy that causes painful feet. In many cases, the dose is arbitrary: many people start on a low dose and have the dose increased as necessary. Side effects are common, but usually not severe enough to stop treatment. The main side effects are drowsiness, weakness, and fatigue; dry mouth; constipation; and low blood pressure and dizziness. These side effects are all dose-related, meaning the higher the dose, the more severe the side effect. Because the drugs cause drowsiness, they are often given before bedtime.

Amphotericin B: The antibiotic amphotericin B is the standard treatment for many infections caused by fungi, including most of the fungi that affect people with HIV infection: *Candida, Cryptococcus, Histoplasma, Coccidioides,* and *Aspergillus.* Amphotericin B, which is given only by vein, is highly effective. Unfortunately, it is also one of the most toxic antibiotics known. The most important side effects include kidney damage, anemia (see below), disturbances in the balance of electrolytes, nausea and vomiting, fever and chills, and phlebitis or inflammation of the vein into which the drug is injected. Many of these side effects can be reduced in severity or eliminated by stopping the drug, by continuing the drug at a lower dose, or by giving other medications at the same time that will counteract the side effects. Because of amphotericin B's toxicity, other drugs, like ketoconazole, itraconazole, and fluconazole, are given when they are considered to be as effective or nearly as effective.

Anemia: Anemia means that the number of red cells in the blood is reduced. Red blood cells are responsible for delivering oxygen to all parts of the body. When the reduction is severe, the result is fatigue. Anemia can be caused by HIV infection itself, by an opportunistic infection, or by several of the drugs commonly taken by people with AIDS. Drugs often responsible include trimethoprim-sulfamethoxazole, other sulfa drugs, pentamidine, amphotericin B, and AZT. When the anemia is severe, it can be corrected with transfusions or a drug called erythropoietin (EPO). When drugs are responsible, the drugs can be reduced in dose or discontinued.

Antiretroviral: HIV is a retrovirus, and drugs that inhibit it are antiretroviral drugs.

Antibiotics: Antibiotics are drugs made from natural substances (as opposed to drugs made artificially) that inhibit the growth of microbes. Antibiotics may be effective against any of the classes of microbes—including bacteria, fungi, parasites, and viruses—that cause infections. Common examples of antibiotics frequently used in people with HIV infection include trimethoprim-sulfamethoxazole, other drugs containing sulfas, pentamidine, ketoconazole, amphotericin B, pyrimethamine, ganciclovir, acyclovir, penicillin, erythromycin, nystatin, clotrimazole, and AZT.

Antibody: Antibodies are proteins and are the part of the complex immune system that attacks any substance—protein or microbe—that is foreign to the body. Certain cells called *B lymphocytes* recognize these substances as foreign and manufacture antibodies that inactivate or eliminate the foreign substance. The foreign substance that the antibodies attack is called an *antigen* (see below). For most antigens, the B lymphocytes take one or two weeks to produce antibodies; for HIV, however, the time required may be months.

Antigen: Antigens are foreign material, including microbes, that the immune system responds to by manufacturing antibodies.

Aphthous ulcer: Aphthous ulcers are ulcers or sores in the mouth and occasionally in the esophagus. They are often extremely painful, they have no clear cause, and they are often cleared up by corticosteroids (see below) or other medications.

ARC: ARC stands for AIDS-related complex. ARC is a collection of conditions associated with HIV infection that do not meet the diagnostic definition of AIDS. There is no official definition of ARC. See *Early symptomatic HIV infection,* below.

Asymptomatic: Asymptomatic means the absence of symptoms. The asymptomatic person feels healthy.

B-lymphocytes: B lymphocytes are the white blood cells—called lymphocytes—responsible for producing antibodies. B lymphocytes are distinct from T lymphocytes (including CD4 cells, also called T4 cells), which are also part of the immune system, but which work against a different group of microbes using different mechanisms.

Baclofen: Baclofen is a drug used to control muscle spasms. The most common side effect is drowsiness and, in large doses, severe sedation, lack of coordination, and lowered functioning of the heart and lungs.

Barbiturates: Barbiturates are drugs commonly used to treat insomnia, anxiety, and seizures. Examples of barbiturates are amobarbital (or Amytal), pentobarbital (or Nembutal), phenobarbital, and secobarbital. All barbiturates affect the central nervous system: low doses cause mild sedation, and high doses can lead to deep coma. When barbiturates are used for sedation, they remain effective for only about two weeks. As a result, alternative drugs are generally preferred to treat insomnia. Barbiturates' most important role may be for controlling anxiety.

The major side effects are symptoms of central nervous system depression, including drowsiness, depression, lethargy, and hangovers. People who take barbiturates should be aware that the drug may impair their ability to perform hazardous activities. Prolonged use of high doses of the drug can cause physical dependence, psychological dependence, and tolerance (that is, higher doses of the drug are required to produce a similar effect). Discontinuing barbiturates can cause withdrawal symptoms that are similar to the withdrawal symptoms an alcoholic has when abruptly discontinuing alcohol. Other side effects include stomach pain, allergic reactions, and fever.

Benzodiazepines: Benzodiazepines are a class of drugs commonly used to treat anxiety, insomnia, seizures, and painful muscles. Examples of benzodiazepines include alprazolam (or Xanax), diazepam, flurazepam hydrochloride (or Dalmane), lorazepam (or Ativan), midazolam maleate, oxazepam (or Serax), prazepam (or Centrax), temazepam (or Restoril), and triazolam (or Halcion). In general, all benzodiazepines act in similar ways and seem to be equally effective.

Most physicians prefer benzodiazepines for treating anxiety and tension. Compared to barbiturates and meprobamate, and when given at the doses that relieve anxiety, they are less addictive and produce less sedation. The major side effects are drowsiness, loss of coordination, confusion, dizziness, and fainting. People taking benzodiazepines should be aware that the drug may impair their ability to perform activities that require mental alertness and physical coordination. Benzodiazepines can also cause physical dependence and symptoms of severe withdrawal if the drug is stopped suddenly after being used regularly for a long time.

Biopsy: Biopsy is a procedure for obtaining a piece of tissue for examination under the microscope. The microscopic changes in tissue often provide a diagnosis, and stains and cultures for microbes will often reveal the infecting organism. The biopsy may be obtained using lidocaine to deaden the skin to avoid pain. The biopsy may be performed on an outpatient basis when the area to be biopsied is near the surface or when it is in the lungs or gastrointestinal tract and can be reached through an endoscope, an instrument passed through the mouth or anus. Alternatively, the biopsy of organs deep within the body may require an operating room procedure.

Bleach: Chlorine bleach is highly effective in killing HIV within minutes. It is available at most grocery stores and is commonly recommended for killing any virus or other microbe that may be in such body fluids as blood, saliva, and stool. Bleach is usually diluted 1:10, or one part of bleach in ten parts of water. This dilution can be applied to surfaces or in the washing machine for clothes.

Blood count: Blood is composed of red blood cells (erythrocytes) which carry oxygen to all parts of the body, white blood cells (leukocytes) which help make up the immune system, and platelets (or thrombocytes) which are required for blood clotting. All three kinds of cells can be counted under a microscope. A low red blood cell count is called *anemia* (see above); a low white blood cell count is called *leukopenia* (see below), and a low platelet count is called *thrombocytopenia* (see below). People with HIV infection commonly have low red counts, low white counts, and low platelet counts. A blood count is a routine procedure for clinical laboratories; it is a relatively simple, inexpensive, and standard test to evaluate people with HIV infection.

Bone marrow: Bone marrow is the tissue in the central portion of many bones where blood is manufactured. Bone marrow can be withdrawn (by placing a needle in the hip bone) and analyzed to detect abnormalities in the production of red blood cells, white blood cells, or platelets.

Buyers' clubs: Buyers' clubs are groups, or even individuals, that make drugs available to people with HIV infection. The drugs may be unlicensed in the United States; they may be considered experimental and may be available only by participating in a clinical trial; or they may be licensed drugs available in pharmacies. Some drugs are purchased in foreign countries or through other quasilegal mechanisms; some of these are essentially the same as those purchased in the United States, but at substantially reduced prices. Other drugs are made at home without the usual manufacturing safeguards, and may be useless or dangerous.

Candidiasis: Candidiasis is an infection caused by the fungus *Candida albicans.* People with HIV infection commonly have candidiasis in the mouth (thrush), in the esophagus (candidal esophagitis), or in the vagina (vaginal candidiasis). The diagnosis can be confirmed by microscopic examination of the patches. Candidiasis is common in people who do not have HIV infection. In people who do have HIV infection, candidiasis is especially common, sometimes severe, and likely to recur. Treatment is with topical drugs (drugs placed in contact with the infection, such as nystatin or clotrimazole) or pills such as ketoconazole, fluconazole, or itraconazole.

CD4 cells: The blood contains several kinds of white cells, each of which plays a specific role in the immune system. CD4 cells (other names are T4 cells and T-helper cells) are the cells that HIV selectively infects. The number of CD4 cells frequently indicates the stage of HIV infection. Healthy people without HIV infection usually have around 1,000 CD4 cells in every milliliter of blood; counts of 400–700 are considered abnormally low, but not alarming. People with AIDS usually have counts of less than 200. In fact, the newest definition of AIDS applies to anyone with a CD4 cell count less than 200. This new definition includes many who feel well and have no opportunistic infections. Nevertheless, counts of less than 200 suggest severe weakening of the immune system. The CD4 count is a relatively expensive test (usually $50–$150), but it is an important way of monitoring the state of the immune system. In any one person, however, the count varies considerably: the same laboratory performing the test on the same specimen can show counts that vary by as much as 20–40 percent. This means that if the true count is 500, the lab may report any value between 300 and 700. The CD4 count is also influenced by a variety of other medical conditions independent of HIV infection. As a result, although the CD4 count is frequently used to assess progressive disease, changes in the count are sometimes difficult to interpret, and it is advisable not to attach too much credibility to a single test. The test should be repeated if there are big changes that are not readily explained.

Centers for Disease Control (CDC): The Centers for Disease Control is a federally funded institution located in Atlanta, Georgia. It has three responsibilities: to serve as an epidemiologic and public health resource for state and local health departments; to investigate epidemics; and to keep track of contagious diseases and other diseases important to public health. The CDC has about 4,000 employees, including 800 physicians and Ph.D.'s. In the past, the CDC has been responsible for much of what we know about Lyme disease, tuberculosis, Legionnaires' disease, and toxic shock syndrome. More to the point, the CDC provided much of the early epidemiologic data that identified the symptoms of AIDS, the kinds of behavior that risked AIDS, and how AIDS was transmitted—in fact, the CDC was responsible for the name *AIDS*. At present, the CDC is the storehouse for all reported cases of AIDS in the United States. It provides guidelines for disease prevention and gives advice on safety for health care providers. It is responsible for funding state and local agencies that test for HIV, counsel, and collect data.

Chloral hydrate: Chloral hydrate is a sedative used to treat insomnia. It is usually taken fifteen to thirteen minutes before bedtime. Using chloral hydrate regularly for more than two weeks often reduces its effectiveness. Major side effects include stomach irritation, residual sedation, or a hangover. Chloral hydrate should be used with great caution in people who are depressed, who may commit suicide, or who have a history of drug abuse.

Clostridium difficile: People who take antibiotics often develop diarrhea as a side effect. A relatively common and particularly severe cause of this diarrhea is a microbe called *Clostridium difficile*. Almost any antibiotic can cause this complication, but the most frequent causes are ampicillin, amoxicillin, clindamycin, and a group of drugs called cephalosporins that includes cefixime (or Suprex), cefuroxime, cephalexin (or Keflex), and cefaclor (or Ceclor). People who have diarrhea while taking these or any other antibiotics should stop taking the antibiotics and call their physicians. A test of stool will determine if *Clostridium difficile* is the cause. If it is, it can be treated with metronidazole or vancomycin hydrochloride. Vancomycin is preferred for serious cases of diarrhea, but it costs about $200 to $300. Metronidazole is less expensive—$10 to $20—and equally effective unless the person has severe colitis.

CMV: CMV, which is short for cytomegalovirus, is a virus commonly found in people without HIV infection. Usually the immune system holds CMV in check, and it remains dormant in the body without causing any serious disease. With a severely weakened immune system, however, CMV may cause serious infection. The site of the infection can be in the eye, lung, liver, gastrointestinal tract, bone marrow, brain, or widespread in many of these areas. The virus can be detected by cultures of blood, cultures of urine, or biopsies of any of the organs that are affected. About 15 to 20 percent of people with AIDS develop CMV retinitis, which is a CMV infection of the eye. This is a serious infection because it will progress and cause loss of vision, sometimes in both eyes. Treatment of CMV retinitis and other forms of CMV infection is with ganciclovir or foscarnet, drugs that are given by vein.

Co-factor: A co-factor is anything—microbes, proteins, hormones, genes—which makes a disease progress more rapidly. With HIV infection, co-factors are only suspected but may include other viruses (like cytomegalovirus), age, and genetic resistance or predisposition.

Colon: The gastrointestinal tract—which starts at the mouth and ends at the rectum—includes the esophagus, stomach, small intestine, colon, and rectum. The colon and the small intestine are commonly the sites of infections that cause diarrhea. To diagnose problems in the colon, common procedures are colonoscopy and sigmoidoscopy. These procedures permit visualization and biopsy of the colon by passing a tube through the rectum. Colonoscopy is expensive ($1,200 to $1,800) and is usually done by a specialist called a gastroenterologist.

Combination treatment: Combination treatment means taking two or more drugs against HIV. The goals of combination treatment are (1) to reduce side effects by using lower than standard doses of each drug; (2) to "gang up" on HIV with a double whammy attack; and (3) to prevent resistance, since a microbe can develop resistance most easily to one drug at a time. The down side to combination treatment is that it may be more toxic, and microbes may develop resistance to both drugs and leave fewer options for treatment.

Community-based organizations (CBOs): Community-based organizations are also called AIDS-advocacy organizations and AIDS service organizations (ASOs). They are organizations and agencies that provide services to people with HIV infection, as well as education and prevention programs for the whole community. The leaders of community-based organizations are lay people, ordinary people who do not come from the government or from organized medicine—although many community-based organizations have physicians as advisers, and most receive public funds.

Examples of community-based organizations dealing with other diseases are the American Lung Association, the American Heart Association, and the American Cancer Society. There is no similar nationwide organization for people with HIV infection or AIDS. Nevertheless, most cities have one or sometimes several such organizations: examples include Shanti in San Francisco, the Gay Men's Health Clinic in New York City, and HERO in Baltimore. The types of services offered vary but may include counseling, crisis support, financial assistance case management, a buddy system, transportation, meals, housing, support groups, legal aid, social services, education, psychological support, hotlines, buyers' clubs, and medical services (see "Resources," which follows Chapter 12). Most of these organizations have a paid professional staff but rely heavily on volunteers. Funding usually comes from state governments, corporations, foundations, and local fundraising events.

Computerized tomography scan (CAT scan): CAT scans are a particular kind of x-ray that provide a three-dimensional view of the body. Conventional x-ray tests provide a two-dimensional view of the body; CAT scans use computers to stack a series of two-dimensional x-rays together to form a three-dimensional image of the body. CAT scans can be done of the entire body or of parts of it. The person receiving a CAT scan often receives an injection of what is called contrast material—material that shows up under x-rays. Some people have allergic reactions to contrast materials and should not receive them again. The person receiving the CAT scan is next put into a chamber with a scanner that circulates around the body, producing three-dimensional images in parallel sections of about an inch or less. CAT scans, first developed in the 1970s, are an excellent method for detecting tumors, infections, or other changes in the anatomy of the brain, chest, abdomen, or other parts of the body. They are also expensive, usually costing around $300 to $800.

Constitutional symptoms: Symptoms caused by the impact of an illness on the entire body or constitution are frequently referred to as constitutional symptoms. Included are fatigue, achiness, weight loss, fever, and night sweats. Constitutional symptoms are present in many types of infectious diseases, tumors, and other medical conditions ranging from the serious to the trivial. For people with HIV infection, constitutional symptoms may be a result of HIV infection itself or the result of such opportunistic illnesses as pneumocystis pneumonia, tuberculosis, or widespread CMV infection.

Contagious: A disease that is *contagious* can be passed from one person to another. A disease that is *infectious* is caused by a microbe. All diseases that are contagious are also infectious; but some diseases, like toxic shock syndrome, are infectious and not contagious. HIV is both infectious and contagious, but is contagious only with specific types of contact.

Corticosteroids (also known as steroids, glucocorticosteroids, prednisone, and cortisone): Corticosteroids are drugs used to reduce the immune response. Numerous preparations are available that can be taken intravenously, by mouth, or in an ointment applied to the skin. Using high doses of corticosteroids for a long time can be dangerous: they reduce the immune system's defenses against certain infections. Corticosteroids are sometimes considered especially dangerous for people with HIV infection, whose immune defenses are already weakened. Nevertheless, many of the complications of HIV infection appear to result from an overly abundant but misdirected immune response. As a result, these complications of HIV infection respond well to corticosteroids, though the drug should be taken at the lowest doses for the shortest period.

Cryptococcis: Cryptococcis is an infection caused by the fungus *Cryptococcus neoformans*. This fungus can cause infection in otherwise healthy people. In people with HIV infection, however, it is especially severe, frequently causing meningitis. Common symptoms include headaches, fevers, vision problems, and seizures. The diagnosis is usually made by analyzing cerebrospinal fluid obtained with a *spinal tap* (see below). The disease is treated with amphotericin B given by vein or fluconazole given by mouth; when treatment is stopped, the disease tends to recur so that long-term treatment is generally necessary.

Cryptosporidiosis: Cryptosporidia are parasites that infect the intestine and cause diarrhea. This infection, called cryptosporidiosis, can occur in otherwise healthy persons, but the diarrhea generally does not last long and is not severe. Cryptosporidiosis in people with HIV infection often causes devastating diarrhea that persists for months. People with cryptosporidiosis may lose large amounts of fluid and nutrients and, consequently, become severely malnourished. The diagnosis is usually established by simply examining the stool under a microscope to detect the parasite. There is no universally accepted form of treatment except to replace the lost fluids and nutrients.

Culture: A culture, in medical terms, is a medium in which microbes can grow. HIV is grown in cultures containing lymphocytes. If a sample of a person's blood is put into such a culture, and HIV grows, the person is infected with HIV. Other blood tests for HIV are *polymerase chain reaction* (see below) or the *P24 antigen test* (see below). The usual blood test for HIV detects antibodies to the virus instead of the virus itself. The antibody test is usually preferred because it is less expensive, better standardized, and more readily available.

Cytomegalovirus: See *CMV,* above.

Dantrolene (or *Dantrium*): Dantrolene is one of several muscle relaxants. The most common side effect is muscle weakness that usually disappears after taking the drug for several days. Other side effects include *hepatitis* (see below), diarrhea, gastric intolerance, depression, insomnia, and frequent urination.

Dementia: See *HIV-associated dementia,* below.

Dextroamphetamine sulfate (or *Dexedrine*): Dextroamphetamine sulfate, along with methylphenidate hydrochloride (or Ritalin Hydrochloride), stimulates the brain. It is usually given to people with HIV infection with *HIV-associated dementia* (see below) to counter the symptoms of apathy and social withdrawal. The most common side effects are nervousness and insomnia. Both side effects can usually be controlled by decreasing the dose and by avoiding taking the drug late in the day.

Dormant: See *Latency,* below.

Dysphagia: Dysphagia means difficulty with swallowing. The most common cause of dysphagia is an infection by *Candida albicans,* a fungus that can be easily treated (see *Candidiasis,* above). Less frequent causes are infections with herpes or CMV. In some people dysphagia has no readily apparent cause. The usual method of finding the cause of dysphagia is endoscopy, a procedure in which a tube is placed in the esophagus to visualize and biopsy the lesions. X-ray examinations are another means of viewing the esophagus. In many cases, neither of these tests is done, and the person is presumed to have a *Candida* infection if he or she also has *thrush* (see below) and if swallowing is painful.

Early symptomatic HIV infection: Early symptomatic HIV infection, also called AIDS-related complex, or ARC, is the stage of HIV infection at which the first signs of a weakened immune system occur. The most common infections at this stage are thrush, oral hairy leukoplakia, shingles, vaginitis, idiopathic thrombocytopenic purpura, and various constitutional symptoms which include chronic fever, weight loss, and chronic diarrhea. All these infections and symptoms occur in people without HIV infection, but in people with HIV infection, the infections tend to be chronic, that is, they persist for weeks or months. People in this early stage usually have CD4 cells counts below 300, occasionally even below 50.

ELISA test: The ELISA (pronounced eelissa) is a blood test done to detect antibodies to certain microbes, among which is HIV. The ELISA is the first of two standard tests done together to detect antibodies to HIV. The test is extremely sensitive but not very specific. Sensitivity means that the test is able to detect HIV infection; specificity means that the test specifically detects a particular infection and no other. In other words, with ELISA, people who have HIV infection will rarely have a falsely negative test, but people who do not have HIV infection will commonly have a falsely positive test. As a result, the ELISA is used as a screening test, and those who are positive have a second test on the same blood sample called a *Western blot.*

The Western blot test, combined with an ELISA, is over 99 percent accurate in both sensitivity and specificity. The combination of tests is generally offered free of charge from most health departments and at a cost of $50 to $150 from commercial laboratories. The test offered may be *anonymous,* meaning that the person receiving the test cannot be identified, or it is *confidential,* meaning that privacy is honored but a record is kept identifying a specific person with the test result. The ELISA is easily performed, but the Western blot is more complicated and often done only by reference laboratories or on certain days of the week. For this reason, the results may not be available for several days or even weeks. The test results are usually either positive or negative, but occasionally people have Western blots that can not be clearly interpreted and the test results are considered indeterminant. The usual recommendation for people with indeterminant results is to have the test repeated in two or three months. People at a low risk for HIV and with indeterminant results almost never have HIV infection, and the cause of the indeterminant results is not known.

Encephalitis: Encephalitis is an infection of the brain. (Meningitis, by contrast, is an infection of the meninges, the membrane surrounding the brain and spinal cord—see *Meningitis,* below.) Encephalitis commonly causes headaches, fever seizures, and neurologic problems. The diagnosis is frequently made on the basis of the person's symptoms, combined with procedures to examine the brain such as *computerized tomography scan (CAT scan)* (see above); *magnetic resonance imaging (MRI)* (see below); or electroencephalogram (EEG). Diagnosis can also be made by analyzing the cerebrospinal fluid obtained by a *spinal tap* (see below). In people with HIV infection, the usual causes of encephalitis are infection with HIV itself or such opportunistic illnesses as toxoplasmosis or lymphoma.

Endoscopy: Endoscopy is a diagnostic procedure in which an instrument is passed through the mouth or rectum to examine an internal organ or to obtain a *biopsy* (see above). In people with HIV infection, the most common types of endoscopy are bronchoscopy to examine the lungs and endoscopies to examine the digestive system. Upper endoscopy of the intestine involves passing an endoscope through the mouth to examine the esophagus, stomach, or upper small intestine. Lower endoscopy of the intestine involves passing an endoscope through the rectum to examine the large intestine or colon. Endoscopes are flexible and can turn corners. Endoscopy requires the expertise of a specialist, can be done on an outpatient basis, and usually costs $1,200 to $1,800, except in New York City, where everything costs more.

Enteritis: Enteritis is an inflammation of the small intestine; the most common symptom is diarrhea. In people with HIV infection, the microbes that usually cause enteritis are cryptosporidia, microsporidia, *Mycobacterium avium,* and CMV. These microbes can be detected by examining stools under a microscope or with a biopsy of the small intestine done with an endoscope (see above, under *Endoscopy*), a tube that is placed through the mouth and into the small intestine.

Epidemic: An epidemic is a disease that occurs in many more people than would be expected during a given time. *Epidemiology* is the study of the factors that determine the frequency and distribution of diseases.

Fluconazole (or *Diflucan*): Fluconazole is used to treat fungal infections, primarily those caused by *Candida albicans* (thrush or candidal esophagitis) and *Cryptococcus neoformans* (cryptococcal meningitis). Fluconazole can be taken by mouth or by vein. Side effects are unusual; occasional problems are nausea, rash, or hepatitis.

Foscarnet: Foscarnet is a drug used to treat CMV infection, especially CMV retinitis. It is given only by vein. The most important side effects are kidney failure and changes in blood electrolytes that may cause tingling, jitteriness, or seizures.

Ganciclovir: Ganciclovir is used to treat infections caused by cytomegalovirus and occasionally for infections caused by herpes simplex and other viruses. It is given only intravenously. The most important side effect is a low blood count, especially neutropenia, which predisposes the person to bacterial infections (see *Blood count,* above, and neutropenia, below, under *Leukopenia*). If neutropenia is severe enough, the dose of the drug should be reduced, or the drug should be temporarily stopped.

HAD: See *HIV-associated dementia,* below.

Hemophilia: A person with hemophilia lacks a protein that helps the blood to clot. Hemophiliacs bleed easily, even with a trivial cut; many have severe hemorrhaging into the joints and eventually get joint disease. Hemophilia is inherited, and only by men; the gene for hemophilia is carried by women, who do not get the disease but who can pass the gene on to their sons.

Hemophilia has two forms, hemophilia A and hemophilia B; each form lacks a different clotting protein, called a *clotting factor.* Hemophilia is treated by substituting a commercial clotting factor for the clotting factor the blood lacks. The commercial clotting factor is extracted chemically from blood donated by hundreds or thousands of people. As a result, hemophiliacs are exposed to the blood of thousands of donors. Between 1978 and 1985, from the time HIV was introduced into the United States until the time the blood banks screened for HIV, hemophiliacs had a high risk of being infected with HIV. Approximately 70 percent of men with hemophilia A and 30 percent of men with hemophilia B acquired HIV infection from infected commercial clotting factors.

Since 1985, the risk of being exposed to HIV through clotting factors has dropped to practically nil. One reason is that donated blood is now screened for HIV; another reason is that clotting factors are heated and purified by detergents and biochemicals which kill HIV. The Centers for Disease Control found that between 1985 and 1988, only 18 hemophiliacs acquired HIV, an annual rate of under 1 per 1,000.

Hepatitis: Hepatitis is an inflammation of the liver. Many people have no symptoms and are unaware of having hepatitis. The symptoms, when people do have them, are loss of appetite, vomiting, yellow discoloration of the skin and eyes (jaundice), dark urine, sore stomach, and fever. Hepatitis is usually caused by a virus called *hepatitis B virus* (see below) or *hepatitis C virus,* both of which may be transmitted by sexual contact or blood-to-blood transmission. Since these are the same mechanisms of transmitting HIV infection, the same people who are likely to be infected with HIV infection are also likely to be infected with the hepatitis B virus and hepatitis C virus. People with HIV infection are also prone to hepatitis caused by CMV and *Mycobacterium avium*. Alcohol and drugs, including AZT, ddI, ddC, pentamidine, ketoconazole, trimethoprim-sulfamethoxazole, and INH, may also cause liver inflammation. The diagnosis of hepatitis is easily made with blood tests to determine liver function and to detect specific microbes, including hepatitis B, hepatitis C, and hepatitis A viruses. When the cause is unclear, it is sometimes helpful to obtain a biopsy of the liver or to do tests of the gall bladder.

Hepatitis B virus: The hepatitis B virus is one of the microbes that causes hepatitis. Hepatitus B infection may be acute and cause serious symptoms that last up to a few weeks (see above, under *Hepatitis*); it may be chronic with occasional symptoms and abnormal liver tests that last for months or years; or it may cause no symptoms at all and may only show up on a blood test. About 5– 10 percent of people with hepatitis B infection become chronic carriers of hepatitis B virus; they continue to carry the virus and can transmit it to others for years. The hepatitis B virus is transmitted the same way HIV is, by sexual contact or blood-to-blood transmission. Hepatitis B is transmitted far more efficiently than HIV, so that a person exposed by a needlestick accident involving a person with both infections is about twenty times more likely to develop infection with the hepatitis virus. The blood supply used for transfusions is screened for the hepatitis B virus and is therefore an unlikely source of this infection.

There is little evidence that hepatitis B is any different in people with HIV infection than in people without HIV infection. However, the presence of liver damage or ongoing inflammation may complicate the use of certain drugs that (like AZT) require the liver for metabolism or that (like AZT and pentamidine) may occasionally cause further liver damage (see *Hepatitis,* above). Once infection takes place, treatment to eradicate the virus is very difficult. Infection may be prevented, however, by a vaccine. The vaccine is recommended for the people at risk for this infection: people who share needles to inject drugs, people who practice unsafe sex with gay men, family members who live in the same household, sex partners of people known to be hepatitis B carriers, and health care workers. Three injections are required, at a cost of about $150–$200 for all three doses.

Herpes simplex virus: Herpes simplex is a virus that commonly causes infections of the mouth and genitals. There are actually two different viruses: though similar in many respects, one kind seems mostly likely to infect the mouth and other, the genitals. The symptoms of both infections are blisters on the mouth or genital area that first contain clear fluid, then become filled with pus, finally form scabs, and eventually disappear. Herpes simplex is a persistent virus: the virus remains dormant most of the time and then causes recurrent symptoms intermittently over a period of years. The initial infection with herpes simplex virus is often severe with large areas of blisters, occasional fevers, and pain and tingling in the area involved. Subsequent attacks are usually milder. The virus is transmitted to others by contact with the mouth or genitals, especially when the blisters are present.

Both the oral and the genital form of herpes are common infections in the general population; in people with HIV infection, however, the blisters are likely to be more severe, be spread over relatively larger areas, and, most importantly, persist for longer periods of time. In a person with HIV infection, herpes blisters that persist over one month constitute an AIDS-defining diagnosis. Treatment with a drug called acyclovir usually heals the blisters, prevents recurrences, and reduces the risk of transmitting the virus to others. Acyclovir is available as an ointment to put on the blisters and as tablets to be taken by mouth. In people with AIDS who have severe herpes infections, acyclovir is also given intravenously; once the infection is under control, the tablets are often given for extended periods to prevent recurrences.

Herpes zoster: Herpes zoster is caused by the same virus that causes chickenpox. The virus persists in the body and may cause symptoms decades after the original infection. Attacks after the first infection are called shingles, or herpes zoster. The skin sores with herpes zoster are similar to those of chickenpox and those of herpes simplex. The sores begin as red spots that become blisters filled with water; the blisters break down into sores with pus, finally scab over, and eventually disappear. Unlike herpes simplex infections or chickenpox, however, the later recurrences of herpes zoster are usually restricted to the area served by a single nerve. In other words, the blisters are restricted to one side of the body, usually in a band across the face, chest, abdomen, back, or leg.

In many people, recurrences of herpes zoster are accompanied by post-herpetic neuralgia, a pain at the site of blisters that may persist for months after the blisters are gone. Post-herpetic neuralgia is fortunately infrequent among people with HIV infection. Herpes zoster is more common and more severe in people with HIV infection. It does not, however, necessarily mean that the immune system is weakening, and it clearly does not indicate AIDS. The diagnosis is generally made with a microscopic examination and culture of blisters, but the appearance of the blisters is usually all a physician needs to make a diagnosis. Acyclovir appears to hasten healing, but high doses of the drug must be given by mouth or by vein.

Hickman catheter: People who require long courses of drugs given by vein will often have a tubing called a Hickman catheter. The catheter is inserted by a specialist, usually a surgeon, through the skin of the chest, and then tunneled under the skin to a vein in the chest. The end of the catheter comes out the chest wall above the breast. Drugs can be injected into the catheter as necessary. The advantage of a Hickman catheter is that it permits access to the vein without re-peated needlesticks in the arms. Other devices are also available, including a type that is placed below the skin so that no tube comes out the chest wall.

It is important to know that the area around any catheter in a vein can become infected. Symptoms of infection of the area where the catheter is located are redness and pain, and sometimes pus. Symptoms of infection around the catheter inside the body are fever and chills. Anyone with a Hickman catheter and these symptoms should tell a physician right away. Antibiotics should be given imme-diately, and sometimes the catheter needs to be removed.

HIV: HIV stands for the human immunodeficiency virus. HIV has had several names. It was first called lymphadenopathy associated virus (LAV) by Luc Montanier in France in 1983, and next called human T-lymphotropic virus III (HLTV-III) by Robert Gallo in the United States in 1984. HIV is now the official international name of this virus. HIV is the virus responsible for AIDS. There are occasional arguments that perhaps HIV does not cause AIDS or is responsible for AIDS only in combination with other viruses, but at present, the great majority of scientific authorities accept HIV as the sole cause of AIDS. They have several reasons for this: virtually all people with AIDS have evidence of HIV infection; people with HIV infection followed for prolonged periods develop AIDS; people exposed to HIV through needlesticks and transfusions acquire the virus and go on to develop AIDS; and HIV infects CD4 cells, which are the cells responsible for nearly all complications that characterize AIDS. In addition, despite ten years of intense pursuit, the only other identi-fied cause of AIDS is the closely related virus HIV-2 that is responsi-ble for a very few cases of AIDS, primarily in Africa. (See *Idiopathic CD4 lymphocytopenia,* below.)

HIV-associated dementia (HAD): HIV-associated dementia is the dementia that appears to result from HIV infecting the brain. HAD was previously called AIDS dementia complex, or ADC. Dementia means the loss of intellectual abilities, including the loss of memory, judgment, and concentration. HAD is relatively common in HIV infection but usually only in the late stages.

Idiopathic CD4 lymphocytopenia (ICL): ICL is a new syndrome, described from a small number of people whose low CD4 cell counts and opportunistic infections suggested AIDS but whose blood tests were negative for HIV. *Idiopathic* means that the causes are unknown; CD4 lymphocytes are the cells affected; and *-penia* means that the numbers of those cells are low. The number of cases of ICL, since it was first described in 1992, has been low. ICL appears to have little similarity to AIDS except for an analogous type of immune deficit. Most people with ICL do not have the usual risk factors for HIV. Their spouses show no evidence of disease, suggesting that ICL is not transmitted sexually. The cause of ICL is obviously unclear. Many suspect that ICL is an enigmatic immune deficiency condition that has been around forever but remained undiscovered until the AIDS epidemic when physicians began taking CD4 cell counts for the first time.

Idiopathic thrombocytopenia purpura (ITP): See both *Platelets* and *Thrombocytopenia*, below.

Immune system: The human body is defended against a multitude of microbes by a complex system called the immune system. The principal components of the immune system are cells called *B lymphocytes, neutrophils,* and *T-lymphocytes.* B lymphocytes make antibodies, the proteins that attack bacteria and viruses; neutrophils envelop and kill bacteria; and T lymphocytes provide communication between the parts of the immune system. Although these three components are somewhat interdependent, each takes primary responsibility for defense against certain types of microbes. For this reason, people deficient in different components are prone to infections with quite different microbes.

   The cell type that is primarily affected in people with HIV infection is a type of T lymphocyte called a *CD4 cell* (see above). The most common infections encountered in people with few CD4 cells are called by *Pneumocystis carinii,* cytomegalovirus, *Mycobacterium avium,* herpes simplex virus, herpes zoster, *Candida albicans, Toxoplasma gondii, Cryptosporidium, Cryptococcus, Salmonella,* and the bacterium that causes tuberculosis. People with immune systems weakened by HIV are not only subject to high rates of infections with these organisms, but the infections tend to be severe, prolonged, and recurrent. At the same time, many other microbes that commonly cause infections in everyone do not appear to be unusually common or severe in people with HIV, presumably because the other components of the immune defenses remain relatively strong.

Incubation period: The incubation period of a disease is the time interval between infection with a microbe and the first symptoms of disease. For influenza and common colds, the incubation period is usually several days; for measles, chickenpox, mumps, and infections caused by many other viruses, the incubation period is two to three weeks. An unusual feature of HIV infection is that the first symptoms of a weakened immune system usually do not occur until several years after the infection takes place.

Infectious: See *Contagious,* above.

Influenza vaccine: The influenza vaccine varies in effectiveness, depending on whether the strain of virus in the vaccine is related to the virus which is causing the influenza. The effectiveness of the vaccine changes every year. In most years, however, the vaccine probably prevents about 70 percent of the cases of influenza, and those who become infected despite having been vaccinated usually have less severe symptoms. Influenza does not seem to be unusually common or severe in people with HIV infection. The only problem specific to people with HIV infection is that the symptoms of influenza can be confused with the symptoms of other pneumonias such as pneumocystis pneumonia (see *Pneumocystis carinii,* below), a confusion it would be nice to avoid. Therefore, the CDC's Advisory Committee on Immunization Practices recommends that people with HIV infection routinely get the influenza vaccine every year.

Informed consent: Informed consent is a form of protection for people considering taking an HIV antibody test or undergoing certain medical procedures (like an operation) or considering participation in a clinical trial. Before taking the test, undergoing the procedure, or participating in the trial, the person or the person's representative must sign an informed consent form stating that he or she has been informed about the purpose, benefits, risks, and alternatives to the test, procedure, or trial, and that he or she consents to it. In the case of participation in a clinical trial, the informed consent form explains the purpose of the trial, what will be done, the risks of participation, the benefits of participation, what other treatments are available, and the right of the participant to leave the trial at any time.

Inoculum size: Inoculum size is a term used in the field of infectious diseases to describe the number of microbes necessary to cause an infection. In HIV infection, for example, a certain number of viruses is required before infection takes place. The specific number is not known. What is known is that the probability of transmitting HIV with the transfusion of one unit (or 500 milliliters) of infected blood is 80 to 90 percent. The probability of transmitting HIV with a needlestick injury, which injects only a fraction of a milliliter of blood, is 0.4 percent. This difference in the probabilities of transmission is most likely due to differences in inoculum size.

Interferons: Interferons are proteins that cause cells to resist attack by certain viruses. Interferons are usually produced by the body, but they are also made artificially and used as medications. For people with HIV infection, interferons are mainly used to treat Kaposi's sarcoma. Interferons may also kill HIV, but only when given intravenously in very large doses, and the side effects are severe. An oral form of an interferon, called Kemron, was once fashionable among some people with HIV infection, based on preliminary studies done mostly in Africa. Kemron, however, is not absorbed into the body when taken by mouth; the doses used seem far too low; and clinical trials in the United States have so far failed to show any benefit. The major side effects of injected interferon are the achiness and fever that accompany flu: it is the interferon produced by the body that causes these symptoms during flu.

Isoniazid (INH): Isoniazid is the standard drug used to treat and prevent tuberculosis. Isoniazid is usually recommended for any person with HIV infection who has tuberculosis or who has a positive tuberculosis skin test. The usual dose is 300 milligrams, taken by mouth. The most important side effect is hepatitis, including jaundice (yellowish skin and eyes), dark urine, nausea, and abdominal pain. This side effect is more likely in people who already have liver damage for other reasons, and in older people. People taking isoniazid and having these symptoms should stop taking the drug immediately and call their physicians. INH tends to cause a vitamin B_6 deficiency, so INH and vitamin B_6 are often given at the same time.

Kaposi's sarcoma: Kaposi's (pronounced kaposhee's) sarcoma is a tumor of blood vessels. Next to the pneumocystis pneumonia, it is most likely to be the first AIDS-defining diagnosis that people have; approximately 20 percent of all people with AIDS have Kaposi's sarcoma. The symptoms of Kaposi's sarcoma are purplish nodules, usually a quarter of an inch to an inch in diameter, anywhere on the skin. The nodules will grow in size and number. They sometimes occur on internal organs like the lung, brain, and gastrointestinal tract, though they often cause no specific symptoms at these sites. Some nodules are painful. The face and legs may swell if the lymph channels nearby are blocked. If Kaposi's sarcoma becomes extensive, people may have fever, weight loss, and severe fatigue.

The diagnosis can be established by a biopsy of the nodules. Biopsies are easy to do with nodules on the skin, but more difficult when the nodules are on internal organs. The main reason to do the biopsy is that the nodules might possibly turn out to be something other than Kaposi's sarcoma; and if they are Kaposi's sarcoma, they are an AIDS-defining diagnosis. Therapy is controversial: Kaposi's sarcoma is rarely life-threatening, and treatment is neither easy nor universally effective. If the nodules are painful, disfiguring, or complicated by swelling, they can be treated with radiation, laser treatment, injections, or interferon; if the nodules have spread widely over the skin or into internal organs, causing symptoms, they can be treated with the same drugs given to people with cancer.

Ketoconazole: Ketoconazole is a drug given by mouth for infections caused by *Candida albicans* and other fungi. Ketoconazole requires acid in the stomach to be absorbed into the system. People should therefore not take other medicines that neutralize stomach acids until at least two hours after the dose of ketoconazole. Side effects include nausea, vomiting, hormonal problems (menstrual problems and reduced sex drive), rash, headaches, and liver damage.

Late symptomatic HIV infection: See *AIDS.*

Latency: Latency and dormancy (which literally means sleeping) mean the same thing: a microbe is in the body but is not actively reproducing, not invading any tissues, and not causing symptoms. Examples of microbes that are latent or dormant in many or most healthy people are: *Pneumocystis carinii, Toxoplasma gondii,* herpes simplex virus, the virus that causes herpes zoster, and cytomegalovirus. Once in the body, these microbes remain in the body. They remain latent or dormant until something tilts the balance in the immune system and permits them to become active.

Leukopenia: Leukopenia means a low number (or penia) of white blood cells (or leukocytes—*leuko* means white), the cells of the immune system that fight infection. Leukocytes include lymphocytes (cells that recognize foreign material) and neutrophils (cells that gobble up microbes). The normal leukocyte count is 4,000 to 8,000 per milliliter of blood. In people with certain infections, especially with bacterial infections, the leukocyte count is high (leukocytosis). In people with viral infections, including HIV infection, the leukocyte count is low (leukopenia). Having a low count of lymphocytes is called *lymphopenia;* lymphopenia is the expected result of HIV infection. A low count of neutrophils is called *neutropenia;* neutropenia can be caused by HIV itself or by some of the drugs commonly taken during HIV infection. Neutropenia becomes worrisome if the count is less than 750 per milliliter; if the count is less than 500 per milliliter, the person is prone to bacterial infections.

Lumbar puncture: See *Spinal tap,* below.

Lymph glands: The lymphatic system is a widespread network, like the blood circulation, of channels that carry lymph. Lymph is a clear fluid containing lymphocytes, or white blood cells (including CD4 cells), that are a part of the immune system. Lymph is manufactured in the lymph glands, which are clumps of lymphatic tissue distributed widely throughout the body. When lymph glands are near the surface of the skin, they can be felt as bumps below the skin's surface. The usual locations where they can be felt are the back of the neck, below the jaw, under the armpits, and in the groin. Lymph glands are commonly swollen and sometimes painful and tender when they are infected. Many infections involve the lymph nodes. In HIV infection, swollen lymph glands are likely to occur in three different circumstances: with *persistent generalized lymphadenopathy,* or *PGL* (see below), in which many lymph glands are swollen for months; with infection of the lymph glands by certain opportunistic diseases; and with lymphomas, which are tumors of the lymphatic system seen more frequently in people with HIV infection than in the general population. Swollen lymph glands may require diagnostic tests: the usual is a biopsy of the lymph gland or removal of the whole gland to permit microscopic examination of the lymphatic tissue.

Lymphadenopathy: Lymphadenopathy means swollen lymph glands. Swollen lymph glands are most common at the back of the neck, along the jaw, in the armpits, and in the groin. The lymph glands may feel like rubbery, discrete nodules that are rarely tender to touch and often pea-sized; glands of this description are common in everyone and in several conditions unrelated to HIV infection. If they are swollen to abnormal size for longer than a month in at least two different areas, they constitute *persistent generalized lymphadenopathy (PGL)* (see below).

Lymphoma: Lymphoma is a cancer of the lymphatic system. Lymphoma occurs most frequently in people without HIV infection, but people with weakened immune systems, including those with HIV infection, have lymphomas about forty times more frequently than normal. About 3 percent of people with AIDS have lymphomas, and for people with AIDS, lymphomas are classified as opportunistic tumors. There are many types of lymphomas: some progress extremely slowly, cause few symptoms, and require minimal treatment; some are more severe. People with AIDS generally have lymphomas called non-Hodgkin's lymphomas of B cell origin. These lymphomas tend to be severe, and they also tend to involve unusual areas of the body like the brain, liver, kidneys, intestines, and lungs. The diagnosis is usually established with a biopsy. Treatment is variable and often requires the assistance of a specialist in cancer treatment using cancer chemotherapy or radiation treatment.

Magnetic resonance imaging (MRI): Magnetic resonance imaging is a technique used to make a three-dimensional image of the interior of the body. Though the technique is somewhat different from a CAT scan (see *Computerized tomography scan,* above), the images are similar. The person getting an MRI is placed inside a large tubular structure and remains motionless for thirty to sixty minutes: the worst problems are boredom, noise, and claustrophobia. During that time, the person's body is bathed in a magnetic field, which causes the atoms in different tissues to give off tiny radio signals. The signals are different depending on the kind of tissue. An MRI is better than a CAT scan at detecting diseases of the brain and spinal cord. MRI is painless, harmless, and does not involve exposure to radiation; the body is not exposed to any kind of potentially harmful radiation. MRIs are also expensive, from $500 to $1,000.

Megestrol Acetate (Megace): Megestrol is a drug that stimulates the appetite. The drug has virtually no serious side effects, even with doses as high as 800 milligrams daily.

Meningitis: Meningitis is an infection of the meninges, the membrane that envelops the brain and spinal cord. The most common cause of meningitis in people with HIV infection is *Cryptococcus* (see under *Cryptococcis,* above).

Meprobamate (e.g., *Equanil, Miltown*): Meprobamate is a drug that acts on the central nervous system much as barbiturates do. Meprobamate is used most commonly to treat anxiety. As with barbiturates, meprobamate can cause drowsiness, lethargy, and lack of coordination. Continued use for weeks or months may cause tolerance—that is, increasing doses are required for the same effect. Continued use may also cause psychological and physical dependence. Withdrawing the drug suddenly after prolonged, regular use may cause severe reactions. Other side effects can include stomach irritation and allergic reactions.

Methadone hydrochloride: Methadone is an opiate that is commonly used to control narcotic withdrawal symptoms and to maintain people addicted to morphine-like drugs, particularly heroin. Methadone maintenance is permitted only in programs approved by the Food and Drug Administration and the designated state authority. Methadone can be given by mouth or by vein. Side effects are those shared by all morphine-like drugs that depress the central nervous system: dizziness, mental clouding, depression, and sedation. Methadone may cause physical dependence. If it is stopped abruptly after prolonged and regular use, it can cause withdrawal symptoms.

Metronidazole (e.g., *Flagyl*): Metronidazole is an antibiotic taken by people with HIV infection for common intestinal infections and common dental problems like gingivitis (inflammation of the gums) and periodontitis (infection of the structures that support the teeth). The drug is given by mouth or by vein. Side effects are unusual, primarily nausea and stomach pain. The side effects can improve if the drug is taken with meals or if the dose is reduced. Taking this drug for periods of months may cause pain in the feet that resembles the pain of HIV *neuropathy* (see below). The pain usually goes away when the drug is stopped.

Microbes: Microbes are organisms so small they require a microscope to be seen. They can be bacteria, viruses, parasites, or fungi. HIV is one example of a virus. Microbes cause infectious diseases. The microbes that commonly cause the opportunistic infections that accompany HIV infection are as follows:

Viruses: Cytomegalovirus, herpes simplex, herpes zoster, molluscum contagiosum

Bacteria: *Mycobacterium avium, Mycobacterium tuberculosis* (the cause of tuberculosis), *Salmonella, Nocardia*

Parasites: *Toxoplasma gondii, Pneumocystis carinii, Cryptosporidium, Isospora*

Fungi: *Cryptococcus, Histoplasma, Candida albicans*

Mycobacterium avium (MA): MA is related to the bacterium that causes tuberculosis, though it is not contagious and is more difficult to treat. In the late stages of HIV infection, infection with MA is spread widely throughout many organs in the body. It can cause fever, pneumonia, diarrhea, hepatitis, and many other complications.

National Institutes of Health (NIH): The NIH is a federal organization located in Bethesda, Maryland, that funds scientific research. The NIH is the world's largest research organization. With a budget of over $10 billion a year, the NIH is responsible for funding about a third of all research in the biomedical sciences, including research related to HIV infection, in the United States. Some of the research sponsored by NIH is intramural, that is, it is conducted by the approximately one thousand researchers inside NIH; most of the research is extramural, at universities and medical schools throughout the country. Extramural research grants are awarded on the basis of priority, as determined by expert review of proposals. The NIH is divided into fifteen different institutes, each with a different scientific specialty: the National Institute for Allergy and Infectious Diseases (NIAID) is responsible for most of the research into HIV infection. The NIH is not related to the *Centers for Disease Control* (see above), except that both are federally funded agencies with somewhat different roles in combating HIV and other diseases.

Funding for research into HIV infection from sources other than NIH comes from other federal agencies (Department of Defense, National Science Foundation, Veterans Administration, and the Centers for Disease Control), pharmaceutical companies, local governments, and private foundations. Funding for this research escalated rapidly in the late 1980s until the total HIV research budget exceeded the funding for heart disease research at a time when heart disease was responsible for twenty times more deaths than AIDS was. Some view this as inappropriate, given the relative impact of the two; others feel AIDS research is underfunded, given its importance as a public health problem and as a prototypic disease for many other conditions.

Neuropathy: Neuropathy is an illness involving the nerves. Nerves are responsible for (among other things) the movement of muscles and the sensation of touch, including the sensation of pain. The symptoms of a neuropathy can therefore be weakness of a muscle or pain and tingling. In people with HIV infection, the most frequent symptoms of neuropathy are painful feet and legs. These may be the result of HIV infection or a side effect of some drugs, especially ddI and ddC.

Nucleoside analogs: Nucleoside analogs are a chemically related group of drugs used to inhibit HIV. Examples include the first drugs approved to treat HIV infection: AZT, ddI, ddC. They all work by the same mechanism, by inhibiting an enzyme called reverse transcriptase that is critical for HIV's survival. Nucleoside analogs often seem to have time-limited benefit, that is, after prolonged use they stop working. This may be because HIV develops resistance to a particular nucleoside analog. Nevertheless, HIV remains sensitive to other nucleoside analogs, which can then be substituted.

Opportunistic infections: In all infectious diseases, the body's defenses are, for a while, inadequate to control microbial invasion. Many microbes can cause disease in people who are otherwise healthy. Other microbes, however, are fairly harmless and can cause disease only in people whose immune defenses are weakened. These microbes are called opportunistic microbes because the microbe takes the opportunity offered by a weakened immune system to cause disease. The opportunistic microbes that most frequently infect people with HIV infection are summarized under *Microbes.*

Opportunistic tumors: Opportunistic tumors, like opportunistic infection, occur primarily in people with weakened immune systems. In people with HIV infection, the major opportunistic tumors are Kaposi's sarcoma and certain types of lymphoma.

Oral hairy leukoplakia (OHL): The symptoms of oral hairy leukoplakia are white (leuko) patches (plakia) on the tongue and elsewhere in the mouth. It usually produces no symptoms, but may distort taste or cause pain. It is caused by the same virus that causes infectious mononucleosis. These patches often appear similar to those of thrush; in fact, oral hairy leukoplakia is often diagnosed when people who appear to have thrush do not respond to the usual treatment. It can also be diagnosed with a biopsy of the patches. Oral hairy leukoplakia seems to occur exclusively in people with HIV infection. It generally indicates progressive weakening of the immune system; without treatment for HIV, the first AIDS-defining diagnosis is likely in the next two or three years. Most people have no symptoms, but when they do, the usual treatment is high doses of acyclovir.

P24 antigen test: The P24 antigen test is, like the PCR test (see *Polymerase chain reaction,* below) and a *culture* (see above) for HIV, a test that detects the presence of HIV in the blood. P24 is one of the several proteins (the protein with a molecular weight of 24,000) that make up HIV. An *antigen* is anything that causes the immune system to identify it as foreign and to manufacture antibodies against it. A P24 antigen test detects P24 and therefore HIV. Unlike PCR and HIV cultures, however, the P24 antigen test is not especially sensitive, and most people with HIV infection have tests for the P24 antigen that are negative.

Levels of P24 are highest both early and late in the disease; the numbers of HIV are likewise highest at the same times. Some physicians therefore suggest that the P24 antigen test might help track the course of the disease in people with HIV infection. That is, it might identify people with HIV infection who are likely to develop symptoms and who are most likely to transmit the virus to others; and it might help evaluate how people are responding to antiviral drugs.

Pancreatitis: Inflammation of the pancreas, an organ in the abdomen that makes insulin and digestive enzymes. Symptoms are abdominal pain, nausea, and vomiting. Pancreatitis is a potentially serious complication of alcoholism and of some drugs used to treat HIV infection, like ddI and ddC.

Pentamidine: Pentamidine is a drug used to treat or prevent pneumocystis pneumonia. Pentamidine is actually used only when someone cannot take the best drug, trimethoprim-sulfamethoxazole. To treat pneumocystis pneumonia, pentamidine is given by vein for three weeks. To prevent pneumocystis pneumonia in people whose CD4 count is less than 200, pentamidine is given by aerosol directly into the lungs, at monthly intervals. When given by vein, pentamidine often has such side effects as low blood pressure (causing fainting), low blood sugar, high blood sugar (diabetes), kidney failure, liver disease, low blood counts, or inflammation of the pancreas. These side effects are common when the drug is given by vein. They are rare or don't occur at all when pentamidine is taken as an aerosol, since so little of the drug gets into the system.

Persistent generalized lymphadenopathy (PGL): A diagnosis of PGL means that lymph glands are swollen for at least one month and at two different sites of the body, not counting the groin area. PGL often occurs early in HIV infection. Lymph glands are the location of HIV multiplication at a time when the patient feels well. (See *Lymph glands* and *Lymphadenopathy,* above.)

Platelets: Platelets are the component of blood that facilitates clotting. The number of platelets is often low in people with HIV infection— sometimes so extremely low that the person is prone to bleeding. The cause of the low platelets may be HIV infection itself, or it may be the drugs that are used to treat people with HIV infection.

Pneumococcal vaccine: The most common cause of bacterial pneumonia in people without HIV infection is a bacterium called *Streptococcus pneumoniae* or pneumococcus. Pneumococcus is also a common cause of pneumonia in people with HIV infection. Pneumococcal vaccine is recommended for people with HIV infection, since they are prone to frequent or severe infections by pneumococcus. It is best to take this vaccine relatively early in the course of the disease when the immune system is strong.

Pneumocystis carinii: *Pneumocystis carinii* is a parasite that commonly causes lung infection and pneumonia in people with HIV infection. *Pneumocystis carinii* pneumonia (PCP) is the most frequent serious opportunistic infection in people with HIV infection. When there is no explanation for immune suppression other than HIV infection pneumocystis pneumonia is an AIDS-defining diagnosis. The symptoms are cough without sputum, shortness of breath, and fever. These symptoms usually evolve over a period of several days or, more commonly, weeks. The diagnosis is generally established by a chest x-ray or studies of lung function, combined with a microscopic examination of respiratory secretions to show the parasite. Treatment with several drugs—most commonly trimethoprim-sulfamethoxazole and pentamidine—is successful. Treatment is most successful when started relatively early in the course of the infection.

Pneumonia: Pneumonia is an infection of the lungs. The usual symptoms are cough, fever, and shortness of breath. The causes of pneumonia vary, and the treatment depends on the cause.

Polymerase chain reaction (PCR): Polymerase chain reaction is a very sensitive test, developed in the late 1980s, for detecting tiny quantities of HIV (see *Retrovirus,* below). Unlike the standard blood test for HIV infection which detects antibodies to HIV, the PCR detects HIV itself. The test is very accurate; over 95 percent of people with HIV infection will test positive on a PCR test. The great majority of people who take the standard antibody test for HIV infection need not take the PCR test. PCR is most useful when the results of the antibody test are ambiguous and in research studies. PCR is similar to a *culture* (see above) for HIV but is substantially less expensive. Neither PCR nor cultures for HIV, however, are available in most laboratories.

Progressive multifocal leukoencephalopathy: Progressive multifocal leukoencephalopathy is a viral infection deep in the brain that is found only in people with severely weakened immune systems, including, occasionally, people with HIV infection. Progressive multifocal leukoencephalopathy has a distinctive appearance on CAT or MRI scans of the brain, but a diagnosis can be established definitely only with a biopsy. The infection tends to be progressive, and no therapy is known to be effective.

Prophylaxis: Prophylaxis is treatment to prevent a disease, as opposed to treatment to eliminate a disease already present.

PWA: PWA is the abbreviation for people with AIDS. The PWA Coalition is one of several national organizations that provides newsletters, lists of resources, and research updates to people with HIV infection and AIDS.

Pyrimethamine (Daraprim): Pyrimethamine is an antibiotic used to treat or prevent *toxoplasmosis* (see below). The full treatment usually combines pyrimethamine with a sulfa drug like sulfadiazine or clindamycin. Pyrimethamine is taken by mouth. The major side effect after prolonged use is anemia. To avoid anemia, another drug, leucovorin, is given at the same time. Other side effects include gastric intolerance, allergic reactions, and hepatitis. Many of these reactions are the result of the sulfa drug that is taken with pyrimethamine.

Research: See *National Institutes of Health,* above.

Resistance: Resistance, when used in medicine, means that a drug is not effective because the microbe being treated has been able to change its chemistry so it is no longer susceptible to the drug. The result is either that the drug does not work in the test tube against this person's microbe, or that the person stops getting better; usually both results are found together.

Retinitis: Retinitis means an inflammation (itis) of the retina, the layer of cells at the back of the eye that collects and send images to the brain. Retinitis usually causes some loss of vision. The earliest symptoms are pain in the eye, "floaters" across the field of vision, or a blind spot, which is the loss of part of a visual field. In people with HIV infection, the most common cause of retinitis is infection with *cytomegalovirus* (see above).

Retrovirus: Retroviruses are a type of virus. Retroviruses do not have DNA, the molecule that holds the genetic code which cells use to reproduce themselves. Instead, retroviruses have RNA and an enzyme called reverse transcriptase, which turns RNA into DNA. When a retrovirus invades one of the cells of the body, it uses reverse transcriptase to turn its own RNA into DNA. This DNA then becomes part of the cell's DNA. When properly stimulated, the DNA then makes more retrovirus instead of more cells. Many different kinds of retroviruses infect many different kinds of animals. HIV is the most important retrovirus to infect humans; it causes disease in no other animal species except for certain types of monkeys. On the whole, it is not easy for retroviruses to pass from one species to another.

Risk factor: A risk factor is a condition or behavior that makes it likely that a person with the risk factor will develop a condition—in this case, HIV infection. The major risk factors for HIV infection are needle-sharing with intravenous drug users and sexual contact with a person who has or may have been exposed to HIV. Another risk factor is having received blood products between 1978—when HIV infection was first known to exist in the United States—and May 1985, when the blood supply was first screened for HIV. Another risk factor is promiscuous or casual sexual contact without precautions. Still another is to be born to a woman with HIV infection: approximately 30 to 35 percent of women who are infected with HIV will pass the virus to the unborn infant. A minor risk factor is needlestick injuries in health care workers who care for people with HIV infection. Less than one percent of all people with HIV infection in the United States have no clearly defined risk factor, although many of these people either are too sick to provide adequate information or are providing information that is suspect.

Safer sex: Safer sex is a qualitative term. To be absolutely safe, sexual contact cannot involve an exchange of any body fluids—specifically, semen or vaginal secretions. The term safer sex recognizes the likelihood of human error and the inexactness of human knowledge. Safer sex refers to sexual intercourse using a condom and spermicide, or sexual practices that do not involve exchange of body fluids.

Seizure: A seizure is a convulsion, uncontrolled movements of the arms and legs accompanied by unconsciousness and inability to control urine or stool. The usual cause of seizures in people with HIV infection is an opportunistic infection or an opportunistic tumor of the brain, including toxoplasmic encephalitis, cryptococcal meningitis, or lymphoma. Less commonly, seizures are caused by an imbalance of electrolytes or by medications. Recurrent seizures can usually be controlled with drugs like Dilantin and phenobarbital. Anyone with recurrent seizures should be careful about his or her physical circumstances: be careful working on ladders, for instance, or driving. In many states it is illegal for a person with seizures to drive until seizures have been controlled for at least one year.

Seroconversion: The immune system usually takes several days or weeks to recognize a foreign substance like a virus to produce antibodies to it. Six to twelve weeks after HIV enters the body, antibodies to HIV usually appear in the blood. Physicians call the appearance of antibodies in the blood *seroconversion*. That is, the result of a test for antibodies in the blood serum converts from negative to positive.

Shingles: Synonymous with *herpes zoster* (see above).

Sinusitis: The sinuses are air sacs next to the passageway from the nose. Sinusitis is an infection of the sinuses, usually as a result of a cold or an allergy. Sinusitis is common in everyone, and is especially common in people with HIV infection. The reason for this is obscure. Symptoms are pus drainage from the nose, headache, face pain, and fever. The usual treatment is with antibiotics taken by mouth, such as trimethoprim-sulfamethoxazole, amoxicillin, erythromycin, cephalexin (or Keflex), ciprofloxacin (Cipro), or tetracycline. Some people do not respond to these drugs, and their sinuses need to be drained, a procedure done by a specialist called an *otolaryngologist* (ear, nose, and throat specialist).

Spinal tap: A spinal tap, also called a *lumbar puncture,* is a procedure for obtaining cerebrospinal fluid, the fluid that surrounds the brain and the spinal cord. The procedure involves inserting a needle into the middle of the back and into the meninges, a membrane that contains the cerebrospinal fluid. The cerebrospinal fluid is then analyzed for evidence of infection of the brain or spinal cord. Despite sounding unpleasant and risky, a spinal tap is a well-established medical procedure and is rarely associated with any important complications. The most common complaint is a headache following the spinal tap, a complaint made less likely by lying flat once the spinal tap is completed.

T-helper cells: Synonymous with T4 cells, T4 lymphocytes, and CD4 lymphocytes. (See *CD4 cells,* above).

T-suppressor lymphocytes: T-suppressor lymphocytes are another class of T lymphocytes (see *Immune system,* above). T-suppressor lymphocytes are synonymous with T8 cells, CD8 cells, and T8 lymphocytes. All T lymphocytes participate in the body's defenses. T8 cells primarily regulate antibody formation by the B lymphocytes. The laboratory test called the T-cell subset analysis is a count of the various types of T lymphocytes. At one time, the proportion of the number of T4 cells to the number of T8 cells was believed to show where the person was in the course of HIV infection. This proportion was commonly referred to as the *T-helper/T-suppressor ratio*. More recent work indicates that only the number of T4 cells (CD4 cells) is important, and counting T4 cells alone is usually far less expensive than doing the total subset analysis.

Thrombocytopenia: Thrombocytopenia is a low count (penia) of thrombocytes (or platelets), cells in the blood which facilitate clotting. The usual count of thrombocytes is 150,000 to 300,000 per milliliter of blood. Lower counts of 80,000 to 120,000 per milliliter are common in people with HIV infection. When the count is very low, from 5,000 to 25,000 per milliliter, bleeding problems may occur. People with HIV infection have thrombocytopenia because their bodies produce antibodies against their own platelets. Some people have no symptoms but must still be careful to avoid cuts or anything that could cause bleeding. Other people have excessive nosebleeds, excessive bleeding from cuts, and red spots the size of pinheads that come from tiny hemorrhages into the skin. Treatment is with drugs—*corticosteroids* (see above), AZT, gamma globulin given intravenously, alpha interferon—or with a splenectomy, the surgical removal of the spleen.

Thrush: Thrush is an infection of the mouth caused by the fungus *Candida albicans.* The symptoms are white patches along the gums, on the inside of the cheeks, on the roof of the mouth, or on the tongue. Thrush is extremely common in people with HIV infection, and is considered part of AIDS-related complex, or ARC (see above). Thrush is easily treated with nystatin, clotrimazole, ketoconazole, or fluconazole.

Toxoplasmosis: Toxoplasmosis is an infection caused by the parasite *Toxoplasma gondii. Toxoplasma gondii* is found in cat excrement and in rare meat, both of which are common sources of infection. About 20–30 percent of all adults in the United States have *Toxoplasma gondii* in their bodies, but the majority are unaware of it. The parasite remains dormant (see *Latency,* above) and rarely causes disease unless the immune system is weakened. In people with HIV infection, the most common form of toxoplasmosis is an infection of the brain called toxoplasma encephalitis.

Tuberculosis (TB): Tuberculosis is an infection, usually in the lungs, that is far more frequent in people with HIV infection than in the general population. The bacterium that causes TB can either be dormant (inactive TB) or active (active TB). In active TB, the usual symptoms are fever and cough. People with either active or inactive TB will have skin tests that are positive for TB. In people with HIV infection, the skin test is less reliable, especially in the later stages of HIV infection, when the immune system is weakened. People with HIV infection and inactive TB should receive treatment—a drug called isoniazid—to prevent active TB. People with HIV infection and active TB should receive a combination of drugs that include isoniazid and rifampin. A new form of tuberculosis is resistant to one or both drugs. This new tuberculosis occurs most commonly in people who do not complete the standard treatment and in people living in New York City.

Vaccine: A vaccine is a substance, given by mouth or by an injection, that stimulates the immune system to form antibodies to some microbe. The polio vaccine, for instance, stimulates the immune system to form antibodies against the polio virus. These newly formed antibodies now protect the person against any subsequent exposure to that microbe. Some vaccines work better than others: with the polio vaccine, protection is nearly 100 percent; with the influenza vaccine, protection is about 70 percent. Vaccines for HIV infection are being tested in people with and without HIV infection. For people without HIV infection, a vaccine could hopefully work like any vaccine, that is, it could stimulate antibodies that protect you if you are exposed to HIV. For people with HIV infection, a vaccine could hopefully stimulate the immune system to make greater numbers of antibodies.

Vaginitis: Vaginitis is infection of the vagina. Symptoms are abnormal vaginal discharge and severe itching. Vaginitis has three common infectious causes: (1) "yeast," or the fungus *Candida,* which is treated with antifungal drugs like Gyne-Lotrimin or fluconazole; (2) "trick," short for the parasite *Trichomonas vaginalis,* which is treated with metronidazole (Flagyl); and (3) certain bacteria also treated with metronidazole. The most common cause of vaginitis in women with HIV infection is yeast infection. This form of vaginitis is more likely to occur if you are taking antibiotics.

Varicella zoster: Varicella zoster is the virus that causes chickenpox (varicella) and herpes zoster (shingles). See *Herpes zoster,* above.

Virus: A virus is a tiny microbe that, unlike bacteria, can neither survive nor reproduce unless it lives in a cell. HIV is a virus that lives in CD4 lymphocytes in humans.

Wasting: Wasting is the term given—somewhat unfortunately—to the weight loss and malnutrition that often accompany HIV infection. The causes of wasting vary; they may include opportunistic infections and tumors. Some people burn more calories because their metabolism increases, usually because of fever and common infections. These people may eat a lot and still lose weight. Other people have malnutrition due to starvation because of sores in their mouths, or depression, or apathy, or side effects of drugs that prevent them from eating. In some cases, wasting is caused by diarrhea; the condition is then called the *diarrhea-wasting syndrome.* Wasting can be an AIDS-defining diagnosis: according to the criteria of the Centers for Disease Control, an unexplained loss of at least 10 percent of the usual body weight accompanied by diarrhea or fever for 30 days, is diagnostic of AIDS.

Western blot: The Western blot is a test for specific antibodies, in this case, for antibodies to HIV. (See above, under *ELISA.*)

Acknowledgments

This book owes a lot of its substance and spirit to the following people who supplied information, answered endless questions, and read and reread drafts. We are grateful to Donna Sorenson and the Nutrition Clinic at Johns Hopkins Hospital for advice on nutrition and the diets that sooth problems with the digestive system; to Varda Fink and Meg Garrett for advice and information on legal, financial, and insurance matters; to Richard Carpenter for advice on the psychological welfare of people with HIV infection; to Gloria Fairhead and Susan Rucker for information on insurance matters and on the social service system, and for advice on the emotional, familial, and social concerns of people with HIV infection and their caregivers; to Fred Schaerf for information about AIDS dementia complex and for his insight into the minds of people with HIV infection; and to the people with HIV infection themselves, and to their caregivers, who told us in detail how to persist in living well, both physically and emotionally.

We are also grateful to Colleen Townsley for typing and overtime; to Marguerite Barbacci for information on resources; to Jo Leslie for her attitude toward dying; and to Jackie Wehmueller for close and concerned editing.

We thank, with particular warmth, Jean Bartlett and Cal Walker.

Index

For definitions of many of these entries, see the Glossary.